The Textbook of Non-medical Prescribing

Edited by

Dilyse Nuttall

MSc (by research), PGDip, BSc (Hons), RN, RHV
Nurse Prescriber, Nurse Teacher, NMC registrant, Fellow of Higher Education Academy, Senior Lecturer, School of Nursing and Caring Sciences, University of Central Lancashire, Preston, Lancashire

and

Jane Rutt-Howard

MSc, BSc (Hons), Dip HE, RGN
Nurse Prescriber, NMC registrant, Associate Fellow of Higher Education Academy, Senior Lecturer, School of Nursing and Caring Sciences, University of Central Lancashire, Preston, Lancashire

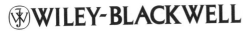
WILEY-BLACKWELL

A John Wiley & Sons, Ltd., Publication

This edition first published 2011
© 2011 Blackwell Publishing Ltd

Blackwell Publishing was acquired by John Wiley & Sons in February 2007. Blackwell's publishing program has been merged with Wiley's global Scientific, Technical and Medical business to form Wiley-Blackwell.

Registered office: John Wiley & Sons Ltd, The Atrium, Southern Gate, Chichester, West Sussex, PO19 8SQ, UK

Editorial offices: 9600 Garsington Road, Oxford, OX4 2DQ, UK
The Atrium, Southern Gate, Chichester, West Sussex, PO19 8SQ, UK
2121 State Avenue, Ames, Iowa 50014-8300, USA

For details of our global editorial offices, for customer services and for information about how to apply for permission to reuse the copyright material in this book please see our website at www.wiley.com/wiley-blackwell.

The right of the author to be identified as the author of this work has been asserted in accordance with the UK Copyright, Designs and Patents Act 1988.

Library of Congress Cataloging-in-Publication Data

The textbook of non-medical prescribing / edited by Dilyse Nuttall and Jane Rutt-Howard.
    p. ; cm.
Includes bibliographical references and index.
  ISBN 978-1-4051-9935-3 (pbk. : alk. paper)
  1. Drugs–Prescribing. 2. Nurses–Prescription privileges. 3. Nurse practitioners–Prescription privileges. I. Nuttall, Dilyse. II. Rutt-Howard, Jane.
  [DNLM: 1. Drug Prescriptions–Great Britain. 2. Allied Health Personnel–Great Britain. 3. Clinical Competence–Great Britain. 4. Medical Staff Privileges–Great Britain. 5. Nurses–Great Britain. 6. Pharmacists–Great Britain. QV 748]
  RM138.T49 2011
  615′.1-dc22

                                                                            2010040971

A catalogue record for this book is available from the British Library.

Set in 9/12.5 pt Interstate Light by Toppan Best-set Premedia Limited
Printed and bound in Malaysia by Vivar Printing Sdn Bhd

1 2011

Contents

Contributor List

Jane Alder, PhD, BSc(Hons)
Lecturer in Pharmacology, School of Pharmacy, UCLAN, Preston, Lancashire

Gillian Armitage, BSc(Hons), RN
Nurse Teacher, NMC registrant , Senior Lecturer, School of Nursing and Caring Sciences, UCLAN, Preston, Lancashire

Alison Astles, BPharm(Hons), Dip Pres Sci, MRPharmS
Pharmacist Practitioner/Teacher Practitioner, School of Pharmacy, UCLAN, Preston, Lancashire

Ruth Broadhead, LLM (Master of Laws, Medical Law & Bioethics), BA(Hons), RGN, PGCert, DipHE (Specialist Practitioner)
V300 Independent & Supplementary Prescriber, NMC registrant, Senior Lecturer, UCLAN, Preston, Lancashire

Janice Davies, MSc, BSc(Hons), MRPharmS
Pharmacist Practitioner/Teacher Practitioner, School of Pharmacy, UCLAN, Preston, Lancashire

Dawn Eccleston, MSc, BSc, RN, RHV, PGCertEd, NP
NMC registrant, Fellow of Higher Education Academy, Senior Lecturer, School of Nursing and Caring Sciences, UCLAN, Preston, Lancashire

Anne Fittock, MSc, BPharm(Hons), PGD, PGCertEd, MRPharmS
Fellow of Higher Education Academy, Senior Pharmacist, Medicines Management Team, Public Health Offices, East Lancashire PCT

David Kelly, MPharm, MRPharmS
Independent Prescriber, Pharmacist Practitioner/Teacher Practitioner, School of Pharmacy, UCLAN, Preston, Lancashire

Val Lawrenson, BA(Hons), MEd, CPT, RN, DN, NP
Nurse Teacher, NMC registrant, Senior Lecturer, School of Nursing and Caring Sciences, UCLAN, Preston, Lancashire

Anne Lewis, MSc, BNurs, RN, RHV, DNcert
NMC registrant, Trust Prescribing Lead, Central Lancashire PCT, Preston, Lancashire

Dilyse Nuttall, MSc (by research), BSc(Hons), PGDip, RN, RM, RHV
Nurse Prescriber, Nurse Teacher, NMC registrant, Fellow of Higher Education Academy, Senior Lecturer, School of Nursing and Caring Sciences, UCLAN, Preston, Lancashire

Joseph Quinn, MSc, BScPharm(Hons), MRPharmS
Member College Pharmacy Practice, School of Pharmacy, UCLAN, Preston, Lancashire

Jane Rutt-Howard, MSc, BSc, Dip HE, RGN
Nurse Prescriber (V300), NMC registrant, Assoc. Fellow of Higher Education Academy, Senior Lecturer, School of Nursing and Caring Sciences, UCLAN, Preston, Lancashire

Jean Taylor, MSc, BA(Hons), RN, RM, RHV
Nurse Teacher, NMC registrant, Fellow of Higher Education Academy, Principal Lecturer, School of Nursing and Caring Sciences, UCLAN, Preston, Lancashire

Samir Vohra, BPharm, MRPharmS
Lecturer in Clinical Pharmacy Practice, School of Pharmacy, UCLAN, Preston, Lancashire

Acknowledgements

Sincere thanks are given to the Non Medical Prescribing Team (David, Dawn, Gill, Janice, Jean, Ruth, Val), our colleagues from the School of Pharmacy (Alison, Jane, Joseph and Samir) and from clinical practice (Anne and Anne), for their valuable contributions to this book.

Special thanks also to our families for their patience and support without which this would not have been possible.

Dilyse would like to thank her husband Paul and her children James, Jack, Robert and Rebecca for their eternal support, encouragement and inspiration.

Jane is truly grateful for the unwavering belief, encouragement and patience shown to her by her family. Thank you Glyn, Ben, Noah and Jenny.

Introduction

Dilyse Nuttall and Jane Rutt-Howard

The *Textbook of Non-Medical Prescribing* has been developed to provide the reader with an insight into the key issues relating to prescribing in the UK today. The book's team of authors have vast experience in the development and delivery of non-medical prescribing programmes. This book has been developed in response to needs of health professionals undertaking the non-medical prescribing programme, and to the views of qualified non-medical prescribers and their colleagues.

The aim of the book is to:

1 provide a foundation on which non-medical prescribing students (V100, V150 and V300 including nurses, pharmacists and allied health professionals) can build their knowledge around the key areas and principles of prescribing
2 act as a continued source of information for qualified non-medical prescribers
3 provide a key source of information for non-prescribing health professionals who need to learn about the concept and context of prescribing in modern healthcare (e.g. pre-registration student nurses, pre-registration paramedics)
4 provide a key source of information for prescribing health professionals, including doctors considering acting as designated medical practitioners, who need to understand more about their role and the context of non-medical prescribing.

This book provides information essential to enable safe and effective prescribing. It also supports and directs the development and expansion of the reader's knowledge base, using generic principles to underpin specialist practice. The introduction has a dual purpose: to introduce the reader to the evolvement of non-medical prescribing and its position in a modern, multidisciplinary health service and to provide guidance on using the book effectively.

The development of prescribing

It had long been recognised that nurses wasted a significant amount of time visiting general practitioner (GP) surgeries and/or waiting to see the doctor in order to get a prescription for their patients. Although this practice produced the desired result of a prescription being generated, it was not an efficient use of either the nurses' or the GPs' time. Furthermore, it was an equally inefficient use of their skills, exacerbated by the fact that the nurse had usually assessed and diagnosed the patient and decided on an appropriate treatment plan. The situation was formally acknowledged in the Cumberlege Report (Department of Health and Social Security 1986) which initiated the call for nurse prescribing and recommended that community nurses should be able to prescribe from a limited list, or formulary. Progress was somewhat measured but *The Crown Report* of 1989 (Department of Health (DH) 1989) considered the implications of nurse prescribing and recommended suitably qualified registered nurses (district nurses (DN) or health visitors (HV)) should be authorised to prescribe from a limited list, namely the nurse prescriber's formulary (NPF).

Although a case for nurse prescribing had been established, progress relied on legislative changes to permit nurses to prescribe. Progress continued to be cautious with the decision made to pilot nurse prescribing in eight demonstration sites in eight NHS regions. In 1999, *The Crown Report II* (DH 1999) reviewed more widely the prescribing, supply and administration of medicines and, in recognition of the success of the nurse prescribing pilots, recommended that prescribing rights be extended to include other groups of nurses and health professionals. By 2001, DNs and HVs had completed education programmes through which they gained V100 prescribing status, enabling them to prescribe from the NPF. The progress being made in prescribing reflected the reforms highlighted in *The NHS Plan* (DH 2000), which called for changes in the delivery of healthcare throughout the NHS, with nurses, pharmacists and allied health professionals being among those professionals vital to its success. The publication of *Investment and Reform for NHS Staff – Taking forward the NHS plan* (DH 2001) stated clearly that working in new ways was essential to the successful delivery of the changes. One of these new ways of working was to give specified health professionals the authority to prescribe, building on the original proposals of *The Crown Report* (DH 1999). Indeed, *The NHS Plan* (DH 2000) endorsed this recommendation and envisaged that, by 2004, most nurses should be able to prescribe medicines (either independently or supplementary) or supply medicines under patient group directions (PGDs) (DH 2004).

After consultation in 2000, on the potential to extend nurse prescribing, changes were made to the Health and Social Care Act 2001. The then Health Minister, Lord Philip Hunt, provided detail when he announced that nurse prescribing was to include further groups of nurses. He also detailed that the NPF was to be extended to enable independent nurse prescribers to prescribe all general sales list and pharmacy medicines prescribable by doctors under the NHS, together with a list of prescription-only medicines (POMs) for specified medical conditions within the areas of minor illness, minor injury, health promotion and palliative care. In November 2002, proposals were announced by Lord Hunt, concerning 'supplementary' prescribing (DH 2002). The proposals were to enable nurses and pharmacists to prescribe for chronic illness management using clinical management plans. The success of these developments prompted further regulation changes, enabling specified allied health professionals to train and qualify as supplementary prescribers (DH 2005).

From May 2006, the nurse prescribers' extended formulary was discontinued and qualified nurse independent prescribers (formerly known as extended formulary nurse prescribers) were able to prescribe any licensed medicine for any medical condition within their competence, including some controlled drugs. Further legislative changes allowed pharmacists to train as independent prescribers (DH 2006) with optometrists gaining independent prescribing rights in 2007. The momentum of non-medical prescribing continues, with 2009 seeing a scoping project of allied health professional prescribing, recommending the extension of prescribing to other professional groups within the allied health professions and the introduction of independent prescribing for existing allied health professional supplementary prescribing groups, particularly physiotherapists and podiatrists (DH 2009). As the benefits of non-medical prescribing are demonstrated in the everyday practice of different professional groups, the potential to expand this continues, with consultation being recently undertaken to consider the potential for enabling other disciplines to prescribe (DH 2010).

Using *The Textbook of Non-medical Prescribing*

Overview

Each of the nine chapters contained within this book addresses a different issue; all of the issues are directly relevant to non-medical prescribing, so it is therefore recommended that the reader peruses all the chapters to gain a full insight into non-medical prescribing. However, it is not necessary to read the chapters in numerical order. The issues and principles considered within each chapter are generic to all prescribing and it is anticipated that the reader will apply this theory to his or her own practice. This will be helped by undertaking the activities incorporated within each chapter. Where appropriate, and in order to support the reader's understanding, references are made within individual chapters to other chapters in the book.

Core themes

The book has three core themes – public health, social and cultural issues and prescribing principles – which are considered significant both to safe and effective prescribing and to modern healthcare in the UK. The core themes are incorporated into the main body of each chapter and considered at the end of every chapter in a Key themes and considerations box. These core themes are:

Public health
Social and cultural issues
Prescribing principles

It is pertinent at this point to introduce the prescribing principles (National Prescribing Centre (NPC) 1999) because it is recognised that this may be a new concept to the reader. These were developed originally to support the first nurse prescribers in their decision-making but have continued to be an essential tool in supporting prescribers from all health professional groups able to prescribe. The 'seven good principles of prescribing' were developed by the NPC (1999) with the aim of providing a structured approach to the *process* of prescribing.

The principles are 'a stepwise approach' and are widely used both theoretically and practically. They are diagrammatically represented within the original *Prescribing Nurse Bulletin* (NPC 1999) as a pyramid. It could be suggested that the use of a pyramid to illustrate a 'stepwise approach' is not particularly representative. The connotation of a pyramid suggests a hierarchy of activity. All the principles of prescribing are as important as each other and may be better represented by the use of a staircase – there is an order to the principles (Figure I: 1).

Each of the seven principles requires the practitioner to have specific skills to support the prescribing process and to consider the relevant issues at each stage:

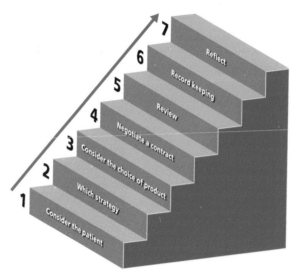

Figure I.1 A 'step wise' diagrammatical representation of the 7 Principles of Good Prescribing (NPC 1999).

Principle 1: examine the holistic needs of the patient
This requires the non-medical prescriber to make a thorough assessment in order to determine the appropriate course of action. This is aided by the use of the mnemonic 2-WHAM (NPC 1999):

W – **w**ho is it for/who is the patient?
W – **w**hat are the symptoms?
H – **h**ow long have the symptoms been present?
A – **a**ction taken so far?
M – other **m**edication?

Principle 2: consider the appropriate strategy
This highlights that the generation of a prescription is only one option and other treatment options might be more appropriate than drugs in some instances. Equally, to ensure that a prescribed treatment is most effective, it may need to be used alongside another strategy such as health promotion or referral to another health professional.

Principle 3: consider the choice of product
This prompts the prescriber to ensure that the product prescribed is that most appropriate for the patient, considering the clinical and cost-effectiveness. The NPC (1999) developed the mnemonic EASE to assist this process:

E - how clinically **e**ffective is the product?
A - how **a**ppropriate is the product for this specific patient?
S - how **s**afe is it?
E - is the prescription cost-**e**ffective?

Principle 4: negotiate a contract

This stresses the importance of involving the patient in decision-making in order to achieve concordance with the patient. The treatment option eventually undertaken should be the result of negotiation between the patient and prescriber, taking into account the patient's views, experiences and expectations.

Principle 5: review the patient

This requires that the prescriber maintain prescribing safety by regularly reviewing the patient to ensure that the treatment remains effective and appropriate.

Principle 6: record keeping

This reiterates the importance of accurate and up-to-date records in prescribing.

Principle 7: reflect

This acknowledges the importance of reflection in enabling the prescriber to maintain competence and continue to develop professionally.

Learning objectives

Each chapter has its own set of learning objectives that underpin its content. Achievement of these learning objectives is supported by both engagement with the discussion within the main text of the chapter and undertaking the activities.

Activities

Throughout the book are activities that support the reader in developing a deeper understanding of the theoretical knowledge base and in the application of theory to individual practice. Activities are present throughout the book and are indicated by the blue activity sign:

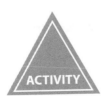

Case studies

The use of this book is supported by case studies at the end of the book. Most of the chapters make reference to a number of the case studies provided. This may be as part of the discussion or as an activity within the chapter. The purpose of the case studies is to help the reader to appreciate the benefits of non-medical prescribing both to the patient and to the different professions. Two groups of case studies are included: patients and health professionals. The patient case studies are numbered 1-9 and form the basis of many of the activities. The health professional case studies are annotated A-J and, in the main, serve to provide relevant examples of the use of non-medical prescribing by the different professional groups able to prescribe, from both an independent and a supplementary perspective.

Chapters and content

Chapter 1: Prescribing in context
This chapter defines and discusses the concept of non-medical prescribing in the context of a modern UK heath service. It explores the different qualifications available in non-medical prescribing and discusses their application in the practice of various professionals, including nurses, pharmacists and allied health professionals. This chapter includes explanation of independent, supplementary, community practitioner, V300, V150 and V100 prescribing. It also explores pharmacist and allied health professional prescribing. Comparisons are made between the different types of prescribing to highlight their individual benefits and restrictions.

Chapter 2: Ethical, legal and professional issues in relation to prescribing practice
The development of non-medical prescribing has depended on changes in professional body regulations, legal frameworks relating to medicines, and attitudes of patients and professionals in relation to roles and responsibilities. This chapter explores the ethical issues that impact on safe and effective prescribing. It also identifies the legal frameworks governing prescribing for all professional groups, highlighting the changes undertaken to enable and support non-medical prescribing. The extension of prescribing to other professional groups meant that the professional bodies had to develop existing regulations and guidance to support and govern this element of practice. This chapter explores these issues, identifying common elements of best practice, including prescription writing.

Chapter 3: Factors influencing prescribing
In addition to ethical, professional and legal issues, non-medical prescribing is subject to a variety of other influences that impact on the non-medical prescriber's ability to prescribe safely and effectively. This chapter explores these issues and identifies strategies to overcome related difficulties in order to promote concordance. The issues discussed include patient expectation, media influences, professional conflicts, drug company representatives, competence and training.

Chapter 4: Effective consultation
Chapter 4 discusses the holistic needs of the patient, considering these within the framework of existing consultation models. The various elements of the consultation process are explored, focusing on history taking and physical examination in relation to prescribing. The consultation culminates in the development of a management plan and this chapter explores the strategies used to enable this, including clinical decision-

making. The chapter incorporates an analysis of clinical decision-making models and theories, from both non-medical and medical perspectives. It also explores the consideration that all practitioners will experience a shift in their practice in order to address the novice aspect of prescribing. The deconstruction of their own practice can be difficult to manage both personally and professionally.

Chapter 5: Essential pharmacology

It is recognised that individual practitioners cannot know everything about all medicines but an essential element of good prescribing practice *is learning how to find out what we need to know*, in order to prescribe safely. This chapter directs the reader to trusted resources to develop and maintain knowledge about drugs. It guides the reader through processes to build a relevant knowledge of pharmacology, therapeutics and medicines management to populate his or her own personal formulary. Non-medical prescribing is founded on the principle that practitioners will prescribe only within their competence and scope of practice. It is an essential component of the clinical competence of prescribers to have knowledge of both how the drugs that they prescribe work at their site of action and how the drugs are handled by the body. The significance of co-morbidity and drug interactions is discussed, as are adverse drug reactions (ADRs), in order that the non-medical prescriber can minimise the risk to patients. The drug that the patient doesn't take is the most expensive drug of all. Patients can pay a high price in unresolved illness and lost earnings, while the NHS wastes valuable resources. This chapter discusses issues of concordance and adherence and guides the reader through processes by which negotiated consultations are encouraged.

Note that the principles of pharmacology addressed within this chapter aim to equip those practitioners with limited pharmacological knowledge with a foundation on which to build their understanding of the key issues.

Chapter 6: The multidisciplinary prescribing team

An essential aspect in safe and effective prescribing is recognition that prescribing is undertaken in a multidisciplinary context. This chapter examines the meaning of multidisciplinary team working in prescribing and explores the roles of the team members. The support processes provided by the various prescribing team members to individual non-medical prescribers, in a variety of situations and circumstances, are discussed.

Chapter 7: Clinical skills

Comprehensive and holistic assessment requires the use of appropriate clinical skills in order to support clinical decision-making and diagnosis. This chapter explores those skills recognised as core to safe and effective prescribing, highlighting relevant resources that can be accessed to incorporate these skills effectively. It is also recognises that a vast array of clinical skills, other than those considered core, will be used by non-medical prescribers in order to support prescribing in their specialist area of practice. Strategies to identify and develop these skills are discussed, emphasising the requirement for individual non-medical prescribers to prescribe within their competence.

Chapter 8: Prescribing for specific groups

It is recognised that different groups, such as children, older people, pregnant and breastfeeding women, and those with hepatic and renal impairment, require specific attention to ensure that the physiological differences and related risks are recognised and considered when prescribing. This chapter explores the needs of these individual groups in relation to prescribing, making reference to relevant guidance to support the non-medical prescriber in safe and effective prescribing. In addition to the groups mentioned, it is also recognised that other groups have specific needs that can impact on the ability of the non-medical prescriber to prescribe safely and effectively. These groups include young people, men, travelling families and black and minority ethnic groups. This chapter examines the needs of these specific groups in relation to prescribing practice.

Chapter 9: Enhancing non-medical prescribing

Non-medical prescribing has continued to evolve, enabling more groups of professionals to prescribe a wider range of drugs. However, the development of non-medical prescribing will continue as the number of prescribers increases. To support this process, infrastructures are necessary at all levels. The development of guidelines and policies to enable the non-medical prescriber to practise is only one aspect of a wider organisational approach. This chapter explains this infrastructure and discusses how it supports non-medical prescribing and promotes its development. The continuing professional development of individual practitioners is paramount and supported by reflection, identifying learning objectives and planning for professional development. This chapter explores the strategies in place to support this process.

References

Department of Health (1989) *Report of the Advisory Group on Nurse Prescribing (The Crown Report)*. London: The Stationery Office.

Department of Health (1999) *Review of Prescribing, Supply and Administration of Medicines: Final Report (The Crown Report II)*. London: The Stationery Office.

Department of Health (2000) *The NHS Plan: A plan for investment, a plan for reform*. London: The Stationery Office.

Department of Health (2001) *Investment and reform for NHS Staff - Taking forward the NHS plan*. London: HMSO.

Department of Health (2002) Pharmacists to prescribe for the first time, nurses will prescribe for chronic illness. Press release, 21 November 2002. London: The Stationery Office.

Department of Health (2004) *Extending Independent Nurse Prescribing within the NHS in England*. London: The Stationery Office.

Department of Health (2005) *Supplementary Prescribing by Nurses, Pharmacists, Chiropodists/Podiatrists, Physiotherapists and Radiographers within the NHS in England*. London: HMSO.

Department of Health (2006) *Improving Patients' Access to Medicines: A guide to implementing nurse and pharmacist independent prescribing within the NHS in England*. London: Department of Health.

Department of Health (2009) *Allied Health Professions Prescribing and Medicines Supply Mechanisms. Scoping report*. London: The Stationery Office.

Department of Health (2010) *Proposals to Introduce Prescribing Responsibilities for Paramedics: Stakeholder engagement*. London: The Stationery Office.

Department of Health and Social Security (1986) *Neighbourhood Nursing - A focus for care (the Cumberlege Report)*. London: The Stationery Office.

National Prescribing Centre (1999) Signposts for prescribing nurses - general principles of good prescribing. *Prescrib Nurse Bull* 1(1).

Chapter 1
Prescribing in Context

Dilyse Nuttall

Learning objectives

After reading this chapter and completing the activities within it, the reader will be able to:

1 identify the development and current context of non-medical prescribing in the UK
2 critically analyse the implementation of non-medical prescribing in relation to the different professional groups
3 evaluate the different types of prescribing and identify their appropriate application to practice

Non-medical prescribing has been subject to on-going development ever since its inception. This has resulted in changes in both the types of prescribing possible and the related terminology. This chapter explores the different qualifications available in non-medical prescribing and discusses their application in the practice of various professionals, including nurses, midwives, pharmacists and allied health professionals. The discussion incorporates explanation of independent prescribing and supplementary prescribing, differentiating between specific prescribers and making comparisons to highlight their individual benefits and restrictions.

The prescribing journey

The current position of prescribing is the result of its evolution from its origin in district nursing and health visiting to a well-established element of everyday practice for a range of health professionals. The journey has not been as straightforward as many would have hoped, with individual professions having to undertake a period of limited prescribing before being able to use it in a manner that best supports their practice. The introduction of prescribing to the nursing profession was, in many ways, tentative,

The Textbook of Non-medical Prescribing, edited by Dilyse Nuttall and Jane Rutt-Howard.
© 2011 Blackwell Publishing Ltd

1

with the 1992 Medicines Act enabling only a small group within a very large workforce to undertake the necessary programmes of education. Furthermore, the limited formulary imposed a controlled and constrained introduction of prescribing. Nevertheless, this was a welcome development, the benefits of which became increasingly apparent and, ultimately, led to prescribing becoming available to more nurses and more professions.

Arguably, the caution employed in the introduction of prescribing in nursing was, in part, due to the lack of a robust evidence base to support this new element of practice. Although many nurses' perceived intimation from this cautious approach was that they were more likely to make mistakes, a view unfortunately held by some medical colleagues (Day 2005), the profession was able to develop an increasing evidence base to support the expansion of prescribing. Supported by government-led consultations and evidence gathering from other professional groups and professional bodies, the necessity to introduce prescribing to other professional groups dictated the apposite change in terminology from nurse prescribing to non-medical prescribing.

Defining non-medical prescribing

The issue of terminology has often caused discord and confusion. The term 'nurse prescribing' remains an accurate description for nurses, with prescriptions continuing to identify nurses as such. Similarly, the terms 'pharmacist prescriber' and 'allied health professional prescriber' are used by the professional bodies governing these groups (Health Professions Council (HPC) 2006, Royal Pharmaceutical Society of Great Britain (RPSGB) 2006). Furthermore, the Departments of Health in England, Scotland, Wales and Northern Ireland (Department of Health (DH) 2006a, 2006b, Department of Health, Social Services and Public Safety (DHSSPS) 2006, Scottish Executive Health Department (SEHD) 2006, Welsh Assembly Government 2007, NHS Scotland 2009) continue to differentiate between prescribers. As a result, these terms are reiterated in the names of education programmes and in the evidence base supporting prescribing. Indeed, there is much benefit in this differentiation, from both a safety and a professional development perspective. However, these individual practitioner titles are components of the

 Activity box 1.1

Go to the government website relevant to your practice area and search for documents that outline the implementation of non-medical prescribing for your professional group. Consider their content in relation to your practice:

- www.dh.gov.uk
- www.scotland.gov.uk
- www.wales.gov.uk
- www.dhsspsni.gov.uk

broader context of prescribing by those health professionals who are not doctors or dentists. The inclusive term 'non-medical prescribing' is now widely used to represent these prescribers. It may be argued that the use of yet another term serves only to add further confusion, particularly to those unfamiliar with the concept of non-medical prescribing. However, the disadvantage of making reference only to individual titles is that there is much potential to support a profession-based approach that detracts from the multidisciplinary approach required for safe and effective prescribing, highlighted in Chapter 6.

The non-medical prescribing vision

In considering the context of non-medical prescribing, it is of benefit to revisit the origins of nurse prescribing to consider its early ethos and vision. The *Review of Prescribing and Administration of Medicines: Final Report* (DH 1999a) identified five key principles within the terms of reference (Table 1.1). On examining these principles and making comparison to policy and guidance supporting the current position of non-medical prescribing, it is evident that these principles remain steadfast. The Department of Health (2008a), in the document *Making the Connections: Using healthcare professionals as prescribers to deliver organisational improvements*, clearly identified the benefits of non-medical prescribing and the opportunities for healthcare professionals to enhance their practice by making effective use of prescribing. The benefits of non-medical prescribing presented for patients included increased access, increased capacity and improved choice for patients. This was supported by the professionals' ability to manage and complete episodes of care for patients, in a variety of settings, reiterating the messages from *Medicines Matters* (DH 2006b). Although the terminology and focus may have shifted slightly, the underpinning principles remain the same: safe and effective prescribing.

The complex nature of good prescribing was identified by the National Prescribing Centre (NPC) when they released their first *Nurse Prescribing Bulletin* (NPC 1999). The seven principles of good prescribing identified within this bulletin have provided a core framework for prescribers in their education and development for the past decade. However, it is important to recognise that, although these remain relevant, since their introduction, non-medical prescribing has moved forward significantly, in terms of both the range of treatments prescribable and the range of expertise and settings in which prescribing can now take place. As such, the seven principles should be seen as a foun-

Table 1.1 Key principles of the Crown Report

Patient safety
Effective use of resources
Skills and competencies of various health professionals
Changes in clinical practice
Public expectations

Department of Health (1999a).

dation on which to build rather than as a measure on which to base effectiveness. The NPC (2001, 2004a, 2006), the UK health departments (DH 2006a, 2006b, DHSSPS 2006, SEHD 2006, WAG 2007, NHS Scotland 2009) and the professional bodies (HPC 2006, Nursing and Midwifery Council (NMC) 2006, RPSGB 2006) have all identified the need to develop and maintain competency in prescribing beyond qualification, developing relevant frameworks and continuing professional development (CPD) strategies. These are discussed further in Chapter 9.

Attitude shifts

The evolution and success of non-medical prescribing should not merely be measured from the context of its magnitude. It is recognised that the process has required many legal, professional and ethical changes, as discussed in Chapter 2. Fundamentally, the increase in non-medical prescriber numbers and the strategies employed to support this development have relied on a change much more difficult to measure. It would, therefore, be inappropriate to consider the context of non-medical prescribing without addressing the significant and ongoing shifts in attitude that have enabled non-medical prescribing to flourish. The processes involved in enabling legal and professional changes have often highlighted the concerns and objections of individuals and groups from both the medical profession and colleagues in other health professions. These concerns have ranged from questions of safety to issues of boundaries within professional roles (Day 2005). Importantly, the evidence base developed has addressed many of these concerns. Data from the National Patient Safety Agency (NPSA 2007) identified that, although prescribing errors still occur, most medication errors arise from administration and supply. There is no indication that non-medical prescribing activity results in an increase in prescribing errors. Interestingly, most errors reported to the NPSA (2007) occurred in the acute setting. However, data held by the professional bodies about professionals with a non-medical prescribing qualification indicate that numbers currently remain lower in secondary care than in primary care.

Many of these prescribing errors have been attributed to junior doctors but the cause of these errors has been found to be multifactorial in nature (Velo and Minuz 2009). It is unproductive to utilise the junior doctor as a diversion from the concerns raised regarding non-medical prescribing, but it does highlight issues that should provide some reassurance to those raising the concerns. Significantly, a need for specific education for all prescribers has been identified (Schachter 2009) and the content of this education suggested by Likic and Maxwell (2009) reflects that already undertaken by non-medical prescribers. It is important that this information should not be seen as a defence of non-medical prescribing, but as evidence of good practice from which others may learn.

Attitudes towards prescribing are becoming increasingly positive, with the benefits brought to specialist roles being recognised (Avery and Pringle 2005). The role of doctors has not diminished as a result of non-medical prescribing, but instead there are numerous examples of how non-medical prescribing can be used by professionals to work alongside doctors to improve the patient experience (Thomas et al 2005, Courtney and Carey 2008). The health professional case studies provide some clear examples of this issue.

It is important also to consider the attitudes of those practitioners undertaking non-medical prescribing and the impact on the team (both the immediate healthcare team and the wider organisation). Prescribing can increase a practitioner's confidence and result in greater job satisfaction but any change in role and attitude of an individual within a team can have an impact on the team dynamics as a whole (Bradley and Nolan 2007). Although this can often be a positive change in dynamics, it is important to recognise that the journey is not always straightforward and change should be supported by ensuring that the team is informed and involved.

The success of non-medical prescribing not only has required an attitude shift by professional colleagues but, possibly more importantly, also has been reliant on its acceptance by patients. A recent study investigating the views of the Scottish general public found that there was a significant awareness of non-medical prescribing (Stewart et al 2009). Interestingly, respondents from Stewart et al's (2009) study reported that they were more comfortable with pharmacist or nurse prescribing than with other non-medical groups, a finding that could, at least in part, be due to familiarity with, and experience of, the public with those professionals. The study identified that the public required reassurance regarding clinical governance issues, reiterating the need for both a strong evidence base and effective channels of communication, to ensure that the public develop an awareness of advancements in non-medical prescribing.

Non-medical prescribing, medical prescribing or prescribing

As acknowledged above, safety and efficacy have remained the key objectives for non-medical prescribing, an ethos that has been fundamental to its success. However, all health professionals would surely argue that these are essential principles that underpin their practice as a whole and, indeed, any aspect of healthcare provision. The professional and ethical codes that serve to regulate the practice of health professionals (RPSGB 2007, HPC 2008, NMC 2008a) remain as relevant to prescribing as they do to other aspects of their practice.

Therefore, the debate should perhaps focus on the need to differentiate prescribing from any other element of healthcare practice. It would be inept to fail to recognise that prescribing presents specific challenges and potential problems that require specific guidance and standards. As such, all relevant professional bodies have developed curricula and standards to ensure that education programmes prepare students to practise as non-medical prescribers within the boundaries of their professional ethical code (NPC 2004a, NMC 2006, 2009, General Pharmaceutical Council 2010).

In recognising that prescribing requires specific consideration, the relationship between non-medical prescribing and medical prescribing must be considered. It has been established that the concepts of safety and efficacy are pertinent to all healthcare practice, including medical prescribing. It is logical to consider that some practices which support safety in prescribing, such as standards for writing prescriptions (British Medical Association (BMA) and RPSGB 2010), were originally developed for medical prescribing, before the advent of non-medical prescribing.

Therefore, it is reasonable to question the necessity to even differentiate between medical and non-medical prescribing. The potential for medicines to result in harm to patients is well acknowledged by the existence of agencies responsible for monitoring this throughout the UK (see Activity box 1.2). The data collected by these agencies reiterate the message that patient safety must be paramount, regardless of who is prescribing. The strategies, used to support patient safety and efficacy, are explored throughout the chapters of this book and adopt a holistic approach to prescribing.

This approach requires non-medical prescribers to consider all factors influencing their prescribing practice, including consultation skills, patient expectations, the clinical evidence base and CPD, in order to achieve the safest and most effective outcomes possible for the individual patient. This approach is reflected in non-medical prescribing education programmes throughout the UK. However, at present, although the objectives of medical and non-medical prescribing are fundamentally consistent, there remain stark differences in the standardisation of education with regards to prescribing between these two groups. The medical profession has shared a wealth of knowledge and skills with other health professionals as designated medical practitioners, to support them through their education and beyond. This has been invaluable in moving non-medical prescribing forward. However, it is evident that the benefits of the formalised and structured approach to providing education focused on prescribing would be relevant and valuable to all prescribers.

Activity box 1.2

The UK has dedicated agencies to address patient safety. Go to the appropriate agency website and, by accessing their resources, identify the recommendations for promoting patient safety in relation to your prescribing practice. Critically reflect on your practice and identify strengths and weaknesses in relation to patient safety:

National Patient Safety Agency (England, Northern Ireland and Wales): www.npsa.nhs.uk
Scottish Patient Safety Alliance: www.patientsafetyalliance.scot.nhs.uk
Healthcare Inspectorate Wales: www.hiw.org.uk
Health and Social Care Safety Forum (N. Ireland): www.hscsafetyforum.com

Changes in clinical practice

One of the major drivers behind the increasing development of non-medical prescribing has been the significant changes that have taken place in clinical practice. These changes have been a direct response to the recognition of the changing health needs of the population. The DH (2007a), in its operating framework, identified priorities for

2008-9 which also evolved as a result of an ageing population. This, in turn, has resulted in an increase in the number of people with long-term conditions. In order to address the demands on services, health care must aim to reduce both hospital admissions and the subsequent lengths of stay. The priorities set by the DH (2007b) maintain the public health approach, identifying access and inequalities as target areas. In addition, the need to reduce healthcare-associated infections and to prepare for emergencies were set as priorities, while also identifying the need to improve patient experience and staff satisfaction. The workforce continues to be subject to significant changes in response to these priorities, resulting in new challenges and demands (DH 2006c, 2008b, DHSSPS 2006, SEHD 2006, WAG 2007). Implementation of current health policy involves a fundamental shift of care into the community arena (DH 2008b) with both primary and secondary care evolving in response. Non-medical prescribing has long since ceased to be a primary care phenomenon, with independent prescribing developing rapidly in the hospital setting, responding to reductions in the working hours of junior doctors and emerging new and specialist roles. The expansion of non-medical prescribing into new areas brings not only many benefits and opportunities (Goswell and Siefers 2009) but also new challenges for all those involved (Clegg et al 2006, Cooper et al 2008a, Pontin and Jones 2008).

The role of non-medical prescribing

The skills and expertise of health professionals has been recognised as a valuable resource that could be used more effectively to support development of healthcare services (DH 2000, 2002, 2006a, Scottish Government 2008a). This has resulted in the development of new roles throughout the healthcare professions, including advanced practitioners, pharmacists and allied health professionals with specialist roles, community matrons and specialist midwife roles. This, in turn, has required a redefinition of many existing roles. In response to these developments and the changes that it has elicited, it has been recognised that health professionals need further education to meet the demands of both new and existing roles (Pooler and Campbell 2006). Arguably, non-medical prescribing not only has proved useful in these developments but also in some cases has been identified as an essential component of the health professional's role, clearly indicated within the job description. In considering the vision for modern UK healthcare in providing an equitable service, which meets the needs of service users and staff, it is clear that the ability for individual practitioners to complete episodes of care is paramount. It is important to acknowledge that it would be unrealistic to suggest that prescribing, as an isolated skill, would enable practitioners to complete every episode of care. However, in the context of prescribing representing an additional skill possessed by experienced and competent practitioners, it is fair to suggest that it would enable a significant number of consultations to be successfully concluded. The principles of prescribing (NPC 1999) and subsequently the competency frameworks supporting prescribing (NPC 2001, 2004a, 2006) have reiterated the message that writing a prescription is only one aspect of the multifaceted process of prescribing practice. As such, the skills acquired by health professionals in enabling them to reach a prescribing decision, whether or not it results in the generation of a prescription, means that those consultations that require referral can proceed in a more efficient and appropriate manner. Therefore, it is clear that, in an evolving healthcare service, non-medical prescribing is, and will continue to be, an essential component.

The economic context

The majority of prescribing activity undertaken by non-medical prescribers in the UK is undertaken by National Health Service (NHS) employees, with the cost of the treatment met by the NHS budget. The extent of spending on prescription items can be demonstrated by making reference to the document *Prescription Cost Analysis for England 2008* (NHS Information Centre for Health and Social Care 2009). In 2008, 70 million prescription items and £650 000 000 worth of payments were processed per month. The magnitude of this is compounded by the knowledge that this related only to prescriptions generated within the community.

The NHS prescribing budget, as with all areas of NHS provision, is a finite resource. As such, non-medical prescribing exists within the context of a service where resources must be used appropriately, efficiently and effectively in order that patients benefit from the full potential of the service. The consequence of this is that, in order for prescribing practice to be safe and effective, prescribers must consider issues of cost-effectiveness as part of the decision-making process. The issue of cost-effectiveness must be regarded in relation not only to the use of treatments but also to the many associate resources that compliment and support prescribing practice.

The achievement of an appropriate balance between cost-effectiveness and clinical effectiveness is an aspect with which many non-medical prescribers struggle. The reasons for this are numerous, influenced by professional, legal and ethical issues. Concordance issues, patient expectations, media influences and practitioner professional development issues are just a small selection of the factors that might impact on the choice of treatment and the balance of cost-effectiveness against clinical effectiveness. Case study 1 provides an example of how local formularies have been used effectively to address some of these issues.

Local formularies and guidelines (e.g. antimicrobial guidelines) can provide clear frameworks for non-medical prescribers and are often an important consideration in aiding decision-making about treatments. However, their use has been identified by some non-medical prescribers as restrictive (Hall et al 2004). Unfortunately, the drive for cost-effectiveness can easily be mistaken by an inexperienced prescriber as a necessity to always prescribe the cheapest treatment available. It is important that local formularies are not unfairly perceived as tools to limit prescribing to the cheapest options available. An engagement with national and local medicine management processes will support the non-medical prescriber in developing an understanding of the benefits of these formularies. It is worth noting that, within individual trust policy, there is usually an option to prescribe outside the formulary (where there is a clear rationale for doing so). Maintaining knowledge and competence in relation to their specialist field, particularly in relation to national guidelines and treatment options, is essential in enabling non-medical prescribers to work effectively with local formularies, while having the expertise to challenge them when appropriate.

Activity box 1.3

Access and summarise national guidelines for a condition for which you could prescribe. Access your local formulary and guidelines and compare these to the national guidelines. Answer the following questions:

- Are there any differences?
- Is there a rationale for the differences?
- Do you know the protocol for prescribing outside your local formulary?

The private sector

Although most non-medical prescribers practise within the NHS, there are a significant and increasing number of prescribers who work within private or independent practices. Each individual practitioner is responsible for ensuring that they practise in accordance with the regulations of their professional body and, of course, this includes a requirement to practise within, and to maintain, one's own competence. This remains the case, regardless of the sector in which they are employed. In order to provide and maintain quality and standardised care, the NHS requires that nationally determined standards are adopted and implemented within individual trusts and that these in turn are implemented within individual practices. Although many private sector practices ensure that comprehensive policies and protocols are in place, others have limited and/or inadequate governance procedures in place. The DH (2006a, p. 19) recognised the potential for differences in clinical governance systems and therefore made the following statement to promote safety, regardless of the setting in which non-medical prescribing is undertaken:

> Nurse and Pharmacist Independent Prescribers who work outside NHS settings where clinical governance systems may be different or may not be applied in the same way, must ensure they comply with requirements to demonstrate their competence to practice. For example, they must be able to show how they audit their practice, keep up-to-date with current guidance, and how they safeguard the patients in their care.

One related concern has been identified in relation to injectable medicines, such as Botox® and Vistabel®, used in cosmetic procedures. The receipt of wholesale supplies of these medicines by nurses, and remote prescribing by doctors, are just two issues that have prompted the need for guidance. The Medicines and Healthcare products Regulatory Agency (MHRA 2008) provided clear direction which also incorporated the position of the NMC in relation to nurses, based on *The Code: Standards of conduct, performance and ethics for nurses and midwives* (NMC 2008a) and *Standards for Medicines Management* (NMC 2008b). In undertaking a non-medical prescribing programme, health professionals are required to analyse their practice and become aware of their responsibility and accountability. This can be seen only as a positive outcome that will support safe and effective practice. The NMC (2007) acknowledged that some nurses were also moving into this area of practice after completion of a non-medical prescribing programme which prompted the identification of additional content for programmes to ensure that issues relevant to this area of practice are addressed.

The public health context

Public health was determined as a core theme of this book, due to its significance in modern UK healthcare. Addressing public health issues was clearly intended to be one of the key functions of non-medical prescribing, with health promotion being identified as one of the four original areas suitable for prescribing from the extended formulary (DH 1998). Although this categorisation has long ceased to be used, the need to consider health promotion and public health in non-medical prescribing practice remains essential.

UK public health policy

Current UK public health policy incorporates strategies to meet targets rather than simply addressing specific diseases and significantly focuses on tackling inequalities. This is due in part to the recognition that poverty and its associated health inequalities originally identified in the Black Report (Black et al 1980) and reiterated by Acheson (1998) and Wanless (2004) remain a key factor in the health of the population. As such, tackling health determinants has consistently been identified as an essential concept in UK health policy (DH 1999b, 2004, Scottish Government 2008b). The health agenda described by DH (2004) identified long-term key target areas (Table 1.2) with the objective of supporting and empowering the public to make healthier and informed choices.

This approach is reflected in the definition of public health provided by Acheson (1998):

Table 1.2 Choosing health key target areas

Accidents
Alcohol
Diet and nutrition
Inequalities
Mental health
Physical activity
Sexual health
Substance misuse
Tobacco

Source: Department of Health (2004).

The science and art of preventing disease, prolonging life and promoting health through the organised efforts of society ...

It is significant that this definition recognises the organised, multiagency partnership approach necessary for tackling health determinants. This reflects the messages in Chapter 6, supporting the need for a team approach to prescribing, in order that safety and efficacy are maximised. Acheson (1998) and Wanless (2004) stress that we all have a responsibility for our public health. This responsibility is both personal and professional, as individuals with responsibility for our own health (DH 2004) and as health professionals with responsibility to provide services that support public health (DH 2002).

It has been argued that every prescribing situation has a potential opportunity to promote health and address public health issues, but relies on individual practitioners developing an awareness of the current health issues, national and local targets, and factors determining health. Furthermore, it requires non-medical prescribers to recognise and embrace the opportunities to impact on public health targets elicited within the prescribing situation (Nuttall 2008).

Need and expectations

The public health focus of modern health care requires that the needs of the population are clearly identified and met. *Bradshaw's Taxonomy of Needs* (Bradshaw 1972, cited in Bradshaw 1994) considers categories of need that, although rudimentary, provide a useful framework for consideration. In relating this categorisation to both the health needs of the UK population and non-medical prescribing practice, links to policy developments, health provision and, indeed, public expectation can be clearly identified. The first category of 'felt need' relates to issues or factors that members of the population feel constitute a need. These needs are felt but not articulated. Once these needs are articulated, they fall in to the second category of Bradshaw's taxonomy: 'expressed need'. The third category of 'normative needs' refers to issues and factors that health professionals have identified as needs within the population. These needs are usually based on epidemiological data and population profiles that identify key health issues in the population as a whole but also in specific communities within the wider population. The final category of 'comparative need' refers to the needs that are determined by making comparisons between individuals within the same community or population. In a health service where the philosophy is to ensure that the patient and his or her individual needs are placed at the centre of the care provided (DH 2006c), it is essential that all these needs be considered.

Current national health targets are largely based on normative needs, which are targeted more specifically at local level. However, although normative needs are generally an accurate representation of broad health needs, they can often differ from those felt and expressed by users of the health service. The disparity may in part be due to differences in prioritisation between service users and service providers. To ensure that non-medical prescribing is meeting the needs of the population, it must not only target public health issues previously identified but also ensure that patients and carers have the ability to express their felt needs.

The DH commissioned a study by the University of Southampton in 2005, to evaluate extended formulary independent nurse prescribing. This study did seek the views of patients, as well as those of nurses and doctors. However, the number of patients involved was unclear and the summary of their responses was broad. The DH has commissioned a further study with Southampton and Keele Universities (Keele University 2009), which will evaluate nurse and pharmacist independent prescribing. This again has an element of patient focus, though it is still unclear if this will enable patients to express their needs. It remains essential to ensure that subsequent research and consultation seeks the views of service users as well as those governing or providing the service.

On an individual level, non-medical prescribers have a responsibility to ensure that the processes and strategies used with individuals enable the patient and carers to receive a service that meets their needs. This may be achieved through a number of measures, not least through the strategy fundamental to safe and effective prescribing – that of the holistic assessment. Concordance, which is discussed in depth in Chapter 5, relies on negotiation between the patient and the non-medical prescriber. For any negotiation to be effective, it must take in to account the needs and views of the individuals involved and there is an expectation that these needs will be adequately considered.

Activity box 1.4

Take time to reflect on your practice and consider the following questions:

- Do you allow patients to express their needs?
- Are there any barriers to this?
- What strategies could you employ to improve the ability of patients to express their needs?

Differentiating between prescribers

The first part of this chapter explored the wider context of prescribing in the UK. However, it is important to identify how individual practitioners apply non-medical prescribing within the context previously examined. The terms 'independent' and 'supplementary' used in relation to prescribing cover a range of professions and a range of prescribing activity. Therefore, the latter part of this chapter differentiates between independent prescribing and supplementary prescribing. It also explores the application of both types of prescribing within the practice of different health professionals.

Independent prescribing

The term 'independent prescribing' has been (and still is) used in a variety of contexts, all presenting differences in its meaning and application. This may cause confusion to those new to the concept of non-medical prescribing, not least because of the use of the term both as a title identifying prescribing activity by a particular type of prescriber and as a method of prescribing in itself. It is important to clarify these issues, recognising that independent prescribing is a core concept that underpins prescribing practice by many professional groups.

Independent prescribing was identified as one of two types of prescribing recommended in the final report of the *Review of Prescribing, Supply and Administration of Medicines* (DH 1999a). It was originally anticipated that independent prescribing would address undiagnosed conditions. However, the current working definition has evolved beyond this.

Independent prescribing is defined by the Department of Health (2006b, p. 2) as:

> ... prescribing by a practitioner responsible and accountable for the assessment of patients with undiagnosed or diagnosed conditions and for decisions about the clinical management required, including prescribing ...

This definition is clearly underpinned by legal, professional and ethical principles, with responsibility and accountability at its centre. It identifies a method of prescribing where the individual professional undertaking prescribing practice must be able to make a prescribing decision and support this with a clear rationale. This, of course, reflects professional practice requirements, while recognising the specific factors supporting safe and effective prescribing. The DH (2006b) definition is significant in that it recognises three important factors in relation to independent prescribing:

1. Assessment is fundamental to safe and effective prescribing.
2. Practitioners who prescribe independently may do so for undiagnosed and/or diagnosed conditions.
3. Independent prescribing involves making a decision about clinical management, which may or may not require a prescription to be generated.

Assessment

A deeper exploration of these factors highlights fundamental practice issues that are frequently identified by both training and practising prescribers. The key elements of assessment are considered in depth in Chapter 4 of this book, with the link to safe and effective prescribing clearly identified. Indeed, independent prescribing requires that assessment is a key component of the process, with the prescriber responsible and accountable for this. Essentially, independent prescribing is a process that relies on the information gleaned from an assessment in order that a diagnosis and/or clinical management decision can be reached. In most instances, the assessment will be an integral element of the consultation process. However, this raises the question of whether or not the prescriber must undertake the assessment.

One of the issues highlighted by *Saving Lives: Our healthier nation* (DH 1999b) was that nurses were undertaking assessments and making decisions about clinical management of patients' conditions. Doctors were then issuing prescriptions based on the judgement of these nurses. Not only did this highlight the often unrecognised knowledge and expertise of many nurses, but it also identified safety issues in relation to these practices. One of the main advantages of non-medical prescribing was therefore that it enabled the same practitioner who had undertaken the assessment, and who was in possession of all the relevant information, to prescribe treatment if necessary. However, some practitioners will argue that this is not always possible or indeed necessary. This again raises further issues, which often relate not only to the individual prescriber's practice but also to the expectations of colleagues.

Ultimately, the independent prescriber is responsible and accountable for the assessment of the patients for whom he or she will make a decision about clinical management. There may be an expectation by some health professionals that their prescribing colleague will issue prescriptions on their request. Of course, in some instances, non-medical prescribers may work alongside colleagues who are competent in assessment and diagnosis of specific conditions, and in whose ability they are very confident. However, the NMC (2008b) has considered the issue of remote prescribing, and has determined that it is only acceptable in exceptional circumstances. Practice issues such as these often highlight other areas that need to be addressed. Although many health professionals may be competent in assessment in order to reach a diagnosis, it is possible that their assessment does not address all issues relevant to making a safe prescribing decision. Furthermore, if these practitioners are competent, there is an expectation that they should be identifying, within their own practice, the need to prescribe themselves, and as such should endeavour to undertake the appropriate programme of education.

Diagnosed and undiagnosed conditions

The Department of Health's (2006a) definition of independent prescribing significantly included diagnosed conditions within its remit, an element missing from previous definitions. This change recognised the fact that non-medical prescribers who prescribed independently may do so in a variety of situations, treating a wide range of patients and conditions. As such, some non-medical prescribers will treat only patients who have been previously diagnosed, whereas others would be making the initial diagnosis and prescribing for that condition. Many non-medical prescribers will prescribe for both previously diagnosed and undiagnosed conditions. As practitioners preparing to undertake a non-medical prescribing education programme, individuals will have a clear indication into which category they fall. However, in reality, the boundaries are arguably more difficult to define, e.g. the practitioner whose case load includes only patients who have previously been diagnosed may find that they present with side effects of treatments that may require short-term treatment. Equally, patients may also present with an unrelated complaint for which the non-medical prescriber is still competent to prescribe.

The prescribing decision

In considering the context of independent prescribing, it is important to reiterate the message set in the prescribing principles (NPC 1999), reinforced in the competency frameworks (NPC 2001, 2004a, 2006), and embedded in the Department of Health's (2006a) definition, that prescribing a drug is only one option available to the practitioner prescribing independently. Indeed, it would be inappropriate to prescribe a drug without providing some health promotion, whether that be advice on physical measures to be taken to support the drug treatment, e.g. dietary advice when prescribing cholesterol-reducing drugs, or preventing accidents such as overdose by giving clear instructions for taking the drug. Strategies used to reach a prescribing decision are discussed at length in Chapter 4 but the key message is that it is not a requirement that independent prescribing results in a prescription. The processes and strategies used will enable an appropriate prescribing decision to be made which may mean that only health promotion advice is necessary or that referral is needed, either in isolation or in support of a drug treatment. The practitioner trained as an independent prescriber will have developed skills that reach far beyond simply being able to write a prescription. The decision to prescribe or not will be made within the context of a holistic and multidisciplinary approach to consultation and treatment options.

Who are independent prescribers?

The process of independent prescribing requires appropriate professionals to undertake the activity. Non-medical prescribers hold a recognised qualification, which is annotated on the relevant professional register, and continue to demonstrate competence in assessment, diagnosis, decision-making and treatment of specific conditions (DH 2006b). The conditions for which they prescribe may be limited to one or may be wide ranging. These professionals are referred to as *independent prescribers*. Unfortunately, the terminology does not lend itself to a simplistic interpretation of the role. Not only is the term 'independent prescriber' used to describe the professional undertaking independent prescribing but it is also a title given to specific prescribers, recorded as such by their professional bodies. This, in essence, means that although a range of professionals undertake the processes highlighted within the DH (2006a) definition, and as such undertake independent prescribing, they would not necessarily be referred to as independent prescribers. Supplementary prescribing is more distinct and it is anticipated that understanding the differences between supplementary and independent prescribing will provide further clarity when considering the role of prescribers within individual professional groups.

Activity box 1.5

Look at case study 1 at the back of this book and consider the following questions:

- Is non-medical independent prescribing the appropriate method for this patient to access medicines?
- What is your rationale for your answer?
- Would there be any potential barriers to you undertaking non-medical independent prescribing for this particular patient?

Supplementary prescribing

Supplementary prescribing, in common with independent prescribing, has evolved from the recommendations made in the final report of *the Review of Prescribing, Supply and Administration of Medicines* (DH 1999a). The original reference was to 'dependent prescribing' where a dependent prescriber would be responsible for the continuing care of patients who had initially been assessed by an independent prescriber. Although the terminology and, indeed, the definition have altered, the core principles have remained very much the same. The current definition of supplementary prescribing is:

> ... a voluntary partnership between an independent prescriber (a doctor or dentist) and a supplementary prescriber to implement an agreed patient-specific clinical management plan (CMP) with the patient's agreement ...

> DH (2005, p. 8)

Undertaking supplementary prescribing therefore requires application of the key principles underpinning it. One key principle of supplementary prescribing is that of partnership. The dynamics of supplementary prescribing are different to those of independent prescribing in that the non-medical prescriber takes on the role of supplementary prescriber, with a doctor (or dentist) adopting the role as independent prescriber. This means that the doctor (or dentist) takes responsibility for a diagnosis, or a decision relating to the review of an existing diagnosis, at the time of the development of a CMP. The supplementary prescriber is then able to review the patient and manage the longer-term care of the patient. This crude interpretation is not a complete reflection of supplementary prescribing because it understates the partnership context that is crucial to its success.

The role of partnership

Partnership in supplementary prescribing is essential in order to effectively achieve the following fundamental requirements of supplementary prescribing:

- Agreement on which patients will be suitable for supplementary prescribing
- Obtaining the patient's agreement to being treated under a CMP
- Agreement of an individual CMP
- Maintenance of communication in relation to review and prescribing.

However, the necessity for partnership extends beyond this. In addition to the responsibility for the diagnosis, the independent prescriber is responsible for the boundaries of the CMP (DH 2005). To effectively set boundaries within which the supplementary prescriber will prescribe, it is crucial that there is an honest exchange to determine the competence of the supplementary prescriber and to ensure that the expectations of the independent prescriber remain within the parameters of that competence. Furthermore, the independent prescriber has a responsibility to provide support and advice to the supplementary prescriber as required (DH 2005). Arguably, this relies in part on the confidence of the supplementary prescriber's ability to seek and receive this support as necessary. Equally, the independent prescriber will have expectations that the supplementary prescriber accepts responsibility, and is accountable, for his or her own prescribing practice (see Chapter 2).

The concept of partnership in supplementary prescribing extends beyond the relationship between the independent prescriber and the supplementary prescriber. In actual fact, the whole concept of supplementary prescribing relies on a three-way partnership, with the patient completing the tripartite collaboration. The patient must be aware of, and agree to, the intention to facilitate his or her care through a CMP, and his or her agreement to receive care via supplementary prescribing must be documented (DH 2005).

The clinical management plan

As already stated the CMP is an essential component of supplementary prescribing and as such must be drawn up before prescribing begins. The CMP may be hand-written or completed electronically but must be relevant to the specific patient and his or her specific condition(s) (DH 2005). Table 1.3 identifies the information that the Department of Health (2007c) determines must be included within a CMP and an example of a completed CMP can be seen in case study 9.

So that supplementary prescribing is utilised efficiently and safely, CMPs need to be relatively quick and simple to complete (NPC 2007). However, there is often confusion about their completion and this has contributed to the notion that their development can be time-consuming. Although the information that must be included may seem extensive at first glance, there are acceptable methods of reducing the magnitude of this information on the CMP, provided that the full details are easily accessible, e.g. as indicated in Table 1.3, it is not necessary to list every medication and every possible regimen on the CMP if it directly reflects that stated in a recognised published guideline. Instead, it is perfectly acceptable to indicate that treatment will be given in line with the guidelines (identifying specific sections where appropriate) named on the CMP, provided that they are readily available to both the independent prescriber and the supplementary prescriber. Similarly, detailed patient information, available to both pre-

Table 1.3 Essential Information to be Included on a clinical management plan (CMP)

Patient's name
Condition(s) for which the supplementary prescriber may prescribe
Start date for CMP
Date for review by the independent prescriber
Identification of medicines or appliances that may be prescribed under the CMP[a]
Identification of limitations or restrictions of identified medicines, including strength, dose, period of use[a]
Indications for referral back to the independent prescriber
Allergies, sensitivities and difficulties relating to medicines or appliances
Arrangements for notification of adverse reactions and incidents of potential or actual serious harm from appliances

[a]Reference to relevant parts of published guidelines may be made instead provided that they clearly identify the required information and are easily accessible.
Department of Health (2007c).

scribers in shared records, does not need to be recorded on the CMP unless there is a specific need to do so.

In addition to the information necessary on a CMP, there is a need for clarity about responsibility for its completion and the signatures required. Although the CMP must be agreed by both prescribers, either may take responsibility for composing it. A CMP that contains the signatures of both the independent and supplementary prescribers provides clear evidence that it has been agreed and, therefore, could be considered preferential. However, it is not always possible for the CMP to be signed by both pre-scribers and, as such, it is not an essential requirement. However, agreement to the CMP must be recorded in the patient's record (DH 2005). Similarly, although the patient's agreement must be obtained if he or she is to be cared for using a CMP, it is not necessary for the patient to sign it. However, a record that a discussion has taken place, and that the patient has agreed, must be recorded in the patient's records (DH 2005).

A further consideration in relation to CMP use is the potential for more than one supplementary prescriber to be involved in the patient's care. If more then one health professional, who is able to prescribe as a supplementary prescriber, is involved in the care of the patient in direct relation to the condition(s) indicated on the CMP, then he or she is able to prescribe from it, provided that (DH 2005):

- they agree to the CMP
- they are named on the CMP
- they have agreed strategies of communication between all prescribers
- they have access to consult and use the same part of the common record.

Termination of supplementary prescribing

Partnership working and agreement are fundamental throughout the process of sup-plementary prescribing and this extends to the point at which a CMP may be terminated. As supplementary prescribing relies on the three-way agreement previously discussed, the CMP must be terminated in the event of any circumstances that compromise this partnership (Table 1.4). The Department of Health (2005) determines that an existing CMP could be used by a replacement supplementary prescriber, provided that he or she agreed to the CMP and was then named on it.

The initial development of a CMP requires an agreement to be made about a date for a joint formal review. This should generally be within a maximum of 12 months unless the stability of the patient's condition indicates otherwise (DH 2005). Essentially, the date of review must be appropriate to the needs of the patient and his or her presenting

Table 1.4 Circumstances for termination of the clinical management plan

At the request of the independent prescriber (IP), the supplementary prescriber (SP) or the patient

If the named SP is unable to continue in this role and is the only named SP

At the set review date (unless agreement has been made to continue)

Department of Health (2005).

condition(s). The CMP will be terminated at the set review date unless it is agreed at the review that the CMP is to continue.

Who are supplementary prescribers?

Supplementary prescribing was enabled by changes in legislation in 2003. These changes allowed first level registered nurses, registered midwives and registered pharmacists to undertake supplementary prescribing, following a recognised programme of education. Subsequently, in 2005, further changes in legislation enabled defined professions from the allied health professions to undertake supplementary prescribing. The identified professionals were radiographers, podiatrists, physiotherapists and optometrists. A recent scoping and analysis of services has recommended the expansion of supplementary prescribing to other allied health professions and to enable physiotherapists and podiatrists to prescribe independently (DH 2009). Legislative changes will be required to enable these developments. For detailed explanation of the law in relation to non-medical prescribing, see Chapter 2.

Resistance to supplementary prescribing

The introduction of supplementary prescribing brought with it the expectation that its use would be in the management of long-term conditions, with the inclusion in some instances of acute episodes within these long-term conditions (DH 2005). Indeed, there is much evidence of its usefulness in this area of healthcare (Carey and Courtney 2008). Although having distinct characteristics, the aim of supplementary prescribing reflects the ethos of non-medical prescribing as a whole, in that its intention is to use the skills of health professionals more effectively and enable patients to access medicines more efficiently (DH 2005). The benefits of supplementary prescribing were arguably much clearer at its inception when independent prescribing was limited to a formulary. Supplementary prescribing enabled health professionals to prescribe drugs within the boundaries of a clinical management plan, who, although competent to do so, were legally unable to prescribe as an independent prescriber. The evolution of independent prescribing has eliminated this as a rationale for supplementary prescribing. Many qualified, and even training, non-medical prescribers would argue that, as they would only prescribe for conditions for which they are competent to do so, they would be competent to prescribe for these same conditions independently. However, in many ways, this has clouded the benefits of supplementary prescribing which always extended beyond simply enabling a broader range of medicines to be prescribed.

In attempting to highlight the continued benefits of supplementary prescribing, it is useful to deconstruct the actual and perceived purposes of its introduction. Supplementary prescribing was introduced to treat long-term conditions. This aspect remains unchanged because it would rarely be an efficient use of resources to develop a CMP for a condition that would respond to a short-term, and often simple, programme of treatment. However, the argument remains that, even in the care of long-term conditions, non-medical prescribers are able to make independent prescribing decisions. It is perhaps this argument that has had the greatest impact on the perceived usefulness of the CMP. Yet, it could be argued that, in making the case for independent prescribing in long-term conditions, there is an assumption that all patients are relatively typical, that the progress of the condition is predictable and that the response to treatment is generally straightforward. Furthermore, it also suggests that all non-medical prescribers would be confident and competent to treat any patient provided that they presented with a condition for which they were competent to prescribe. When presented in this manner, the argument seems more fluid.

Realistically, many new non-medical prescribers find the prospect of prescribing very daunting. It is recognised that, for some practitioners, supplementary prescribing is a useful method of allowing them to develop their skills in prescribing and, in turn, increase their confidence (DH 2005). Of course, some patients have a simple medical history and respond well to the routine treatments indicated for their long-term condition. However, many others are much more complex, with multiple medical conditions and/or polypharmacy issues that increase the likelihood of complications. In such instances, the supplementary prescriber may feel that the ability to discuss the patient's needs and to determine a suitable plan of management within predetermined boundaries, enables him or her to prescribe more safely and, indeed, more confidently.

Although pharmacists, nurses and midwives are able to prescribe independently, at present allied health professionals are able to prescribe only as supplementary prescribers, thus requiring a CMP to be in place for any patient for whom they would want to prescribe. As is recognised in nursing and pharmacist practice, supplementary prescribing is not appropriate for every patient, requiring the allied health professional in some instances to refer to an independent prescriber instead. These limitations do not serve to improve the profile of supplementary prescribing by being the only tool available to prescribe. However, they do successfully demonstrate that supplementary prescribing is a useful method of prescribing for some patients but that other methods need to be available to meet the needs of the client/patient group as a whole.

Considering the current UK context of non-medical prescribing, there are limitations that serve to maintain the need for supplementary prescribing. Pharmacists, for example, are unable to prescribe any controlled drugs as an independent prescriber and nurses and midwives able to prescribe can prescribe only a limited range of controlled drugs for specific conditions (note that community practitioner nurse prescribers cannot prescribe any controlled drugs). In instances where controlled drugs are necessary, the CMP enables the non-medical prescriber to meet the patient's needs. It is anticipated, however, that, even without any legal limitations relating to controlled drugs, some non-medical prescribers would choose to use supplementary prescribing as a safety mechanism.

The development of supplementary prescribing and clinical management plans has been hindered by medical apathy and implementation problems (Cooper et al 2008b). Indeed, it has been perceived as a time-consuming process, an issue that for some outweighs any benefits of supplementary prescribing. CMPs do involve an initial outlay of time in their development but, when used appropriately, this is reimbursed through the time saved by enabling the supplementary prescriber to undertake subsequent reviews. Although CMPs must be relevant to individual patients, it is acceptable for prescribers to develop CMPs for specific conditions provided that they are refined for each patient in order to meet their individual needs.

Difficulties in accessing records have also proved problematic for some non-medical prescribers. DH (2005, p. 19) stated that in supplementary prescribing:

The independent prescriber and the supplementary prescriber must share access to, consult, keep up to date and use the same common patient record ...

This has often been misinterpreted to mean that only supplementary prescribers who use the same patient records as the independent prescriber can undertake prescribing. This would eliminate a large number of non-medical prescribers, particularly those who work in areas with limited direct medical input. The requirements in relation to records is that there must be a common record where prescribing is documented. The mechanisms for enabling this must be agreed by the independent prescriber and the supplementary prescriber, so that both prescribers remain aware of the current status of the treatment plan.

A further challenge experienced by practitioners in relation to supplementary prescribing is that of responsibility of diagnosis. Podiatrists, for example, often see patients who have been referred to them by a doctor, in order that they, as the specialist, make a diagnosis and often a decision about treatment. Although this obviously supports the need for independent prescribing for these professional groups, it should not be seen as a barrier to supplementary prescribing. In fact, developing supplementary prescribing partnerships within these circumstances enables effective use of specialist knowledge and skills in a shared decision-making context.

Although it is important to recognise the limitations of supplementary prescribing in an evolving context of non-medical prescribing, it is equally important not to lose sight of the many benefits that remain. To promote an understanding of these benefits, it is pertinent to provide clear examples of when it might be utilised effectively.

Activity box 1.6

Look at case study 9 at the back of this book and consider the following questions:

- Is non-medical supplementary prescribing the appropriate method for this patient to access medicines?
- What is your rationale for your answer?
- Would there be any potential barriers to you undertaking non-medical supplementary prescribing for this particular patient?

Nurse non-medical prescribers

The NMC currently validates courses to train three different types of non-medical prescriber (V100, V150 and V300), all of whom have fundamental similarities, yet some distinct differences.

V100 non-medical prescribers

The history of non-medical prescribing identified that health visitors and district nurses were the first groups of professionals to undertake non-medical prescribing. This pre-scribing was, and still is, limited to a defined formulary. This limited formulary is known as the Community Practitioner Nurse Prescriber Formulary and contains items felt to be relevant to community practitioner practice. Although some prescribers have found the formulary to be limiting (Hall et al 2004), the extent of prescribing undertaken from this formulary and the limited number of health visitors and district nurses who go on to extend their prescribing role would suggest that, in the main, this is an appropriate formulary. However, V100 or community practitioner nurse prescribing is an extended role available to all community practitioners, including school nurses, community mental health nurses, community children's nurses and general practice nurses, provided that they have undertaken and successfully completed a specialist community practitioner programme. The V100 education programme is incorporated into many specialist community public health nursing and community specialist practice programmes as a core component, although the requirement for specific groups within these programmes to undertake the V100 element varies. However, when V100 is not a compulsory element, dictated by either programme specification or local trust requirements, few of these other nursing groups have chosen to undertake V100 prescribing education. The limitations of the formulary are no doubt a significant reason for this apparent lack of interest in prescribing, with its contents still very much relevant to health visitors and district nurses. However, there are also other possible explanations that must be recognised.

Competence is a crucial element in nursing practice and one that is equally important in prescribing. Interestingly, although some practitioners would consider themselves competent to make a decision about a need for treatment with many drugs within the *British National Formulary* (BNF), they would not do so in relation to the drugs within the community practitioner nurse prescribing formulary. For example, a community mental health nurse may assess the patient, decide that an increase of his selective serotonin reuptake inhibitor (SSRI) is necessary and prescribe the treatment (if appro-priately trained) from the BNF. However, the same nurse may not feel competent to make a diagnosis of constipation and so would not prescribe, even though there are drugs available to treat constipation within the community practitioner nurse prescriber formulary. Other legal and ethical issues may also impact on the decision by some specialist community practitioners not to undertake the V100 education programme. Consent is often problematic, for example, for school nurses. Although they may feel that, with further education, they would be competent to prescribe from the formulary, they may argue that the legal and ethical constraints of prescribing for children within the school environment would make it impossible. However, it is worth noting that changing roles for school nurses mean that there is potential to prescribe in other set-tings where the issues are different from those within the school. Day (2007) identified clear benefits of non-medical prescribing within a school nursing role. However, this was limited to a specific setting and supported V300 prescribing rather than V100.

V100 prescribing requires the nurse to make an assessment, diagnose or review an established diagnosis, and decide on the appropriate treatment (which may include prescribing). As such, V100 prescribing can be seen to be representative of independent prescribing. Case study A provides an example of V100 prescribing in practice.

V150 non-medical prescribing

V100/community practitioner nurse prescribing has become well established since it was introduced throughout the UK and, overall, has confirmed the benefits suggested at its introduction. However, the service provided by community nurses has evolved and, as such, the adequacy of V100 prescribing to meet current service needs has been in question. Indeed, it has become evident that, in many areas, developments in community nursing have, unintentionally, had an adverse impact on prescribing. This impact has included limitations on practice caused by the lack of available non-medical prescribers and, as a result, has also often supported poor prescribing practice. Changing roles in district nursing has meant that many experienced nurses have moved to newly developed roles, and teams that once had a number of nurses with a community specialist practitioner qualification now often have only one. These nurses are responsible for leading a team of staff nurses who generally do not hold the V100 qualification and so are unable to prescribe. The obvious impact of this change is a significant reduction in the number of non-medical prescribers within district nursing teams. This, in turn, has meant that, overall, fewer episodes of care can be completed by district nurses. The consequence of this is that alternative strategies have been employed to address the limited numbers of available prescribers within a service that has maintained a need for non-medical prescribers. Although no doubt well intentioned, these strategies have often involved practice that does not conform to the standards supporting safe and effective prescribing. In effect, practices that V100 prescribing aimed to replace have now re-emerged in a new guise.

In recognition of these problems, and of the obvious need for more prescribers, a study of the education needs of community nurses was undertaken by Fitzpatrick et al (2007). The findings from their work led to the introduction of V150 community practitioner nurse prescribing. The V150 prescriber is able to prescribe from the same formulary as the V100 prescriber, but undertakes the education programme as a stand-alone module of study rather than as part of a community specialist practitioner or specialist community public health nursing programme. The differences in context of the education programmes for V150 and V100 have determined the differences in the content of the courses. The V150 education programme incorporates additional study days which aim primarily to consider leadership and related issues that V100 students receive within the wider specialist nursing programme. The requirement for the nurse to assess the patient, reach a decision about diagnosis or outcome of a review, and negotiate treatment means that, as with V100, V150 prescribing can be seen to be representative of independent prescribing.

The introduction of V150 prescribing varies dramatically throughout the UK. The north west of England has already trained significant numbers of nurses and numbers are slowly increasing in other areas of England. V150 education programmes are becoming available in other areas of the UK, subject to the identification of a service need. Hogg and Schelowok (2009) recognise that V150 can be a useful tool in meeting the needs of services where there is a need for more prescribers but where V300 prescribing is not indicated. Case study C provides an example of how V150 prescribing has improved services for patients.

V300 independent/supplementary nurse prescribers

Nurses and midwives who wish to undertake education to prepare them to prescribe as independent prescribers will now access programmes that incorporate both independent and supplementary prescribing. It is worth clarifying at this juncture that V200 extended formulary nurse prescribers were trained as independent prescribers but were able only to prescribe from a specific formulary known as the 'extended formulary'. This has now been replaced by the V300 programme. V200 prescribers are no longer limited to this formulary but may or may not have accessed further education in supplementary prescribing. Supplementary prescribing is considered in detail later.

As with all the aforementioned types of nurse prescribers, V300 independent prescribing incorporates all the elements of independent prescribing previously determined but allows a much more extensive range of medicines to be prescribed. Unlike V100 and V150 prescribers, who are limited to the community practitioner formulary, V300 prescribers can prescribe any drug (including some controlled drugs), for any condition. However, despite the differences in the range of medicines available to the V100, V150 and V300 prescribers, there remains a common restriction that limits the range of medicines actually prescribed. That restriction is enforced by the NMC in its standards for prescribing, which reinforce the need for individual practitioners to prescribe only within the limits of their competence. Furthermore, restrictions may be set locally to address concerns relating to specific areas of practice, e.g. a study conducted in Wales by Jones (2008) identified a view among health professionals that a cautious approach was needed in the implementation of independent prescribing in mental health settings. Studies in both Scotland (Snowden 2008) and Ireland (Wells et al 2009) reflected this, albeit within differing contexts.

The term 'independent prescribing' has been used consistently in relation to V300 prescribing for many years. As a result of this, many people would use the terms 'V300' and 'independent prescriber' synonymously. However, as previous discussion identified, supplementary prescribing is a key strategy in V300 prescribing, the benefits of which are commonly overlooked.

Although it is intended that, when using the term 'nursing' within this book, reference is also being made to midwifery and health visiting, it is important to recognise that the uptake and prescribing needs of these specific professions do not necessarily match those of the wider nursing profession. Non-medical prescribing qualifications recorded by the NMC show that access to V300 education programmes by both midwives and health visitors has been significantly lower than for other nursing professions. The reasons for this vary but may include both service need and benefit-awareness issues. Many health visitors may argue that, although the community practitioners' formulary does not enable them to prescribe everything that they require, the service need does not warrant them undertaking the V300 education programme. However, some health visitors do have specialist skills that would be better used if they were able to prescribe a wider range of medicines. Case study A at the end of the book provides an example of how V300 prescribing can improve the service offered by health professionals and make best use of their skills.

Similarly, midwives have specific exemptions in medicines legislation, which enables them to supply and administer specific medicines in specified circumstances (NHS Education for Scotland 2006, MHRA 2007). Many midwives would suggest that this negates the need for undertaking non-medical prescribing. However, many of the exemptions relate to the period around labour and the childbirth situation, and do not cover many of the situations encountered in the postnatal period in the home. Case study B provides an example of the application of V300 prescribing in midwifery practice.

 Activity box 1.7

Consider the following examples of nursing practice. Decide which type (V100, V150, V300) of prescribing would be most appropriate:

Zoe is a nurse on a rehabilitation ward. She currently has to wait for a doctor to prescribe medicines for conditions that she is competent to treat.

David is a community staff nurse who has undertaken extensive training in wound care. In order to change a treatment, he has to request a prescription from the GP or ask his team leader to review the patient.

Sam is a health visitor. He trained 15 years ago but gave up work for 5 years to care for his child. He completed a return to practice course 3 years ago. He is the only health visitor in his team without a prescribing qualification.

Pharmacist non-medical prescribers

The RPSGB, in response to the legislative restrictions and subsequent changes, has validated programmes of study to train pharmacists as supplementary prescribers and independent and supplementary prescribers, and to enable those trained as supplementary prescribers to become independent prescribers.

Pharmacist supplementary prescribers

Pharmacists who undertook a programme of education in non-medical prescribing before the legislative changes of 2008 were able to train and subsequently practise only as supplementary prescribers. This enabled pharmacists to prescribe any medicine identified within a CMP under the criteria of supplementary prescribing discussed earlier. Pharmacist supplementary prescribers do not have any restrictions on the drugs that they may prescribe or on the conditions for which they may prescribe. This enables pharmacists to prescribe controlled drugs and unlicensed drugs where there is a patient need and has been agreed by the independent prescriber and the supplementary prescriber within the CMP.

Some pharmacist supplementary prescribers have found that supplementary prescribing has improved patient management and their role within it (Johnson et al 2006). However, many pharmacist supplementary prescribers have identified that the ability to prescribe independently would enhance their role further by enabling them to prescribe in situations where supplementary prescribing is inappropriate. These pharmacists have undertaken additional education on conversion courses that focus on the elements particularly significant in achieving safe and effective independent prescribing. Pharmacists undertaking courses validated to encompass the 2008 legislative changes will receive education in supplementary prescribing as part of the independent prescribing programme. It is important again to reiterate the advantages of supplementary prescribing as previously highlighted. The perceived superiority of independent prescribing can detract from the benefits of pharmacist supplementary prescribing (Cooper et al 2008). Case study D provides an example of pharmacist supplementary prescribing.

Pharmacist independent prescribers

Pharmacist independent prescribing incorporates all the elements of independent prescribing previously identified. Pharmacists who have successfully completed a recognised programme of education will be able to prescribe any licensed or unlicensed medicine within their clinical competence. However, independent prescribing for pharmacists has not eliminated the need for supplementary prescribing, nor has it enabled them to prescribe all medicines that they may feel competent to prescribe. Pharmacist independent prescribers are not able to prescribe controlled drugs. Case studies E and F provide examples of pharmacist independent prescribing.

 Activity box 1.8

Consider the following examples of pharmacist practice. Decide which type (independent or supplementary) of prescribing would be most appropriate:

Beth is a community-based pharmacist who reviews patients in a busy GP practice. She sees patients already diagnosed with hypertension and advises on any necessary changes in medication.

William is a hospital-based pharmacist who works in a specialist drug dependency unit. He reviews patients on a methadone programme.

George is a pharmacist specialising in heart failure. He reviews a range of patients who are receiving medicines to treat chronic cardiac failure.

Allied health professional non-medical prescribers

The HPC, in response to the legislative changes in 2005, has validated courses to train eligible allied health professionals as supplementary prescribers. However, this is currently available only to physiotherapists, radiographers, podiatrists/chiropodists and optometrists. As optometrist training includes specific requirements not indicated for other allied health professions, they are considered separately.

Physiotherapist, radiographer and podiatrists/chiropodists supplementary prescribers

Allied health professionals are able currently only to train and prescribe as supplementary prescribers. This enables physiotherapists, radiographers and podiatrists/chiropodists, in line with other supplementary prescribers, to prescribe any medicine identified within a CMP under the criteria of supplementary prescribing discussed earlier. Allied health profession supplementary prescribers also have no restrictions on the drugs they may prescribe or on the conditions for which they may prescribe. This enables physiotherapists, radiographers and podiatrists/chiropodists to prescribe controlled drugs and unlicensed drugs where there is a patient need and where it has been agreed by the independent prescriber and the supplementary prescriber in a CMP (DH 2006b).

The HPC (2008), in line with the NMC (2008a) and RPSGB (2007) have encompassed non-medical prescribing in their ethical and professional codes. This ensures that physiotherapists, radiographers and podiatrists/chiropodists restrict their prescribing practice to those conditions for which they are competent to prescribe.

As identified in pharmacist prescribing, supplementary prescribing does not meet the needs of all allied health professional non-medical prescribers. Patient group directions (PGDs) continue to meet the needs of some patients and there are others where independent prescribing would be the most appropriate option. As a recent scoping exercise (DH 2009) has recommended that independent prescribing should be introduced for physiotherapists and podiatrists, it is likely that further developments will be forthcoming. However, the benefits of supplementary prescribing remain evident for this professional group and it is important that this continues to be recognised, even in the event of independent prescribing rights being granted. Case studies G, H and I provide practice examples of allied health professional supplementary prescribing.

Activity box 1.9

Consider the following examples of allied health professional practice. Decide if supplementary prescribing would be most appropriate:

Darren is a hospital-based physiotherapist, specialising in musculoskeletal conditions.

Yvonne is a podiatrist, specialising in diabetic foot conditions, who regularly has to prescribe long-term antifungal preparations.

Frances is a radiographer who is lead for her hospital's lower gastrointestinal endoscopy unit. Patients often require 'one-off' prescribing of bowel preparations.

Optometrist prescribers

Optometrist prescribing programmes are validated by the General Optical Council (GOC) and are currently limited to three universities in the UK. Non-medical prescribing education for optometrists is somewhat different to the generic programmes offered to other professions, focusing very much on the speciality of optometry. All registered optometrists are able to administer and supply using specific exemptions but these are limited. Those optometrists wishing to administer, supply or prescribe beyond those exemptions must undertake specialist training that must be registered with the GOC (College of Optometrists 2009). In order to achieve this, legislative changes have now enabled optometrists to undertake three routes: additional supply, supplementary prescribing and/or independent prescribing. Additional supply has enabled appropriately qualified optometrists access to an extended list of exemptions. Supplementary and independent prescribing is undertaken using the same criteria identified for other non-medical prescribing professions. Case study J provides an example of optometrist prescribing in practice.

Patient group directions

It is important that clarification is provided in relation to the differences between prescribing and the use of PGDs. Prescribing is undertaken on an individual basis, taking into account the individual needs of a patient, based on a thorough and holistic assessment, resulting, where appropriate, in the generation of a prescription. The use of PGDs does not constitute prescribing, although it could be argued that the processes leading up to both the generation of a prescription and the use of a PGD are similar.

The preferred method by which patients receive medicines is to have them prescribed, on an individual basis, by a health professional who has been trained to do so (NPC 2004b). An alternative to this is the use of a PGD. It is not the intention of this discussion to provide a detailed account of the application of PGDs. Instead, the focus is on the differences between the two and the appropriateness of their use.

A PGD is defined as (NPC 2009, p. 11):

... a written instruction for the sale, supply and/or administration of named medicines in an identified clinical situation. It applies to groups of patients who may not be individually identified before presenting for treatment.

The PGD therefore allows a healthcare professional to supply and/or administer a medicine directly to the patient. This can be done without the patient being required to see a prescriber, although a prescriber may have referred the patient in some instances. The health professional using a PGD is responsible for assessing the patient, just as a prescriber would in order to reach a decision about treatment. The difference in this assessment is that the health professional using a PGD undertakes the assessment against set criteria that determine if the PGD is appropriate (NPC 2004b). In the same situation, the prescriber's assessment would no doubt incorporate many of the criteria used for the PGD but would also incorporate information that is individual to the patient.

As the definition of a PGD states, the medicines are predetermined for an identified clinical situation. Prescribing, on the other hand, enables the health professional to take into account the individual needs of the patient, using these to decide on an appropriate treatment, which may or may not be the same as indicated in the PGD. The prescriber may also support this by tackling the long-term implications of the presenting clinical situation.

The necessity to determine whether the PGD, or prescribing, is most appropriate highlights the reality that many services will function most effectively using a combination of both. Case study 9 provides an example of how the same clinical situation may be dealt with promptly and effectively by both methods, demonstrating a situation where prescribing would be preferable but where a PGD would enable a satisfactory outcome.

Although it is acknowledged that prescribing is the most appropriate option in most instances, it is also recognised that the use of PGDs, in a limited number of situations, can be advantageous for patient care, provided that it does not compromise patient safety (DH 2006b). Immunisation is an example of such a situation. The criteria set within the PGD to determine if a vaccine is appropriate enables health professionals to administer vaccines safely and efficiently within busy clinics, without the necessity of every health professional being a prescriber.

Activity box 1.10

Access the following websites for in depth information on PGDs:

PGD website (England): www.portal.nelm.nhs.uk/PGD/default.aspx
NES PGD website (Scotland): www.nes.scot.nhs.uk/pgds
HOWIS (Wales): www.wales.nhs.uk
MHRA (All UK): www.mhra.gov.uk/index.htm

Patient specific directions differ from PGDs in that they are specific to a named patient. It is important to briefly clarify the link between prescribing and patient-specific directions because many non-medical prescribers will use them within their prescribing role. A patient-specific direction is defined by the Department of Health (2006b, p. 1) as:

> ... the traditional written instruction, from a doctor, dentist, nurse or pharmacist independent prescriber, for medicines to be supplied or administered to a named patient ...

As a non-medical prescriber, a nurse, midwife or pharmacist may direct a relevantly qualified person to administer or supply a medicine. This direction will be based on the independent prescriber's assessment and decision about diagnosis and treatment. An example of this in secondary care would include an instruction given on a patient's ward drug chart.

Access to education programmes

Although many professionals reading this book will either be currently undertaking, or will have completed, a recognised programme of education in supplementary and/or independent prescribing, it is recognised that others will be using it to acquire information to help them to decide whether or not non-medical prescribing is appropriate for them. In many ways, the professional bodies governing the relevant professions have determined criteria that have simplified this decision. It is recommended that any professional considering undertaking an education programme in non-medical prescribing accesses the standards set by their own professional body, the links for which are:

- General Optometry Council: www.optical.org/en/our_work/Standards/index.cfm
- Health Professions Council: www.hpc-uk.org/assets/documents/10002367FINAL copyofSCPEJuly2008.pdf
- Nursing and Midwifery Council: www.nmc-uk.org/aDisplayDocument.aspx? documentID=1645
- Royal Pharmaceutical Society: www.rpsgb.org/pdfs/indprescoutlcurric.pdf

However, a brief explanation of the criteria used in determining access to education programmes is provided below.

Criteria relevant to all

Health professionals must:

- be in a post in which prescribing will enhance their role and make better use of their skills
- be able to identify that the introduction of non-medical prescribing within their role will improve the quality of patient care
- be able to identify that the introduction non-medical prescribing within their role will enable quicker and more efficient access to medicines for patients
- be able to prescribe within their practice area once the education programme is successfully completed
- have the ability to study at a minimum of degree level
- have the support of their employer
- have access to a budget from which the cost of their prescriptions will be met
- have access to continuing professional development
- be able to identify an appropriate doctor who has agreed to act as their designated medical practitioner (note that for nurses, midwives and health visitors undertaking the community practitioner prescribing V100/150 programmes must **instead** be able to identify a practising prescriber who has agreed to act as their practice supporter; this may be another non-medical prescriber).

Nurse, midwife and health visitor-specific criteria

Nurses, midwives and health visitors must do the following.

V100

- Undertake a specialist community public health nurse or community specialist practitioner programme or already hold these qualifications.

V150

- Have practised for a minimum of 2 years in the area in which they intend to prescribe.

V300

- Have at least 3 years of post-registration clinical experience, with the last year being in the speciality/area in which they intend to prescribe.

Allied health professional specific criteria

Allied health professionals must:

- have at least 3 years relevant post-qualification clinical experience.

Pharmacist-specific criteria

Pharmacists must:

- have a minimum of 2 years appropriate patient orientated experience in addition to the pre-registration year after graduation
- be on the practising register.

Optometrist specific criteria

Optometrists must have been practising in the UK for 2 full years before they are eligible to start training for the therapeutic specialty qualifications.

Summary of the context of prescribing

This chapter has examined the context in which non-medical prescribing continues to develop in the UK. It is apparent that, although evolving, non-medical prescribing maintains its original vision of improving patient access to medicines through safe, effective and efficient prescribing. The achievement of this vision has relied on appropriate responses being made to the pressures placed on it. Figure 1.1 serves to highlight that the achievement of safe, effective and efficient prescribing results from a balance between these pressures and responses.

The pressures on prescribing are multiple. The identification of emerging safety issues, new public health targets and the resultant needs of the patient, professional

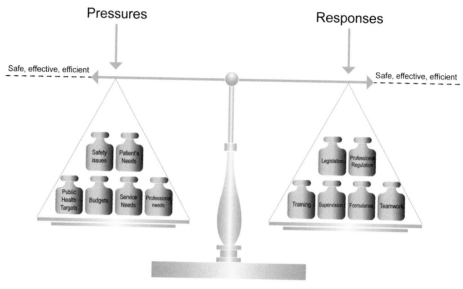

Pressures

Responses

Safe, effective, efficient

Safe, effective, efficient

Safety issues | Patient's Needs

Public Health Targets | Budgets | Service Needs | Professional needs

Legislation | Professional Regulation

Training | Supervision | Formularies | Teamwork

The context of safe, effective
and efficient prescribing

Figure 1.1 The balance between pressures and responses.

and service all require response within a limited budget. To ensure that prescribing is able to form an effective element of the health services' response to these pressures, a teamwork approach is important. CPD, which incorporates not only relevant education but also appropriate and effective supervision, is essential in order to promote evidence-based and cost-effective practice. As the context of prescribing continues to evolve, so must the support provided to prescribers by legislation and professional regulation.

Key themes: conclusions and considerations

Public health

Public health has been shown to be a responsibility of all health professionals. So that inequalities in health in the UK are addressed, public health targets must remain a consideration in all areas of practice. Non-medical prescribing provides an appropriate setting for considering public health issues

Consider how you, as an individual practitioner, can impact on public health targets. Evaluation of your own practice will highlight areas that can be developed to ensure that public health becomes an integral part of non-medical prescribing practice

Social and cultural issues	The current context of non-medical prescribing has evolved from a position where prescribing was seen as the domain of doctors. The process of change has involved social and cultural shifts on the part of both patients and health professionals. Much of this process has relied on effective communication and the development of a sound evidence base
	Consider what measures you can take to further reduce the barriers to non-medical prescribing and to promote it as an effective tool in meeting the needs of the patient and the health service
Prescribing principles	The prescribing principles have continued to support safe non-medical prescribing for over a decade
	Consider each principle individually in order to evaluate how effectively you address them in practice. Dependent upon your experience as a prescriber, the consideration given to the individual principles on a daily basis is likely to differ. Reflecting on and revisiting the prescribing principles will aid both the novice and the experienced prescriber to ensure that their practice remains safe

References

Acheson D (1998) *Independent Inquiry into Inequalities in Health*, London: The Stationery Office

Avery AJ, Pringle M (2005) Extended prescribing by UK nurses and pharmacists. *BMJ* **331**: 1154-5.

Black D, Morris J, Smith C, Townsend P (1980) *Inequalities in Health: Report of a research working group*. London: The Stationery Office.

Bradley E, Nolan P (2007) Impact of nurse prescribing: a qualitative study. *J Adv Nurs* **59**: 120-8.

Bradshaw J (1994) The conceptualisation and measurement of need. In: Popay J, Williams G (eds), *Researching the People's Health*. London: Routledge, Chapter 3.

British Medical Association and Royal Pharmaceutical Society of Great Britain (2010). *British National Formulary* (latest version). Available at: http://bnf.org/bnf.

Carey N, Courtney M (2008) Nurse supplementary prescribing for patients with diabetes: a national questionnaire survey. *J Clin Nursing* **17**: 2185-93.

Clegg A, Meades R, Broderick W (2006) Reflections on nurse independent prescribing in the hospital setting. *Nursing Stand* **21**: 35-8.

College of Optometrists (2009) Therapeutics/Prescribing (on-line). Available at: www.college-optometrists.org/index.aspx/pcms/site.education.Therapeutics.therapeutics_home.

Cooper RJ, Anderson C, Avery T et al (2008a) Nurse and pharmacist supplementary prescribing in the UK - a thematic review of the literature. *Health Policy* **85**: 277-92.

Cooper RJ, Lymn J, Anderson C et al (2008b) Learning to prescribe - pharmacists' experiences of supplementary prescribing training in England. *BMC Med Educ* **8**(57).

Courtney M, Carey N (2008) Nurse independent prescribing and nurse supplementary pre-scribing. *J Adv Nurs* **61**: 291-9.

Day M (2005) UK doctors protest at extension to nurses' prescribing powers. *BMJ* **331**: 1159.

Day P (2007) School nursing independent prescribing in practice. *Br J School Nurs* **2**: 267-71.

Department of Health (1998) *Nurse Prescribing A Guide for Implementation*. London: The Stationery Office.

Department of Health (1999a) *Review of Prescribing, Supply and Administration of Medicines: Final Report*. London: The Stationery Office.

Department of Health (1999b) *Saving Lives: Our healthier nation*. The London: Stationery Office.

Department of Health (2000) *The NHS Plan*. London: The Stationery Office.

Department of Health (2002) *Liberating the Patients: Helping primary care trusts and nurses to deliver the NHS Plan*. London: The Stationery Office.

Department of Health (2004) *Choosing Health: Making healthier choices easier*. London: The Stationery Office.

Department of Health (2005) *Supplementary Prescribing by Nurses, Pharmacists, Chiropodists/ Podiatrists, Physiotherapists and Radiographers within the NHS in England*. London: The Stationery Office.

Department of Health (2006a) *Improving Patients' Access to Medicines: A guide to imple-menting nurse and pharmacist independent prescribing within the NHS in England*. London: The Stationery Office.

Department of Health (2006b) *Medicines Matters*. London: The Stationery Office.

Department of Health (2006c) *Our Health, Our Care, Our Say: A new direction for community services*. London: The Stationery Office.

Department of Health (2007a) *The NHS in England: The operating framework for 2008/9*. London: The Stationery Office.

Department of Health (2007b) *Our NHS, Our Future*. London: The Stationery Office.

Department of Health (2007c) *Clinical Management Plans (CMPs)*. Available at www.dh.gov.uk/en/Healthcare/Medicinespharmacyandindustry/Prescriptions/TheNon-MedicalPrescribingProgramme/Supplementaryprescribing/DH_4123030.

Department of Health (2008a) *Making the Connections: Using healthcare professionals to deliver organisational improvements*. London: The Stationery Office.

Department of Health (2008b) *NHS Next Stage Review: Our vision for primary and community care*. London: The Stationery Office.

Department of Health (2009) *Allied Health Professions Prescribing and Medicines Supply Mechanisms Scoping Project Report*. London: The Stationery Office.

Department of Health, Social Services and Public Safety (2006) *Improving Patients' Access to Medicines: A guide to implementing nurse and pharmacist independent prescribing within the HPSS in Northern Ireland*. Belfast: DHSSPS.

Fitzpatrick M, Hogg D, Schelowok C (2007) Community practitioners want training. *Assn Nurse Prescribing J* **1**: 16-17.

General Pharmaceutical Council (2010) *Standards of Conduct, Ethics & Performance*. London: GPhC.

Goswell N, Siefers R (2009) Experiences of ward-based nurse prescribers in an acute ward setting. *Br J Nurs* **18**: 34-7.

Hall J, Cantrill J, Noyce P (2004) Managing independent prescribing: the influence of primary care trusts on community nurse prescribing. *Int J Pharmacy Pract* **12**: 133-9.

Health Professions Council (2006) *HPC in Focus: Issue 6*. London: HPC.

Health Professions Council (2008) *Standards of Conduct, Performance and Ethics*. London: HPC.

Hogg D, Schelowok C (2009) The need for V150 prescribing. *Nurse Prescrib* **7**: 122-5.

Johnson G, McCaig DJ, Bond CM et al (2006) Supplementary prescribing: early experiences of pharmacists in Great Britain. *Ann Pharmacother* **40**: 1843-50.

Jones A (2008) Exploring independent nurse prescribing for mental health settings. *J Psychiatr Mental Health Nurs* **15**: 109-17.

Keele University (2009) National study launched to measure impact of non-medical prescriptions on patient care. Press release, Keele University.

Likic R, Maxwell SR (2009) Prevention of medication errors: teaching and training. *Br J Clin Pharmacol* **67**: 656-61.

Medicines and Healthcare products Regulatory Agency (2007) *Midwives: Prescribing*. London: MHRA.

Medicines and Healthcare products Regulatory Agency (2008) *Supply and Administration of Botox, Vistabel, Dysport and Other Injectable Medicines in Cosmetic Procedures*. London: MHRA.

National Health Service Scotland (2009) *A Safe Prescription: Developing nurse, midwife and allied health profession prescribing in NHS Scotland*. Edinburgh: NHS Scotland.

National Prescribing Centre (1999) Signposts for prescribing nurses – general principles of good prescribing. *Prescribing Nurse Bull* **1**(1).

National Prescribing Centre (2001) *Maintaining Competency in Prescribing: An outline framework to help nurse prescribers*. Liverpool: NPC.

National Prescribing Centre (2004a) *Maintaining Competency in Prescribing: An outline framework to help allied health professional supplementary prescribers*. Liverpool: NPC.

National Prescribing Centre (2009) *Patient Group Directions: A practical guide and framework of competencies for all professionals using patient group directions*. Liverpool: NPC.

National Prescribing Centre (2006) *Maintaining Competency in Prescribing: An outline framework to help pharmacist prescribers*. Liverpool: NPC.

National Prescribing Centre (2007) *Scoping Study of Supplementary Prescribing*. Liverpool: NPC.

National Patient Safety Agency (2007) *Safety in Doses*. London: NPSA.

NHS Education for Scotland (2006). *Midwives and Medicines*. Edinburgh: NES.

NHS Information Centre for Health and Social Care (2009) *Prescription Cost Analysis England 2008*. Available at: www.ic.nhs.uk/statistics-and-data-collections/primary-care/prescriptions/prescription-cost-analysis-2008.

Nursing and Midwifery Council (2006) *Standards of Proficiency for Nurse and Midwife Prescribers*. London: NMC.

Nursing and Midwifery Council (2007) *Additional Requirements to Include within the Indicative Content of Nurse Independent Prescribing Education and Training Programmes: NMC Circular 10/2007*. London: NMC.

Nursing and Midwifery Council (2008a) *The Code – Standards of conduct, performance and ethics for nurses and midwives*. London: NMC

Nursing and Midwifery Council (2008b) *Standards for Medicines Management*. London: NMC.

Nursing and Midwifery Council (2009). *Standards of Educational Preparation for Prescribing from the Nurse Prescribers Formulary for Community Practitioners for Nurses without a Specialist Practitioner Qualification – Introducing Code V150*. NMC Circular 02/2009. London: NMC.

Nuttall D (2008) Introducing public health to prescribing practice. *Nurse Prescribing* **6**: 299-305.

Pontin D, Jones S (2008) Children's nurses and nurse prescribing: a case study identifying issues for developing training programmes. *J Clin Nurs* **16**: 540-8.

Pooler A, Campbell P (2006) Identifying the development needs of community matrons. *Nurs Times* **102**: 36-8.

Royal Pharmaceutical Society of Great Britain (2006) *Outline Curriculum for Training Programmes to Prepare Pharmacist Prescribers*. London: RPSGB.

Schachter M (2009) The epidemiology of medication errors: how many, how serious? *Br J Clin Pharmacol* **67**: 621-3.

Scottish Executive Health Department (2006) *Guidance for Nurse Independent Prescribers and for Community Practitioner Nurse Prescribers in Scotland*. Edinburgh: SEHD.

Scottish Government (2008a) *Supporting the Development of Advanced Nursing Practice: A toolkit approach*. Edinburgh: Scottish Government.

Scottish Government (2008b) *Equally Well: Report of the ministerial task force on health inequalities*. Edinburgh: Scottish Government.

Snowden A (2008) Quantitative analysis of mental health nurse prescribers in Scotland. *J Psychiatr Mental Health Nurs* **15**: 471-8.

Stewart DC, George J, Diack HL et al (2009) Cross sectional survey of the Scottish general public's awareness of, views on, and attitudes toward nonmedical prescribing. *Ann Pharmacother* **43**: 1115-21.

Thomas M, Motion M, Strickland-Hodge B (2005) Setting up supplementary prescribing clinics can be rewarding and exciting. *Pharmacy Pract* **15**: 319-22.

University of Southampton School of Nursing and Midwifery, on behalf of Department of Health (2005) *Evaluation of Extended Formulary Independent Nurse Prescribing: Executive summary*. London: The Stationery Office.

Velo GP, Minuz P (2009) Medication errors: prescribing faults and prescription errors. *Br J Clin Pharmacol* **67**: 624-8.

Wanless D (2004) *Securing Good Health for the Whole Population. Final report*. London: The Stationery Office.

Wells J, Berginn M, Gooney M, Jones A (2009) Views on nurse prescribing: a survey of community mental health nurses in the Republic of Ireland. *J Psychiatr Mental Health Nurs* **16**: 10-17.

Welsh Assembly Government (2007) *Non-Medical Prescribing in Wales. A guide for implementation*. Cardiff: Welsh Assembly Government.

Chapter 2

Professional, Legal and Ethical Issues in Relation to Prescribing Practice

Ruth Broadhead

Learning objectives

After reading this chapter and completing the activities within it, the reader will be able to:

1 discuss the importance of maintaining professional responsibility and accountability in relation to prescribing practice
2 identify the sources and systems of UK law and its application in healthcare
3 critically analyse the relevance of moral and ethical theory in prescribing practice

A comprehensive understanding of professional, legal and ethical issues is a fundamental component of safe prescribing practice. This chapter therefore explores some of the relevant issues that impact on safe, legal prescribing and identify judicious frameworks that guide and support practitioners in the complex principles of the prescribing process. In particular the chapter aims to identify what is and what is not legally permissible within the prescribing practices of nurses, midwives, pharmacists and allied health professionals. The chapter is divided into three parts: Part 1: professional issues; Part 2: legal issues; and Part 3: ethical issues. However, the topics included in each of these sections have a significant degree of intercorrelation and issues should not be considered in isolation, but be examined concurrently, e.g. when studying aspects of consent or confidentiality, there are professional, legal *and* ethical issues to consider.

UK law is ever changing and legislation is continuously open to shifting interpretation and amendment. Although the statutes, case law judgments and legal guidelines contained within this chapter are correct at the time of writing, a contemporary awareness is advised for non-medical prescribers to keep abreast of changes. The legal rules of England and Wales are generally synonymous, yet Scotland and Northern Ireland have some discernible variants that are highlighted in this chapter where possible. It is, however, individual prescribers' responsibility to regularly update their knowledge of

The Textbook of Non-medical Prescribing, edited by Dilyse Nuttall and Jane Rutt-Howard.
© 2011 Blackwell Publishing Ltd

the current legislation within their respective countries and to incorporate the appropriate legal guidelines into their own prescribing practice. The purpose of this chapter is, therefore, to heighten the awareness of the practitioner to the potential consequences resulting from failure to fully appreciate the significance of adhering to professional regulations, legislation and moral principles rather than transliterate legislation verbatim. A lack of appreciation by the prescriber of the concepts contained in this chapter can result in dire consequences for both the patient and the practitioner and, as such, the overall intention is to inform the non-medical prescriber sufficiently well to prescribe within professional, legal and ethical parameters.

In response to progressive developments in UK healthcare and with the consequential inception of non-medical prescribing, there have been significant requisite changes to the regulations and guidelines determined by the associated professional bodies. Legal frameworks relating to prescribing have been modified to take account of prescribers from disciplines other than medicine and dentistry and, as a result of these amendments, a more acute appreciation of professional accountability has evolved. Furthermore, the continuing expansion of non-medical prescribing has depended on changes being implemented with regard to education, professional regulations, and in the legal frameworks for the prescribing, supply and administration of medicines. Despite the successful augmentation of the non-medical prescribing initiative, prescribers still remain under scrutiny from associated professionals and the general public, not least because of the perceived inadequacy of prescribing training courses to address diagnostic skills (Avery and Pringle 2005, British Medical Association 2005), but also by the newfound litigious culture within the UK. However, educational programmes have responded to this criticism by incorporating into the curricula a major focus on clinical decision-making, professionalism, the legalities of prescribing and the ethical principles of patient-centred prescribing practice. It is now increasingly evident that the changing attitudes of service users and healthcare professionals are positive and remain key to securing the acceptance of this advanced role.

PART 1: PROFESSIONAL ISSUES

The regulatory framework for prescribing

As prescribers, just as we require a structured framework to guide the clinical prescribing process, we need a suitable directive to guarantee that we work to an approved standard in legal and professional terms. Table 2.1 illustrates the sources of professional regulations for practice, current legislation and guiding regulatory bodies that govern non-medical prescribing.

Medicines and prescribing

The Medicines Act 1968, Misuse of Drugs Act 1971 and Prescription Only Medicines (Human Use) Orders 1997 provide legislative guidance on the production, sale and use of medicines, including regulation on prescribing rights.

The Medicines Act 1968 governs the manufacture and supply of medicines and defines three categories of medicines:

Table 2.1 Legal and professional regulatory framework governing

Legislative	Professional	Regulatory
The Medicines Act 1968 Misuse of Drugs Act 1971 Misuse of Drugs Regulations 2001 Prescription Only Medicines Orders (Human Use) 1997 and subsequent Statutory Instruments	Nursing and Midwifery Council (NMC): www.nmc-uk.org General Pharmaceutical Council (GPhC): www. pharmacyregulation. org Health Professions Council (HPC): www.hpc-uk.org	Medicines and Healthcare products Regulatory Agency (MHRA): www.mhra. gov.uk Area drugs and therapeutics committees

1 Prescription-only medicine (POM)
2 Pharmacy medicines (P)
3 General sales list medicine (GSL).

As the name suggests, POMs are only available with a prescription supplied by a qualified, authorised prescriber and are for the use of the patient named on the prescription only. Pharmacy medicines are available from a pharmacist, with over-the-counter advice without a prescription, and GSLs are available at other outlets such as supermarkets. However, supermarkets are legally bound to limit the number of certain drugs that they sell to single customers, e.g. analgesics. The Medicines and Healthcare products Regulatory Agency (MHRA 2010) identifies that:

Under medicines legislation, the general rule is that pharmacy (P) and prescription only medicines (POMs) may only be sold or supplied through registered pharmacies. POMs are subject to the additional requirement that they are sold or supplied in accordance with an appropriate practitioner's prescription. The law also restricts the administration of parenteral medicines which, if not self-administered, must be administered by a doctor or, in certain circumstances an independent nurse prescriber or a supplementary prescriber. Parenteral medicines can also be administered by anyone acting in accordance with the patient-specific directions of a doctor or, again in certain circumstances, an independent nurse prescriber or a supplementary prescriber.

Exemptions under the Medicines Act 1968 include a range of exemptions from these restrictions (MHRA 2010). These exemptions allow certain groups of health professionals such as midwives or paramedics to sell, supply and administer particular medicines directly to patients. The MHRA state that:

The exemptions are distinct from prescribing which requires the involvement of a pharmacist in the sale or supply of the medicine. They also differ from the arrangements for Patient Group Directions (PGDs) as the latter must comply with specific legal criteria, be signed by a doctor or dentist and a pharmacist and authorised by an appropriate body.

Table 2.2 Misuse of Drugs Act 1971 Drug Classification

Class A	Heroin, cocaine, ecstasy, methamphetamine, LSD and psilocybin mushrooms
Class B	Cannabis, amphetamine, codeine and methylphenidate (Ritalin)
Class C	GHB, ketamine, diazepam, flunitrazepam, most other tranquillisers, benzodiazepines and anabolic steroids

The Misuse of Drugs Act 1971 is an Act of Parliament that governs the penalty for possession and supply of narcotics and psychotropic drugs. The Act clearly categorises three separate classes of drugs (Table 2.2).

The responsibility for listing, de-listing and grading of drugs is devolved to the current Home Secretary and offences and penalties under the Misuse of Drugs Act 1971 vary for both the illegal and unlicensed possession of drugs and the possession of drugs with intent to supply. Prescribers are no less likely to be prosecuted under the Misuse of Drugs Act than other members of the healthcare professions or the general public, yet it is suggested that perhaps prescribers should be penalised more severely, due to the position of trust that they hold within society. Non-medical prescribers are responsible for upholding the credibility of their respective professions and are in a privileged position regarding the safe and legal management of medicines. Regulations for the storage, prescribing, supply and administration of drugs in the categories identified in Table 2.2 need to be stringent and those of us who are prescribers or administrators of these drugs should obtain a heightened awareness of the associated legislation and professional guidance. The prescribing of controlled drugs is discussed in more depth in Part 2 of this chapter.

Prescription Only Medicines Orders (Human Use) 1997 and subsequent Statutory Instruments/Amendments are successive modifications to the Medicines Act 1971 and detail contemporary changes to certain aspects of the legislation. Non-medical prescribers are required to keep abreast of these amendments to ensure that they are working in line with current guidelines. Changes can be located at the Office of Public Sector Information (see www.opsi.gov.uk) or from prescribers' respective professional bodies.

The MHRA is responsible for regulating medicines in the UK. This includes ensuring that medicines and medical devices are safe and for bringing prosecutions when medicines legislation has been broken. The MHRA is an executive agency in the Department of Health and its inception in 2003 was as a result of the amalgamation of the Medicines Control Agency (MCA) and the Medical Devices Agency (MDA). A fundamental aspect of the role of the MHRA is to oversee and promote the safe use of medicines and devices. They are also responsible for monitoring adverse drug reactions (ADRs) and taking appropriate action as necessary when they are identified. The Yellow Card scheme is a reporting system that was initiated in 1964 after the thalidomide catastrophe to facilitate a robust and timely information system to highlight potential and actual ADRs. It is a requirement of the scheme that ADRs be reported to the MHRA via the Yellow Card scheme by prescribers as soon as they are suspected. However, anyone can report suspected ADRs to the MHRA.

Area drugs and therapeutics committees are locally appointed groups responsible for overseeing and implementing national guidelines at a local level. Their terms of reference and locally devolved policies can be obtained from each of the committees in the prescribers' area of work.

Activity box 2.1

Find out where your local area drugs and therapeutics committee is located.

Who are the members of this committee?
What policies have been developed by this group?

Professional codes

All non-medical prescribers are required to work within the boundaries of their own codes of conduct with the intention of providing high-quality standards of healthcare, safeguarding the public and promoting professional credibility.

In gaining a prescribing qualification, practitioners should aim to be fully conversant with their codes of practice (Table 2.3), along with the associated legislation and applicable ethical principles. Nurses, midwives, pharmacists and those from allied health backgrounds are duty bound to ensure that their professional development incorporates a robust appreciation of the parameters contained within their professional codes of practice because it is these codes that act as a principal set of rules and standards to guide clinical practice, including the prescribing process. It is perhaps significant to add here that anecdotal evidence suggests that familiarisation with the content of codes of conduct is poor or completely lacking in many potential prescribers, leaving them exposed to potentially intractable, but avoidable, problems. It could be argued that with the recent advent of an abundance of web-based information and the relevant documents being easily accessible for each profession, a lack of awareness would be an unsatisfactory defence should prescribing practice be questioned. As the professional codes of practice provide practitioners with a regulatory framework for prescribing, it is suggested that the acquisition of this additional skill should be founded on this inaugural knowledge.

Activity box 2.2

Obtain a copy of your own code of conduct. Look at the standards contained therein and:

- Write down how you can ensure that you meet these standards as a qualified prescriber
- Reflect upon the benefits to your prescribing practice of reviewing the standards

Table 2.3 Non-medical prescribers' professional codes of practice

Nurses	*The Code: Standards of conduct. Performance and ethics for nurses and midwives* (Nursing and Midwifery Council 2008a)
Pharmacists	*Standards of Conduct, Ethics and Performance* (General Pharmaceutical Council 2010)
Allied health professionals	*Standards of Conduct. Performance and Ethics* (Health Professions Council 2008)

Accountability and responsibility

Accountability is synonymous with components of 'governance', in that organisations and individuals are held *accountable* for assuring quality standards are met in the care they deliver. The Nursing and Midwifery Council (NMC 2010a), the General Pharmaceutical Council (GPhC 2010) and the Health Professions Council (HPC 2008) all recognise clinical governance as 'a framework through which NHS organisations are accountable for continuously improving the quality of their services and safeguarding high standards of care ...'. Therefore it is suggested that organisations place the accountability of prescribing practitioners high on the clinical governance agenda. The practical application of this is discussed further in Chapter 9.

Although it is clear that nurses, midwives, pharmacists and allied health professionals work with a fair degree of professional autonomy, it is evident that holding a prescribing qualification demands a higher measure of responsibility. The term 'accountability' is often misconstrued by healthcare professionals due to its ambiguity and multidirectional connotations, but is generally accepted as being a measure of *liability* for the practitioner's conduct. Savage and Moore (2004) identified that being 'accountable' describes certain relationships such as those with patients, those with organisations and those with oneself. Accountability can imply being responsible *to* someone or something and a resulting, definitive willingness to take the consequences of actions or inactions. Furthermore, as prescribing professionals, being held accountable can both motivate and explain our decision-making, but perhaps more so it allows us to accept or apportion blame for prescribing misdemeanours.

Professional indemnity

As a result of the demands brought about by the advanced role of prescribers, it could be said that there is an increased risk of claims being brought against us for mistakes in our clinical judgement, or indeed for clinical negligence allegations due to inadvertent acts and omissions in practice. Therefore, it is paramount that professional indemnity insurance be in place. Most nurses, pharmacists and allied health professionals such as podiatrists and optometrists obtain indemnity insurance through their recommended unions, most of which offer substantial cover for clinical negligence and legal representation. It is important to note that criminal acts, such as intentionally harming a patient or prescribing large doses of opiates for personal use, are not covered by professional indemnity insurance. The Pharmacists' Defence Association (PDA), the Royal College of Nursing (RCN) and the British Chiropody and Podiatry Association (BCPA), for example, all offer their registered practitioners up to £5000 000 of cover for professional indemnity. The Medical Defence Union (MDU) now offers membership to healthcare professionals other than doctors and dentists, including those undertaking cosmetic procedures such as injecting botulinum toxin. As prescribers, it is essential that, before undertaking this extended role, we ensure that adequate professional indemnity insurance has been secured.

Vicarious liability

If a patient makes a claim for damages, the employer is usually the defendant. As practitioners with new prescribing rights, our professional interest should be drawn to the protection that we hold under vicarious liability. Problems in practice may arise if a patient suffers harm as a result of a prescriber's wrongful act that was not an activity authorised by the employer. It is suggested by British Employment Law (Emplaw) (2010) that there is no legal dilemma if the wrongful act done by an employee *was* in fact authorised by the employer. However, some contracts of employment and job descriptions are vague and it is not always obvious what exactly is authorised. In law, after a wrongful act, the dilemma would be whether or not an employer should be liable. Emplaw (2010) further state that:

> ... until the late 1990's the basic test for deciding whether an employer should be held liable in such a case was to consider:

- whether the employee had used an unauthorised method to do a job he was authorised to do (in which case the employer would be vicariously liable) or
- whether he was simply doing something which was unauthorised (in which case the employer would not be vicariously liable).

However, in 2001 the House of Lords ruled in *Lister and ors v Hesley Hall Ltd* 2001 that:

> ... important legal decisions should not turn on such semantics ...

As a result of the ruling in *Lister* it is now established that the correct test for whether vicarious liability is probable is to examine the connection between:

- the nature of the employment *and*
- the particular wrong *and*
- to ask whether, looking at the matter in the round, it is just and reasonable to hold the employers vicariously liable.

In prescribing terms, therefore, we need to ensure that our prescribing practice is actually authorised by our employers and stipulated as being a legitimate component part of our job description. We should be aware that holding a prescribing qualification does not automatically allow us to prescribe outside of the terms and conditions of our contracts and this should be discussed, agreed and signed up to. Gulliver (2006) suggests that some employment arrangements can be complex and that it would be sensible for non-medical prescribers to check that their contract of employment stipulates prescribing. Complexities in employment contracts may arise if a nurse, pharmacist or allied health professional is working for several GP practices, for example. The practitioner may not be working for any of them formally and may be employed by a primary care trust. It is therefore essential and sensible to ascertain in advance who will be responsible if a claim is made. Emplaw (2010) state that:

> ... more than one employer can share 'joint vicarious liability' in line with Court of Appeal decisions. None of this of course rules out the old traditional test as an aid to deciding whether the employer should be liable for unauthorised wrongful acts of his employees but does put it into a proper perspective.

In conclusion to this section, it is recommended that all non-medical prescribers take steps to:

- ensure that prescribing rights are explicitly detailed in contracts of employment and job descriptions
- confirm that vicarious liability is offered by your employer
- obtain adequate personal profession liability insurance.

Evidence-based practice

It is clearly stated in guidance from each of the non-medical prescribers' codes of conduct that prescribing practice must, wherever possible, be evidence based and in accordance with relevant national and local guidance. The RPSGB (2007) remind us that deviations from these policies must be justifiable and be in the best interest of the patient. This direction is also applicable to nurse and allied health professional prescribers.

As non-medical prescribers, it is good practice, and a professional expectation, to ensure that we are all adhering to the evidence bases, research and guidance available to us, but also maintaining our personal professional development (Department of Health (DH) 2009a). In a court of law, should we be called upon to defend our clinical decision-making, the procedure for ascertaining whether or not we acted appropriately would be judged and scrutinised in great detail, often with some vigour on behalf of the claimant. With all prescribing decisions it is undeniably imperative for us to contemplate our ability to endorse and validate our actions, should they ever be called into question. Gulliver (2006) suggests that with the added clinical responsibility of prescribing comes an inevitable increased risk of liability. One important issue that she highlights is the scope of prescribers' knowledge and the expectations of them if confronted by signs and symptoms that are obvious, but that do not fall within their area of expertise. All non-medical prescribers should bear in mind that, should the practitioner prescribe outside their field of competence, it is likely that a court of law will make instant and unsympathetic judgments against them. This is discussed in more depth in Part 2.

Fraud, criminal behaviour and whistleblowing

Prescribing rights, although well earned by the practitioner, could be seen as a professional privilege. With this licence comes an increase in the accessibility and availability of drugs, which, to those with ulterior motives, could lead to fraudulent behaviour. The Shipman Inquiry (2010) produced six independent reports after the murderous acts of Harold Shipman, and two of these are relevant to us as non-medical prescribers. The Fourth Report (Shipman Inquiry 2004a) was responsible for examining controlled drugs and how they are monitored in the community. The Chairman of the Report, Dame Janet Smith DBE, made recommendations based on her findings including the implementation of systems for the management and regulation of controlled drugs and the conduct of those who operate these systems. The findings and recommendations contained within the Fourth Report are very significant for prescribing practice, particularly for those working in pharmacies, palliative care, the community, intensive care units and accident and emergency departments, for example. The Fifth Report (Shipman Inquiry 2004b) examined safeguarding patients and looked at the lessons learnt from Shipman in order to inform and regulate future practice. Again, the findings contained within it, although largely relevant to the regulation of doctors, are essential reading for all non-medical prescribers. The principles set out in the report guide practitioners on how to identify and raise concerns about serious professional misconduct, and the morality of ignoring such concerns, all of which should be considered by those who prescribe and manage drugs in the course of their work.

Whistleblowing in the NHS has long been a taboo subject and, historically, employees have been reluctant to expose substandard care or professional misconduct due to the fear of victimisation or retribution (DH 1999). More recently however, NHS Employers (2010), as part of the Social Partnership Forum, have agreed to work alongside the main health service unions, the Department of Health and the independent whistleblowing body, Public Concern at Work (PCAW), to produce new guidance for NHS staff. The guidance, due for publication in June 2010, aims to investigate appropriate policy-making and the reluctance of staff to speak out against underperforming colleagues. Despite reassurances from the Department of Health (2003a) that practitioners will be supported, there still remains, however, a distinct element of unwillingness to partake in whistleblowing. This is perhaps increased by examples such as the case of nurse, Margaret Haywood, who spoke out about neglect at the Royal Sussex Hospital and was subsequently removed from the NMC register for breaching patient confidentiality (Staines 2009). As prescribers, it is recommended that we ensure our practice is always trustworthy and wholly defensible. Furthermore, should we ever encounter bad practice, fraud, or criminal behaviour, we should be aware of the policies to guide us with whistle-blowing, in order to protect the interests of our patients and professional credibility.

Remote prescribing

The term 'remote prescribing' is twofold. First it refers to prescribing for patients who are 'physically remote' in the context of not being present with the prescriber in the same vicinity, such as being on the telephone. Second, the term can refer to areas of the country that are described as being 'geographically remote' such as islands in the far north of the UK where healthcare services are poorly accessible and generally provided on the mainland.

The NMC (2008b) published a position statement in support of remote assessment and prescribing to improve access to medicines and enable choice in the delivery of healthcare. The General Medical Council (2008b) also acknowledge that 'from time to time it may be appropriate to use a telephone or other non-face-to-face medium to prescribe medicines and treatment for patients'. Although the latter guidance is aimed at doctors, the principles are analogous with those for other practitioners who prescribe via telephone, fax, email, video link or websites. It is highlighted that the prescriber must be satisfied that alternative means of prescribing for the patient in question are not available to them. It is a stipulation that appropriate dialogue is developed in order for the prescriber to establish a rapport with the patient to elicit a detailed history and gain informed consent. It is further suggested that, if all these conditions cannot be met, remote prescribing should not be undertaken. For some non-medical prescribers, this method of prescribing could become a significant means of providing a service to their patients. However, it may not be appropriate for other non-medical prescribers, particularly if the recommended criteria cannot be met. Kular (2010) highlighted that remote consultations are an important primary care tool, particularly for triage, acute conditions such as respiratory conditions and uncomplicated urinary tract infections, well-controlled chronic conditions such as diabetes or asthma, follow-up after hospital admission, and providing results of diagnostic tests or health promotion.

Activity box 2.3

Within your practice area and considering available policy relating to remote prescribing:

- Identify when remote prescribing via telephone, text or internet may be appropriate
- Consider how you would ensure that you obtain sufficient information from the patient
- Identify how you would gain consent
- Critically evaluate if remote prescribing is equitable

The criteria contained within the NMC and General Medical Council (GMC) guidance relates to generic prescribing yet the MHRA (2008) has produced additional guidance on the supply and administration of Botox®, Vistabel®, Dysport® and other injectable medicines used in cosmetic procedures. They identify the term 'appropriate practitioner' for prescribers undertaking this role and these include a doctor, dentist and ('subject to certain limitations') a nurse or pharmacist independent or supplementary prescriber. There are explicit stipulations in the guidance regarding the supply and administration of these products, and it is recommended that the MHRA document

Table 2.4 Care regulators in the UK

England	Care Quality Commission
Wales	Healthcare Standards Inspectorate for Wales
Scotland	Scottish Commission for the Regulation of Care
Northern Ireland	Regulation and Quality Improvement Authority

should be read in conjunction with this section. Guidance within the NMC (2008b) position statement clearly identifies aspects of clinical governance that are necessary to safeguard the public in remote prescribing of cosmetic treatments and it is advised that any independent organisation using remote/online prescribing commit an offence if they are not registered with one of the bodies in Table 2.4.

Transcribing or transposing

The terms 'transcribing' and 'transposing' are synonymous and represent the action of copying details of an independent prescriber's prescription on to other order forms. It is used specifically to assist in the transition of prescribed treatments to new record cards or documents when original ones are full, or if information needs to be passed from one area to another or from one professional to another. Examples would be on a hospital ward prescription sheet or within instructions from secondary to primary care. There are many similar definitions of transcribing including the NHS Education for Scotland (2010) who define it as:

Any act by which medicinal products are written from one form of direction to administer to another is 'transcribing'. This includes discharge letters, transfer letters, copying illegible patient administrations chart onto new charts (whether hand written or computer generated).

The action of transcribing is definitely not a means of prescribing but allows for information to be copied without directly involving the original prescriber (NMC 2010a, NHS Education for Scotland 2010). Prescribing involves holistic assessment of the patient, reaching a diagnosis and making a clinical decision about treatment, whereas transcribing involves none of these things, just the ability to transpose information from one area to another. Doormaal et al (2009) clearly identify a distinction between prescribing and transcribing, and it is this distinction that needs to be highlighted to both prescribers and transcribers so that the parameters of the guidance are not breached or misunderstood.

The NMC (2010a, page 26) position document Standards for Medicines Management Standard 3 states how registrants may transcribe medication from one 'direction to supply or administer' to another form of 'direction to supply or administer' but only in exceptional circumstances. They further advise that 'any medication that is transcribed must be signed off by a registered prescriber. In exceptional circumstances this may be done in the form of an email, text or fax before it can be administered by a registrant'.

Hospital trusts and primary care trusts (PCTs) should produce their own transcribing protocol such as the example available from East Riding of Yorkshire Primary Care Trust (2007) and is a voluntary activity that can be undertaken only by certain practitioners as part of a holistic patient assessment. Practitioners authorised to transcribe should be competent to do so as assessed by the relevant trust and should have completed and signed a transcribing signature form that is thereafter held in their personnel records. Practitioners that are permitted to transcribe usually include registered community practitioner nurse prescribers, GPs and locality pharmacists, for example. All non-medical prescribers should be aware of their own transcribing protocol to ensure safe and legal practice. It is suggested that, if the requirements are not identical to those that have previously been prescribed, then staff must not transcribe. Furthermore, drugs that have been discontinued or are not clearly legible must not be transcribed. Staff are unable to transcribe the details of schedule 2 or 3 controlled drugs, e.g. opiates, amphetamines, barbiturates, and referral back to an independent prescriber must be made for complete re-writing. Local guidance for paediatric transcribing should be sought, but generally it is not recommended. Glare (2009) identified, in a study of medication errors in medical wards, that over half of the medication orders studied contained a prescribing or transcription error. Transcribing errors were classified as errors in the process of interpreting, verifying and transcribing medication orders; however, the incidence of preventable medication errors was low. In view of this, as prescribers we need to ensure that anyone who is transcribing our prescription orders are appropriately trained and competent to undertake the role safely. In legal terms, transcribing is not a means of prescribing itself, yet it could be perceived as being a component of the complete 'prescribing process' for some patients, e.g. a patient under the care of a non-medical prescribing specialist nurse in hospital could have a medication transcribed in the discharge process. Care should therefore be taken to ensure that transcribing staff understand the difference and practitioners undertaking this role should be accountable for their actions, as should those who delegate it.

Prescription form safety

The NHS Business Services Authority (2009) publishes guidance on the security of prescription forms. This section should be read in conjunction with the document *NHS Security Management Service Security of Prescription Forms Guidance* in order that the different types of prescribers familiarise themselves with the regulations appropriate to their place of work. In association with the above guidance, it is recommended that prescribers seek their own employers' protocols on the safety of prescriptions. It is evident that stolen prescriptions are most often used to obtain controlled drugs for recreational use or to sell for financial gain (NHS Business Authority 2009).

The security guidance available from the NHS Business Services Authority includes:

- Security features displayed on prescription forms including a 10-digit serial number, prescribers' personal details, anti-photocopying safeguards and UV-sensitive message
- Ordering, delivery, safe storage and stock control of forms
- Details of current forms for all types of prescriber
- Information on destroying obsolete forms

- Preventing theft and fraudulent use of prescriptions
- Reporting procedure for theft of prescriptions including where to report, form to use and directions that may be given, e.g. to write in a specific colour (not always red) for a period of usually 2 months. The PCT/NHS trust local counter-fraud specialist (LCFS) will then inform local and surrounding pharmacies to alert them to the potential abuse of the stolen forms.

Prescription forms can be ordered and received only for use by nurses, pharmacists and allied health professionals once the issuing trust receives notification of the appropriate annotation on the register of the prescribers' respective professional bodies. It is the responsibility of all non-medical prescribers to be fully conversant with the regulations and guidance available to them regarding the safety of prescriptions and to ensure that they use only the relevant prescription forms that have been issued to them.

PART 2: LEGAL ISSUES

The UK legal system

The law affects virtually everything we do and almost all activities are legally regulated. The law sets standards of behaviour and can be defined as 'a rule or body of rules'. Within society, rules can both *guide* and set *standards* for behaviour and can be classified as 'legal', 'social', 'ethical' or 'moral' rules. For example, a 'social rule' of the UK is that we drive on the left-hand side of the road or a 'moral rule' is that we do not ignore someone who may be asking for help. In prescribing practice, there are legal, social, ethical and moral rules that we must abide by.

 Activity box 2.4

As a prescriber, think of some examples of:

- legal rules
- social rules
- ethical rules
- moral rules

All rules have the same basic characteristics in that they are:

- general, i.e. they apply to everyone or a specific group
- normative or prescriptive, i.e. they set standards of how things ought or ought not to be
- laying down standards of behaviour with which everyone must comply.

Some rules are ascribed the status of law. These rules must be definitive, consistent and understandable by everyone that they may affect. In other words rules as laws should not be vague or imprecise and they should be openly disseminated in advance, and, most importantly, they must be recognised and enforced by the courts. Therefore, law is a framework of regulations and rules that allow a society to self-govern, yet it is flexible, in that, should society's demands and needs change, the law too will change in order to reflect the current norms and values of a society. As society (or indeed health-care) alters, laws will be reformed in keeping with those changes, e.g. the Mental Health Act 2007 has a new definition of mental disorder and is a re-formation of the Mental Health Act 1983.

In the UK, laws can be the following:

- Formally enacted laws or statutes and are the main source of law
- Customary law or common law (derived from cases, i.e. 'case law'). Case law used to be the most important source of law and dates from the thirteenth century. It origi-nates from local custom and is also known as 'judge-made' law. Case law has signifi-cantly contributed to the development of healthcare law and it develops through a system known as 'precedent' in which the courts examine and interpret similar cases and circumstances resulting in a judgment.

English law derives from three main sources:

1 Legislation (AOP)
2 Common law (Case law)
3 European law.

Legislation is drafted by Parliament and becomes law following royal assent. Statutes are otherwise known as Acts of Parliament or Primary Legislation and refer to specific areas, detailing the law AND the penalties for breaking such laws, e.g. the Medicines Act 1968. Amendments to Acts of Parliament are otherwise known as 'secondary', 'subor-dinate' or 'delegated' legislation and these can be:

- Statutory instruments
- Scottish statutory instruments
- Welsh Statutory instruments
- Statutory rules of Northern Ireland
- Church instruments
- Byelaws.

Secondary legislation is delegated to a person or body under authority contained in primary legislation, typically being conferred on ministers, the Crown or public bodies (e.g. Statutory Instrument 1992 No. 604. The Medicines Act (Amendment) Regulations 1992). Further reading on the UK legal system is recommended from the UK Statute Law Database (2010) at www.statutelaw.gov.uk.

The courts are the focal point of the UK legal system and can be classified in a number of ways:

- House of Lords
- Court of Appeal
- High Court
- Crown Court
- Magistrates' and County Courts
- Coroners' Court
- European Court of Justice
- Court of Human Rights.

The law in the UK is classified into the following types.

Private law

- Deals with the legal relationship between private individuals and organisations
- Includes regulating the provision of healthcare and provides a system of compensation for victims of malpractice.

Public law

- Comprises criminal law and the constitutional and administrative rules
- It governs how public bodies operate, e.g. NHS, local authorities, police force, the courts, civil service
- Protects the civil liberties and rights of citizens.

Further classification is as follows.

Civil law

- Comprises a very large area
- Includes every division of private law
- Includes all of public law *except* criminal law
- Actions in civil law are based on the principle that a *remedy* (usually monetary) be recovered from another party.

Criminal law

- Includes any behaviour (act or omission) that the state considers harmful or disruptive
- Offenders are punished (if caught)
- Some overlap between civil and criminal law may occur, e.g. a non-medical prescriber who treats a patient without consent is committing a *civil wrong* and a *criminal act*. If harm ensues, the practitioner can be both sued under civil law and face criminal charges.

Breaking a law will mean that we are legally blameworthy and deserve appropriate punishment. However, although we can all philosophise about laws, such as those

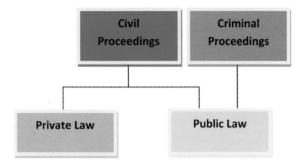

Figure 2.1 Civil law and criminal law proceedings.

around emotive subjects such as drug misuse or euthanasia, we must abide by the law in question, unless we are willing to be punished. As prescribers, for example, the 'law of the land' is that we do not prescribe class A drugs for ourselves to misuse, nor do we prescribe for patients in order to assist their suicide. However, for a crime to be committed, there needs to be two elements:

1 *Actus reus* (or the guilty *act* of prescribing inappropriately for self or others)
2 *Mens rea* (or a guilty *mind* or intention to self-ingest or kill others).

Figure 2.1 demonstrates the classification of law in diagrammatic form to facilitate further understanding. In short, we have two possible directions for proceedings to be brought, i.e. under civil law or criminal law. Within civil law sits all of private law and all of public law except criminal law. Therefore civil proceedings can be brought under both public law and private law, whereas criminal proceedings will be brought under public law only. It is important for prescribers to have an introductory knowledge of the legal system in order that they develop an informative comprehension of how the law may affect them and their practices.

Further reading is recommended and information regarding the UK judicial system can be found on the UK Government website at www.direct.gov.uk.

 Activity box 2.5

Consider your prescribing practice and reflect upon the relevance of law. To support critical reflection, it will be useful to consider the following questions:

● Do you have sufficient knowledge of how the law works?
● Do you feel protected by the law (why/why not)?
● In what instance may a criminal prosecution or civil suit be undertaken?

Negligence and duty of care

Tort law is a component of civil law and includes different types of action such as trespass, defamation, breach of statutory duty, nuisance and negligence. Therefore, clinical negligence is dealt with under the 'law of tort'. The Department of Health (2003b) identify tort as:

> ... an act or omission that causes harm to a person's property, reputation or interests ... and negligence is the specific tort involved in medical litigation.

In prescribing practice, should the practitioner cause harm as a result of his or her clinical decision-making and resultant prescribing, he or she could be held accountable under tort law. The law of negligence has been built up by the courts over years and derives from both *principles* and *precedents*. Judgments are based on specific legislation (statutes) and actual cases (common law). A petitioner who wishes to bring a claim in negligence has to meet the requirements set out by the House of Lords in a landmark case – that of *Donoghue v Stevensen* 1932, in which the 'duty of care' rule was applied. Herring (2008) identifies that most medical litigation is brought under the tort of negligence, but in order to proceed, three criteria need to be met:

1 The professional who is being sued owed the claimant a duty of care
2 The professional breached that duty of care
3 The breach of the duty of care caused the claimant loss.

Any professional owes a duty of care to his or her patient or client and non-medical prescribers are no exception to this. The duty of care by a healthcare professional to a patient is well established and Herring (2008, p. 94) further suggests that 'you owe a duty of care to anyone you may reasonably foreseeably injure'. As prescribers we need to take heed of this in every patient whom we treat and consider whether we could 'reasonably, foreseeably injure' them by our prescribing practice.

Once a duty of care is established, it is necessary to establish a breach of that duty. In law, negligence is ascertained on the balance of probabilities in that the practitioner acted as a 'reasonable person' would. The judgment in *Bolam v Friern Hospital Management Committee* 1957 stated:

> A doctor is not guilty of negligence if he has acted in accordance with a practice accepted as proper by a responsible body of medical men skilled in that particular art.

The *Bolam* test applies to all healthcare professionals and as a prescriber you would be judged against 'a responsible body' of non-medical prescribers undertaking the same role as yourself, should it be deemed that a breach of duty of care has occurred and a loss has resulted. In *Bolam*, the court said:

> Where the case involves some special skill or competence, then the test as to whether there has been negligence or not is ... the standard of the ordinary skilled man exercising and professing to have that special skill or knowledge.

In other words, prescribing is that 'special skill or knowledge' and you would be judged against your fellow prescribing peers. Therefore, negligence by a nurse, pharmacist or allied health professional (AHP) will be determined by the standard of the *ordinary* nurse, pharmacist or AHP. However, if the nurse, pharmacist or AHP professes to have specialist-prescribing skills, then the standard will be that of the *ordinary prescribing* nurse, pharmacist or AHP.

It is important to remember that a duty of care involves all aspects of practice including warning of those side effects, consequences and risks that the reasonably competent professional would have warned of as in *Chester v Afshar* 2005. As a prescriber, a fundamental responsibility of prescribing for others is to ensure that these risks are discussed with the patient or his or her advocate. Furthermore, it is clear that a 'reasonably competent' equivalent professional would not act unlawfully or outside their competence, and a prescriber who does act outside their field of competence is likely to be found guilty of negligence in a court of law should harm ensue.

Claims for clinical negligence are usually dealt with through a legal process resulting in compensation, known in legal terms as a 'remedy' and there have been recent reforms in respect of how such claims are dealt with in the NHS. Following recommendations from the Department of Health Chief Medical Officer's (CMO's) consultation document *Making Amends* (DH 2003b) the NHS Redress Bill (DH 2005a) allowed the Secretary of State for Health to set up a redress scheme to 'apply to cases involving liabilities in tort' occurring from NHS hospital care (DH 2005b). These rules were appropriately placed in secondary legislation so that they could be easily amended in line with future changes within the realms of NHS service delivery, and it was anticipated that the subsequent NHS Redress Act 2006 would secure a fair and honourable system for compensatory resolution to hospital negligence claims. The NHS Redress Act 2006 received Royal Assent on 8 November 2006 and exists as:

An Act to make provision about arrangements for redress in relation to liability in tort in connection with services provided as part of the health service in England or Wales; and for connected purposes.

Although at face value, the Government's proposals for reform seemed commendable, if somewhat overdue, there has been some opposition to the philosophy of the Act in that some see it as a diluted 'quick fix' to addressing claims of negligence. Farrell and Devaney (2007), for example, insisted that a 'golden opportunity' had unfortunately been missed in providing a reasonable and equitable recompense for individuals who have 'suffered harm through medical treatment in the NHS'. However, on examination, it is argued that the Act offers a faster and more easily accessible scheme for numerous patients who are entitled to damages up to a certain value.

Under the NHS Redress Act, the NHS Redress Scheme must meet certain objectives. It should provide the following:

- an offer of compensation
- an explanation
- an apology
- a report detailing how similar cases may be avoided in the future.

So, it would appear that it is the Government's intention not only to provide compensation to the harmed individual(s), but also to take appropriate action to investigate how and why the particular harm ensued in order to improve NHS performance in ensuring the safety of patients. However, any settlement agreement provided under the scheme includes a waiver that prohibits the right of any claimant to bring civil proceedings 'in respect of the liability to which the settlement relates'. On balance, this appears to be a reasonable stipulation but does not take account of the possibility that a claimant may in fact become aware of related and contributory facts regarding their claim for damages after the settlement. Compensation could, in theory, be hastily accepted when in fact the resultant harm could have warranted further monetary remedy. It could be argued therefore that the Redress Scheme is, in effect, relying in part on the vulnerability of patients.

As prescribing practitioners, an awareness of the NHS Redress Scheme allows us to advise our patients if necessary but also to raise our sense of responsibility and vigilance in practice.

Prescription writing

A prescription is a legal document under the Medicines Act 1968. The law dictates which healthcare professionals can and cannot prescribe medicines, yet it also allows local arrangements to be developed to administer medicines by other means, to certain types of patients, in certain circumstances, by using patient group directions (PGD), for example. The use of PGDs is, however, not the same as prescribing. Non-medical prescribers are permitted to prescribe within the parameters of the current guidelines for nurses, pharmacists and AHPs and, at the time of writing, specific prescribing entitlements are as detailed in this section. Prescribers are required to keep abreast of changes in these entitlements as an essential part of safe practice and effective professional development. The National Prescribing Centre regularly updates information for prescribers on their website and includes specific facts on prescribing entitlements. The section 'Prescribing controlled drugs', in Table 3.5, outlines professional annotations and prescribing rights for nurses, pharmacists and AHPs.

The *British National Formulary* (BNF) provides clear guidance on prescription writing and the standard produced by all non-medical prescribers should always reflect the example contained within the current version of the BNF. It is recommended that this part of the chapter should be read in conjunction with the following sections of the BNF:

- How to use the BNF
- Guidance on prescribing
- Prescription writing
- Emergency supply of medicines.

In law, the **only** healthcare practitioners legally permitted to write prescriptions are:

- Doctors
- Dentists

- Suitably qualified independent nurse and midwife prescribers (nurses and pharmacists)
- Supplementary prescribers (nurses, pharmacists and AHPs)
- Community practitioner prescribers (V100 and V150) – limited formulary.

Guidance on 'unlicensed', 'off-label', 'off-licence' medicines

Unlicensed medicines are medicinal products that are not licensed for any indication or age group. An unlicensed medicine is one that does not have a valid marketing authorisation (i.e. licence) in the UK (NMC 2010b). The NMC Circular 04/2010 (NMC 2010b) provides nurse and midwife prescribers with guidance on prescribing unlicensed medicines. It should be noted that the information in this circular replaces Practice Standard 17 (17.1) of the *Standards of Proficiency for Nurse and Midwife Prescribers* (NMC 2006). The circular advises that previous legislation has been amended to allow nurse and midwife independent prescribers to prescribe unlicensed medicines for those in their care on the same basis as doctors, dentists and supplementary prescribers. Furthermore the Pharmaceutical Services Negotiating Committee (PSNC 2010) advise that the Drug Tariff Part XVIIB (ii) has been amended in line with the regulations to clarify that pharmacist independent prescribers may also now prescribe unlicensed medicines for their patients. They do, however, emphasise that optometrist prescribers continue not to be able to prescribe unlicensed medicines.

The NMC (2010b, p. 2) state that certain criteria should be considered before prescribing unlicensed medicines and it is proposed here that pharmacist independent prescribers should follow similar guidance. These guidelines are as follows:

- Practice Standard 17 (17.1) of the Standards of proficiency for nurse and midwife prescribers (NMC, 2006) should be replaced with the following information; You may prescribe an unlicensed medication as an independent nurse prescriber providing:
- You are satisfied that an alternative, licensed medication would not meet the patient's or client's needs.
- You are satisfied that there is a sufficient evidence base and/or experience to demonstrate the medication's safety and efficacy for that particular patient or client.
- You are prepared to take responsibility for prescribing the unlicensed medicine and for overseeing the patient's or client's care, including monitoring and any follow-up treatment.
- The patient or client agrees to the prescription in the knowledge that the medicine is unlicensed and understands the implications of this.
- The medication chosen and the reason for choosing it are documented in patient's or client's notes.
- You seek, as necessary, professional advice, e.g. from a pharmacist or other authoritative clinical guidance to support your prescribing practice and the specification for the unlicensed medicine.
- You must report suspected adverse drug reactions arising from unlicensed medicines to the MHRA and Commission on Human Medicines via the Yellow Card scheme.

Borderline substances

Borderline substances are mainly foodstuffs, such as enteral feeds and foods that are specially formulated for people with medical conditions, but also include some toiletries, such as sun blocks for use by people with conditions such as photodermatosis (NHS Purchasing and Supply Agency (PASA) 2010). A list of ACBS (Advisory Committee on Borderline Substances)-approved products and the circumstances under which they can be prescribed can be found in the BNF. Although this is a non-mandatory list, independent prescribers should normally restrict their prescribing of borderline substances to items on the ACBS approved list.

Emergency supply requests

Community practitioner nurse prescribers, nurse and pharmacist independent prescribers, all supplementary prescribers, doctors and dentists can also request, in an emergency, the supply of a prescription-only medicine that is not a schedule 1, 2 or 3 controlled drug, if they would otherwise be entitled to prescribe that drug. The prescriber must give an undertaking to furnish a prescription within 72 hours (PSNC 2010). Prescribers should always keep abreast of changes in their entitlements and more information on the prescribing rights of different health professionals can be found in the PSNC online Drug Tariff Resource Centre (see www.psnc.org.uk)

Writing the prescription

Writing a prescription is just one of the options that a non-medical prescriber can choose when considering 'What strategy' in the NPC (1999) prescribing pyramid. Figure 2.2 suggests where prescribing and prescription writing fit into the prescribing process and

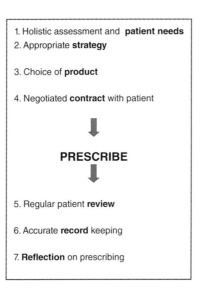

1. Holistic assessment and **patient needs**
2. Appropriate **strategy**

3. Choice of **product**

4. Negotiated **contract** with patient

PRESCRIBE

5. Regular patient **review**

6. Accurate **record** keeping

7. **Reflection** on prescribing

Figure 2.2 Prescribing and the prescribing principles. (Adapted from the National Prescribing Centre 1999.)

it could be vehemently argued that the act of prescription writing should never be considered earlier than this point.

Non-medical prescribers should not undertake this role without supervision until fully conversant with the specific inclusions and definitive configuration of the prescription sheet. Anecdotal evidence suggests that it is habitually misconstrued by students how convoluted prescription writing actually is, and many perceive it as a minor part of the prescribing process. In actuality, students do not always perform this part of the process particularly well. Typical errors include misspelling of drug names, incorrect doses, unclear instructions, missing patient details and illegibility. It is therefore advised that non-medical prescribers perfect prescription writing before qualification and annotation on the register. Table 2.5 summarises the key requirements for safe and accurate prescription writing.

It is suggested by Weaver (2006) that Latin abbreviations should be avoided and, just as we should not abbreviate the names of drugs, nor should we abbreviate the specific instructions to both the pharmacist and the patient. Latin abbreviations as detailed in Table 2.6 cannot be translated completely accurately so good practice is to write the prescription in full, using English language. Weaver (2006) argues that 'the continued use of abbreviations often shortcuts medication safety' and advocates that the use of abbreviations in prescription writing be withdrawn. He suggested that organisations and disciplines that continue to use abbreviations in prescribing practice often do so because it is 'the way it has always been done'. Perhaps it could be suggested here that it is often difficult to change practice, particularly as the use of Latin can and is still deemed an almost elite, exclusive skill and language, used by health professionals, that is difficult to relinquish. Weaver (2006) further identifies rationale for avoiding Latin abbreviations and offers examples whereby misinterpretation can arise to the detriment of patient safety and prescriber credibility.

The following excerpt from Weaver's (2006) article demonstrates the dangers of using abbreviations:

A recommended total daily dose of 2400mg of ibuprofen should be prescribed as 600mg every 6 hours rather than 600mg q.i.d. (quarter in die) for several reasons. With the Latin directions, the patient could take all 4 doses before noon and still feel that he or she was in compliance with the q.i.d. directions. Also, if your handwriting is like that of most busy doctors, the pharmacist or nurse might misinterpret the q.i.d. for q.4 h. (quaque quarta hora). That would result in 6 doses of 600mg in a day and a total of 3600 mg/day of ibuprofen, which is well beyond the recommended adult daily dose of 2400mg. Thus, modern, safe prescribing practices discourage the use of Latin abbreviations such as b.i.d. (bis in die), t.i.d. (ter in die), h.s. (hora somni), p.c. (post cibum), and a.c. (ante cibum) and encourage the use of clear wording such as every 12 hours, every 8 hours, at bedtime, after eating, and before eating a meal, respectively'.

Although it is not illegal to use Latin abbreviations, it should be avoided on prescriptions, particularly if hand-written, unless the prescriber can guarantee that their instructions are clearly legible and that the pharmacist can accurately interpret those instructions. However, it is suggested here that, although the generic use of mutually recognised abbreviations in healthcare as such is an essential form of shorthand for

Table 2.5 Prescription writing guidelines

Only prescribe what you are qualified to within your *own competencies*
Some prescriptions may be computer generated
Write legibly and in indelible ink (black preferably)
State patient's full name, address, age, date of birth (years and months for under 12s is a legal requirement)
Clearly state the name (generic wherever possible) of the prescribed item, its formulation, strength, quantity, dosage and frequency
Do not use abbreviations (see below)
Use a line to distinguish between items
State clear directions
It is good practice to write 'No more items on this prescription' if there is unused space
Block out left-over space with a straight a line or Z
Legible signature (electronic signatures not permitted)
Date the prescription

Dose
For preparations to be taken 'as required', a **minimum dose interval** should be specified (e.g. 4 hourly)
For preparations to be taken 'as required', a **maximum dose** should be specified (e.g. No more than 8 tablets in any 24 hours)
Avoid unnecessary use of decimal points (e.g. 5.0 mg)

Frequency
For preparations to be taken at frequent intervals, a time period between doses should be specified (e.g. 1 capsule every 6 h)
May need to be agreed with the patient/parent/carer depending on normal routine

Quantity
Quantities of 1 gram or more should be written as 1 g, 1.5 g, 2 g, etc.
Quantities of less than 1 gram should be written in milligrams (e.g. 500 mg and NOT 0.5 g)
Micrograms should be written in full and not abbreviated (e.g. 50 micrograms and NOT 50 mcg)
Quantity should generally reflect pack sizes from the *British National Formulary/Nurses' Prescribing Formulary*

Further considerations
Indicate the number of days of treatment required in the box provided on NHS forms
This does not apply to items directed to be used as required – the quantity to be supplied needs to be stated
Although directions should preferably be in **English without abbreviation**, it is recognised that some Latin abbreviations are still used (see Table 2.6)

Adapted from guidance in the *British National Formulary* (BMA and RPSGB 2010).

practitioners, non-medical prescribers, particularly novice prescribers, should learn to write their scripts in full as a matter of course.

℞ The symbol Rx has long been used to represent 'prescription' and its origins are thought to lie in the Latin for 'recipe' or more literally 'to take'. Again, the use of this

Table 2.6 Latin abbreviations in prescribing

a.c.	ante cibum (before food)
b.d.	bis die (twice daily)
o.d.	omni die (every day)
o.m.	omni mane (every morning)
o.n.	omni nocte (every night)
p.c.	post cibum (after food)
p.r.n.	pro re nata (when required)
q.d.s.	quater die sumendum (to be taken four times daily)
q.q.h.	quarta quaque hora (every four hours)
t.d.s.	ter die sumendum (to be taken three times daily)
t.i.d.	ter in die (three times daily)
stat	immediately

symbol is widely used, yet its meaning and that of other abbreviations is open to misinterpretation by the user and the reader. It is suggested that, due to the risk of ambiguity and perhaps detrimental mistakes, non-medical prescribers limit or decline their use.

Activity box 2.6

Using the appropriate template for your professional group (Appendix 1) practice writing safe, accurate and legible prescriptions for the patients below:

1 Write a prescription for Sam, a 45-year-old man who has been smoking 20 cigarettes a day for 30 years and wishes to give up. He has heard about nicotine patches. He is generally well and takes no other medication.
2 You see Ethel, aged 76, in A&E after a fall. She sustained a Colles' fracture and has a plaster of Paris in situ. Write a prescription for some analgesia to take home. She has type 2 diabetes and takes metformin 500 mg three times daily.
3 Sharon, aged 31, presents at the pharmacy with constipation. She is 26 weeks' pregnant and has not had her bowels opened for 5 days. She is extremely uncomfortable. What would you advise? If prescribing, write a prescription.
4 Jack is 18 and is an intravenous drug user. He presents with cellulitis of his left forearm. Apart from intravenous heroin, he takes no other medication. Write a prescription for appropriate treatment of his cellulitis.
5 Mary has recurrent vaginal discharge. It is itchy and has previously been diagnosed as 'thrush'. She has used the cream she was given 6 months ago with no effect. Write a prescription for this woman.

Prescribing controlled drugs

As with the previous section, this element of the chapter should be read in conjunction with the following part of the current BNF:

- Controlled drugs and drug dependence
- Emergency supply of medicines.

The Misuse of Drugs Act 1971 prohibits certain activities in relation to 'controlled drugs', in particular their manufacture, supply and possession. The penalties applicable to offences involving the different drugs are graded broadly according to the 'harmfulness attributable to a drug when it is misused' and for this purpose the drugs are defined in the three classes identified in Table 2.2. Furthermore, there are limitations in the prescribing of controlled drugs, with some non-medical prescribers only being permitted to prescribe controlled drugs under certain circumstances and others being currently prohibited from prescribing any controlled drugs. This is detailed in Table 2.7.

The Misuse of Drugs Regulations 2001 define the classes of *person* who are authorised to supply and possess controlled drugs while acting in their professional capacities, and lay down the conditions under which these activities may be carried out. In these regulations, drugs are divided into *five schedules* each specifying the requirements governing such activities as import, export, production, supply, possession, prescribing and record keeping that apply to them. Occasionally, it may be necessary for a prescriber to request an emergency supply of medicines for their patient. However, the Prescription Only Medicines (Human Use) Order 1997 does not extend to controlled drugs, except for phenobarbital sodium for the treatment of epilepsy.

As the legalities, regulations and nuances of controlled drug prescribing is ever changing, it is suggested that the reader keeps abreast of the amendments by always using the most appropriate guidance for the field of healthcare within which they are employed. Further information can be obtained from the current version of the BNF and accessing contemporary information via professional bodies: the National Prescribing Centre (NPC) publication *A Guide to Good Practice in the Management of Controlled Drugs in Primary Care* (NPC 2009) and the Department of Health's (2007) document *Safer Management of Controlled Drugs*. For those prescribers working within or in partnership with care homes, the Care Quality Commission (2010) produce guidance in their document *Management of Controlled Drugs in Care Homes* that can be accessed via their website (www.cqc.org.uk).

The chapter continues with an examination of some of the legal issues of prescribing that could also be regarded as ethical considerations. Therefore, the reader is guided towards studying the next section from both a legal and an ethical perspective.

Legal aspects of autonomy and gaining consent

Purposeful evaluation of patients' autonomy and their ability to consent or refuse treatment is one of the main principles of prescribing. Anecdotally, prescribers can recoil from this important aspect of prescribing practice, perhaps in part due to a lack of awareness of the concepts or the lack of ability to assess the patient in the absence of transparent guidelines. Many practitioners wrongly assume that the assessment of a patient's mental capacity concerns only those patients with mental illness or learning disabilities. In reality, capacity to consent concerns all of us, and we, as prescribers, should be competent and confident to assess all of our patients' ability to consent at

Table 2.7 Prescribing rights and controlled drugs

V100 nurse
Community practitioner prescriber *with* specialist qualification

Formulary and entitlements
Nurse Prescribers' Formulary for Community Practitioners
- Cannot prescribe controlled drugs

V150 nurse
Community practitioner prescriber *without* specialist qualification

Formulary and entitlements
Nurse Prescribers' Formulary for Community Practitioners
- Cannot prescribe controlled drugs

V300 nurse
Independent and supplementary prescriber

Formulary and entitlements
British National Formulary
- Nurse independent prescribers are restricted by current legislation to independently prescribe only certain controlled drugs solely for specified medical conditions according to BNF nurse prescribers' formulary – nurse independent prescribing
- **Nurse supplementary prescribers** can prescribe any schedule 2–5 controlled drugs for any condition within their competence, as part of a patient specific, written clinical management plan (CMP) agreed with a doctor

Pharmacist
Independent and/or supplementary prescriber

Formulary and entitlements
British National Formulary
- Pharmacist independent prescribers are not yet able to independently prescribe any controlled drugs
- **Pharmacist supplementary prescribers** can prescribe any schedule 2–5 controlled drugs for any condition within their competence, as part of a patient specific, written CMP agreed with a doctor

Optometrist
Independent and/or supplementary prescriber

Formulary and entitlements
British National Formulary
- Optometrist independent prescribers are able to prescribe any licensed medicine for ocular conditions affecting the eye, and the tissue surrounding the eye, within their recognised area of expertise and competence, except for controlled drugs or medicines for parenteral administration
- Optometrist independent prescribers cannot prescribe controlled drugs
- **Optometrist supplementary prescribers** can prescribe any schedule 2–5 controlled drugs for any condition within their competence, as part of a patient specific, written CMP agreed with a doctor

Chiropodist/Podiatrist
Supplementary prescriber

Table 2.7 *(Continued)*

Formulary and entitlements
British National Formulary
- **Chiropodist/podiatrist supplementary prescribers** can prescribe any schedule 2–5 controlled drugs for any condition within their competence, as part of a patient specific, written CMP agreed with a doctor
- **Note:** registered chiropodists with the appropriate annotation to sell, supply and administer medicines may obtain packs of certain wholesale medicines from a registered pharmacy for the chiropodist to sell or supply to their patients. This is different to prescribing (RPSGB 2009)

Physiotherapist/Radiologist
Supplementary prescriber

Formulary and entitlements
British National Formulary
- **Physiotherapist supplementary prescribers** can prescribe any schedule 2–5 controlled drugs for any condition within their competence, as part of a patient specific, written clinical management plan (CMP) agreed with a doctor

Adapted from information from the National Prescribing Centre (2010).

any given time. In view of the complexities of autonomy and consent, a large part of this section is dedicated to this issue.

The NPC's prescribing pyramid (NPC 1999) directs the prescriber to 'consider the patient' in step 1. A component part of 'considering the patient' involves the prescriber respecting the person's autonomy or acting as his or her advocate and assessing willingness and ability to consent. Educational programmes for non-medical prescribers promote the use of the NPC model in order to structure the prescribing process, yet it would seem that although the NPC makes reference to considering the patient 'holistically', the assessment of mental capacity, autonomy or gaining consent appears implicit and therefore could potentially be overlooked or trivialised. It is the prescriber's responsibility to ensure that these principal facets of the consultation are always allowed sufficient consideration.

Paternalism

Traditionally healthcare practice has been dominated by a paternalistic approach to decision-making. Practitioners using a paternalistic approach make decisions on behalf of the patient with little or no consultation or agreement (Maude P, Hawley G 2007, cited in Hawley 2007). In recent years, it is noted that doctors, nurses and other practitioners deemed this approach an appropriate and acceptable means of delivering healthcare. Today, however, with the advent of patient involvement, choice and a greater emphasis on patients' right to autonomy, a paternalistic approach is not as fervently conventional. Jefford and Tattersall (2002) identify that the literature generally suggests that most patients want as much information as possible and will seek it out from various sources, yet, further to this, Jefford et al (2005) argue that, in some circumstances, clinicians may have to adopt a paternalistic approach to information giving when the information that they give may cause detrimental effects to their patient's wellbeing. The example that Jefford et al (2005) use is the withholding of information about unavailable, expensive cancer treatments that the patient could never afford to purchase. As suggested, much of the current literature concerning paternalistic approaches to healthcare does in fact support autonomy rather than paternalism, yet others believe that a paternalistic approach may be welcomed by some patients when developing their treatment plan. Often the patient will respect the practitioner's knowledge and skill in diagnosing their illness and willingly accept their judgement in deciding how to treat the presenting complaint. It could be argued that this approach is not paternalistic, but, in actual fact, an illustration of the trust within the prescriber–patient relationship. In support of this assumption, Edwards and Elwyn (2009) remind us that 'paternalism' is not intended to be 'objectionable per se', but rather that it is motivated by our desire to act with the patients' best interests at heart and is more about the adoption of parental, protective attitudes towards our patients. As prescribers, therefore, we need to acquire the ability to identify when a paternalistic approach to our patients is either inappropriate or justified.

Defining autonomy

Autonomy is a term that is associated with ideas such as self-determination, self-government and choosing one's own moral position (Beauchamp TL 1997, cited in Hendrick 2000) and can be defined as the person having the capacity to think, decide and act independently, without hindrance (Gillon 1985). Respect for autonomy is considered to be one of the most fundamental of moral principles (Hendrick 2000) yet, in relation to prescribing practice, it can be fraught with difficulty. One such problem is that patients are unique, populations are diverse and autonomy is variable, yet there is a significant group of people in whom autonomy is absent, compromised or undeveloped, which immediately presents us with a challenge. From a prescribing perspective, when assessing our patients and gathering information, it can often be assumed by practitioners that autonomy is present, yet it can equally be assumed to be absent in particular individuals such as those with mental illness, elderly people and children. It is suggested here that insufficient attention is paid to patient autonomy in some cases, perhaps because the consultation appears uneventful and straightforward. The utilisation of an appropriate consultation model may go part way to ensuring that autonomy is always assessed.

Dworkin (1989) characterised autonomy as 'the capacity of a person to critically reflect upon, and then attempt to accept or change, his or her preferences, desires, values and ideals'. Although this is a somewhat idealistic view of autonomy, our aim as prescribers should be to capture the essence of Dworkin's (1989) ideal as far as is attainable with our patients, while also recognising that autonomy is unrealistic and unachievable for some individuals such as those with dementing illness, people who are unconscious, mentally impaired individuals or neonates. As prescribers we need to aim to sufficiently respect and protect the autonomy of individuals in prescribing decisions or indeed act with the patient's best interests at heart if self-determination is absent.

The Kantian view of autonomy is that all people have unconditional worth (Beauchamp and Childress 2001) and that each person has the capacity to determine his or her own moral destiny. Immanuel Kant (1724-1804) expressed that an individual's autonomy is violated when he or she is merely treated as a means to achieving another's goals, with no consideration for his or her own personal goals. An example of this theory in today's terms and in prescribing practice is in a situation whereby a carer's goal may be to request that the practitioner prescribes sedating medication to a relative in order to ease the burden of care. Furthermore, patients may be prescribed particular medication in order to satisfy a prescriber's ulterior motives, as in the case of Harold Shipman. It is paramount that prescribers and prescribing practice be monitored appropriately to avoid prescribing that ignores the rights of the patient.

However, putting aside the potential abuse of prescribing rights, it could be suggested that, although Kant's concept of non-violation of a person's right to choose is honourable, it has to be established whether this can always be achieved in prescribing practice. It would be fair to argue that, despite acknowledging the patients' absolute right to autonomy, in healthcare it is possible only to maintain a patient's right to choose up to a certain point. Fallowfield et al (1994) reasoned that, in many circumstances, clinicians are best placed to make the overall decision in a treatment context and the skills and knowledge of non-medical prescribers could be seen as the rationale to underpin this school of thought. Furthermore, Tingle and Cribb (2002) recognised that patients often expect the healthcare professional to make decisions for them, including whether they need to have certain clinical interventions or take prescribed medication. In other words, some patients are quite content to relinquish their autonomy, in favour of the clinician's professional judgement. As prescribers, it could be suggested that this is evident in many, if not most, of our prescribing consultations.

Kottow (2003) recognises that autonomy has previously been 'hailed as the foremost principle in bioethics', but historically patient care has been subject to medical paternalism because the doctor was considered to be better qualified to make medical decisions than the patient, who can, according to Kottow, be 'distracted by illness'. Kottow further argues that the assumption that the sick person is not fully autonomous could be viewed as biased and unsubstantiated. Moreover, he states that, although it is undisputed that healthcare professionals may possess a sound clinical knowledge base, they habitually lack the ethical understanding and qualifications to allow them the prerogative to make decisions for others. It would then be fair to suggest that, in order to function effectively in the role of a non-medical prescriber, it is essential to become fully conversant with the principles of law and ethics.

A further premise is that it is well documented that respect for autonomy cannot always be observed in certain individuals. Our obligations as healthcare professionals to respect autonomy cannot possibly extend to those individuals who are considered non-autonomous, e.g. incapacitated, immature or severely mentally ill individuals. It is the responsibility of the prescriber to identify this inability in their patients and act in the person's 'best interests'. Interestingly, Beauchamp and Childress (2001) list 'drug-dependent persons' as being non-autonomous. This viewpoint is ambiguous and controversial, in that it would be fairer to say that a person 'under the influence of certain drugs' is temporarily non-autonomous. To clarify this argument, a 'drug-dependent' person could be anyone from an individual with one or more chronic diseases who is reliant on certain drugs for continued survival or control of symptoms, to a heroin addict who, although dependent on it, has long periods of lucidity and, hence, the mental capacity to make decisions for himself. Significantly, Gillon (1985) stated that when assessing whether a patient is 'sufficiently autonomous' we should judge the capacity of the *individual* rather than label certain groups as capable of making decisions for themselves. This allows for those less clear-cut cases where an individual's autonomy may be compromised or underdeveloped, such as in unconscious individuals or children. Assessing the person as an individual affords us the authorisation to assess whether the patient is 'sufficiently autonomous' in a certain situation. We need to be aware, as prescribers, that in these situations the capacity to consent is not always static because an individual's autonomy and resulting capacity to consent can fluctuate.

The importance of consent

The following section should be read together with the Department of Health's document *Reference Guide to Consent for Examination or Treatment* (DH 2009b).

Obtaining consent for clinical interventions is a fundamental consideration in healthcare and particularly pertinent to the role of prescribers. Not only does the prescriber have to take a complete and thorough history, but examination of the patient and clinical investigations are often also required to confirm a diagnosis and agree a management plan. In order to perform all aspects of this process, suitable consent must be obtained. It is suggested that patient consent is valid only where the individual is competent to give it, has been properly informed and has agreed without coercion (GMC 2002). It should be made evident for all non-medical prescribers and students that gaining consent is a substantial component of prescribing practice which cannot and should not be superficially considered. To aid our practice, published guidelines in respect of consent are in abundance from each of the respective professional bodies and from the Department of Health, and it is the assimilation of these guidelines that is vital for legal, safe and ethically sensitive prescribing practice.

Dimond (2009, p. 19) identified different forms of consent and states that:

Consent is the agreement by a mentally competent person, voluntarily and without deceit or fraud, to an action which without that consent would be a trespass to the person ...

It is interesting to note that Dimond's definition of consent identifies a number of issues that need to be considered by the prescriber in the first instance: first, there needs to be 'agreement'; second, the patient must be deemed 'mentally competent'; third, agreement needs to be given 'voluntarily'; and fourth the prescriber has to act in a way that does not conceal any 'deceit or fraud'. Should any of these components be missing, the prescriber could be liable to answer to an accusation of 'trespass to the person'. When examined in more depth, the prescriber may feel apprehensive that each of these areas of consent alone is complex and laden with ambiguity, imprecision and possible misinterpretation.

Activity box 2.7

In your own area of practice, and using a model of reflection, write down an example of when you have obtained consent from a patient. Consider the following:

1 Was there satisfactory agreement?
2 Was the person mentally competent?
3 Was consent given voluntarily?
4 Was there any deceit or fraud?
5 In prescribing practice, could your method of gaining consent be deemed robust?

Consent in adults with capacity

There are various terms and distinct categories of consent and, in understanding the differences, the prescriber will feel more confident to assess the ability of patients to consent or refuse treatment. In prescribing it is good practice to document, however laborious, the nature of consent gained (Gulliver 2006).

Implied consent

This is otherwise referred to as 'non-verbal consent' and it is characterised by the patient displaying behaviours of acquiescence to a procedure such as having a blood test or their blood pressure taken by offering their arm. The GMC (2008a) warn, however, that 'you should be careful about relying on a patient's apparent compliance with a procedure as a form of consent. For example, the fact that a patient lies down on an examination couch does not in itself indicate that the patient has understood what you propose to do and why'. The RPSGB (2007c) state that in implied consent 'the patient indicates their consent without writing or speaking, for example, a patient who brings their prescriptions to you for dispensing'. In prescribing practice, it is suggested here that the use of implied consent is limited and unsafe with regards to the actual prescribing of treatments, because, in an ideal situation, a verbal exchange and discussion of those treatments will take place. However, implied consent may be evidently used in the clinical examination of patients, yet the practitioner should always be certain that consent is, in actual fact, bona fide.

Verbal consent

This is the type of consent that is used most readily by healthcare professionals in the course of their work. Nurses, pharmacists and AHPs rely on patients to verbalise their consent in response to the questions that they may ask of them. A resounding 'yes' or 'no' from the patient would quite easily confirm or refute agreement to a plan of treatment and it is this form of consent that would be sought in many prescribing situations. However, as Dimond (2009) highlights, should any discrepancy arise as to whether or not valid consent was gained, in the absence of witnesses, it would be the word of the prescriber against that of the patient. Therefore, in prescribing practice, perhaps we need to consider more robust methods of safeguarding both our patients and ourselves.

Written consent

This is that in which, as the name implies, an agreement is given in writing and this is considered to be the most transparent form of gaining consent. Dimond (2009) suggests that written consent can be viewed as good evidence that the person agreed to the treatment by providing a signature. The GMC (2008b) suggest that 'in cases that involve higher risk, it is important that you get the patient's written consent. This is so that everyone involved understands what was explained and agreed. By law you must get written consent for certain treatments, such as fertility treatment and organ donation and you must follow the laws and codes of practice that govern these situations'.

Written consent forms should include details of the treatment or procedure and it is against this information that the patient agrees or disagrees to it. In supplementary prescribing, the clinical management plan can be viewed as detailing sufficient information for the patient to sign up to it. As part of the tripartite agreement among the independent prescriber, supplementary prescriber and patient, signatures are required to legitimise and seal the plan as a mutually consensual care pathway. However, although written consent is the ideal in supplementary prescribing, and easily orchestrated, it would be unfeasible to obtain written consent in all independent prescribing consultations, mainly due to time constraints. In written consent, in addition to gaining a signature, the patient should be provided with details of any significant risks from the treatment or procedure in order that they can make an informed decision. The BMA (2009), in their guidance, confirm that there is no legal requirement to obtain written consent, but it may be advisable in some cases. As a non-medical prescriber, it is an independent professional judgement that needs to be made depending on the circumstances of the consultation. It is important to remember that the consent form documents only that some discussion about the treatment has taken place and it is advised by the BMA that the nature of any discussion is recorded in the patient's records.

Informed consent

This is a term that is used widely in healthcare law and ethics. Informed consent is defined by the Royal College of Nursing (RNC 2005, p. 5) as 'an ongoing agreement by a person to receive treatment, undergo procedures or participate in research, after risks, benefits and alternatives have been adequately explained to them'. It is, however, a complex principle that many healthcare professionals fail to comprehend in any great depth. Anecdotal evidence suggests that the term 'informed consent' is generally used superficially, even nonchalantly, with very little evidence of an appreciation of its precise meaning among healthcare professionals. It appears that in practice there are varying degrees of detail given to patients before clinical procedures and treatments, and it could be argued that there are a variety of reasons why this is so. As a consequence, it is suggested here that consent is often obtained inadvertently from patients, without the benefit of true understanding of the treatment, procedure or examination. Moreover it is further suggested that, without any prior consideration of the implications for either the healthcare professional or the patient, prescribing would be unsafe. This is completely unsatisfactory, but common practice. Therefore, informed consent is explored in greater depth here to secure sound understanding.

Although much has been written on informed consent and its importance in protecting patient autonomy, a great deal of the literature is unconvincing and supported by poor arguments, yet it remains an essential facet of prescribing practice. O'Neill (2003) acknowledges that there are significant limitations as well as strengths in the procedures that we undertake in order to obtain informed consent, and suggests that all healthcare practitioners should seriously recognise these in order to support their clinical practice and professional accountability. Patients should be given sufficient information, in a way that they understand, to enable them to exercise this right and make informed decisions about the care that they receive. But, as prescribers, we need to assess how much information is sufficient. A further consideration is how we can establish if a patient has truly understood what he or she has been told. A question that we may ask of ourselves in prescribing practice is: Can we actually guarantee that a patient's autonomy is protected when there appears to be no failsafe method of ensuring that consent is indisputably informed? In effect, could we be seen to be proceeding with what should be viewed as 'uninformed consent'.

Jones et al (2005) identified that information giving is variable depending on the individual circumstances of the situation, but confirmed that it is significant enough a dilemma to warrant further exploration. Leading case law provides us with guidance on the limits and extent of information giving and truth telling in the consent process, and non-medical prescribers should not shy away from exploring the law in order to gain a deeper insight into the complexities of their practice. There are leading cases such as *Chatterton v Gerson* 1981 in which it was established that:

> ... once the patient is informed in broad terms of the nature of the procedure which is intended, and gives consent, that consent is real.

However, as Jones et al (2005) highlight, some practitioners may deduct from the above ruling that a limited amount of information is sufficient in interpreting 'broad terms', yet others may decide that significantly more information is required in order to guarantee that consent is truly valid. Perhaps we need to use our own informed clinical judgement to interpret the true meaning of 'broad terms' and apply our judgements accordingly in individual circumstances. In *Sidaway v Bethlem Royal Hospital Governors* 1985, a neurosurgeon failed to disclose a very remote complication of paraplegia (<1%) in the surgical procedure to which the claimant had consented. The patient's claim for damages was rejected and the court held that 'consent did not require an elaborate explanation of remote side effects'. This said, in prescribing, we are duty bound to offer the patient information about the potential side effects of the prescribed treatments. In both step 3 'consider the choice of product' and step 4 'negotiate a contract' of the NPC (1999) *Prescribing Pyramid*, disclosure and discussion of the side effects are an essential component. A patient's consideration of these side effects will often influence their decision to accept or refuse the suggested treatment. Using the judgment in *Sidaway*, it would seem that it is the practitioner's prerogative to determine to what depth the remote side effects of treatments are discussed with individual patients.

It could be argued that patients are protected by the law and the Human Rights Act 1998, and Article 5 of the European Convention on Human Rights and Biomedicine of 1997 ('the Convention') states that 'an intervention in the health field may only be carried out after the patient has given free and informed consent to it' (Garwood-Gowers et al 2001). Not only are we concerned with the ethical principles of upholding the prescriber/patient relationship here, but also the legal implications of the prescriber being liable for not adhering to the required guidelines for obtaining consent, should we fail to do so. Article 5 clearly addresses patient autonomy and recognises that consent can be withdrawn at any time without penalty. However, there are exceptions to this, in that, should consent be withdrawn during a procedure, and withdrawal of consent results in a situation that contravenes a practitioner's professional standards and obligations, then it does not have to be honoured (Garwood-Gowers et al 2001). An example of this may be when a prescriber has commenced life-saving treatment and withdrawal of consent would interfere with their obligation to preserve life. Ethically, we, as prescribers, would need to decide if this would be the right or wrong thing to do, and the ethical principle of deontology is discussed later in the chapter to offer clarity to the argument. This exception to the rule, however, appears to make a mockery of patient autonomy, in that patients are allowed to exercise self-determination only up to a certain point should a practitioner's professional obligations be considered more significant.

Article 6 of the Convention provides safeguards for the protection of those individuals who are unable to consent for themselves to medical interventions. It is stated that, if an individual does not have the capacity to consent to an intervention because of mental disability, disease or other similar reason, then authorisation can be legally obtained from a responsible person or body. However, the opinions of the patient should be taken into account as far as possible. In the case of a child, authorisation is given by the adult who is legally responsible for that child, yet the opinion of the child is increasingly being sought, depending on the age and degree of maturity of the individual. But are children able to make 'informed' decisions? And who is to say that the adult with responsibility for that child is actually acting as their advocate, or in their 'best interest', and not solely just for their own benefit, or to satisfy their own agenda?

Wager et al (1995) acknowledged that, although it is essential to gain patients' consent when entering into a professional relationship, it is not a simple task. This could possibly be explained by the apparent complexity of the issues involved, or even the reluctance of healthcare professionals to look deeper into the intricacies of the principles of consent. Jones (1999), in citing the *Sidaway* case, acknowledges that, despite the numerous cases involving informed consent, judges have remained conservative in their approach to setting standards for the health professions. As such, it would appear that they remain content to allow the continuation of substandard and potentially unlawful practice in some situations. However, common law dictates that the autonomy of the patient should be protected, by ensuring that health professionals satisfy certain standards of disclosure (Kuhse and Singer 2001). These standards of disclosure were developed within the realms of common law over the last two decades in order to guarantee that the healthcare professional had adequately informed the patient in cases where there was some doubt. The standards have been used solely for the purpose of redress within the law, yet there has been some legislative progress in recent years to provide guidance to practitioners regarding what to tell their patients before medical interventions (Appelbaum P, Lidz C and Meisel A 1987 – cited in Kuhse and Singer 2001). Young (R 2001 – cited in Kuhse and Singer 2001, p. 442) suggests there are certain 'elements of disclosure' for informed consent that include:

- the nature of the procedure (or treatment)
- the risks involved
- the alternatives
- the benefits of the proposed treatment.

It would be fair to say that these elements of disclosure should be applied as a *minimum* standard when gaining consent from our patients in a prescribing context. In a landmark case, that of *Chester v Afshar* 2005, the claimant was awarded damages when it was held, in a House of Lords decision by a three to two majority, that insufficient information had been given before surgery which resulted in the potential risks of the particular surgery being realised. The principles of the judgment in *Chester* can be applied effectively to prescribing practice in that it is essential for prescribers to adequately inform patients of the potential risks, interactions, contraindications and side effects of a chosen medication. Failure to provide adequate information would be deemed negligent and prescribers could find themselves in a court of law, defending their practice and decision-making.

Wager et al (1995) further suggest that, before giving consent, patients require information about their illness, the treatments available, the proposed management plan, the effect on their condition and the alternative choices available to them. This does not always happen in practice because anecdotal evidence suggests that the information given to patients is largely dependent on the particular prescriber. There are huge discrepancies in both the *amount* and the *quality* of information that patients receive, despite agreed protocols being in place. As prescribers, we need to consider whether we can ever precisely assess the level of understanding of an individual and whether this can be done with absolute accuracy in all cases. Appelbaum and Grisso (1988, cited in Wager et al (1995), Fitten (1993, cited in Wager et al 1995), Fulford and Howse (1993), Lavelle-Jones et al (1993), Kessel (1994) and the GMC (1998) all acknowledged a multitude of factors that may impact on a patient's level of understanding and suggest that healthcare professionals cannot assume that, because individuals appear to fully comprehend the information given to them, they fully understand the consequences. Furthermore, they advise that the ability of the patient to repeat or regurgitate the information told to them as a means of assessing understanding is not the same as truly appreciating its consequences, and the technique should be used cautiously. For the patients who appear to have a degree of understanding within the realms of their own abilities, but do not understand to the same level of our *own* mental capacity, can it then still be considered ethical to proceed with prescribing, even if they give their consent? Is this truly 'informed consent'? We could argue that it *is* informed consent, because consent has been given within the limitations of their own understanding. As prescribers, if we always endeavour to obtain consent within the sphere and extent of a patient's understanding, we could argue, and defend our judgement by saying that it is truly informed.

Silverman (1989) stated that healthcare practitioners are at liberty to ensure that the process of obtaining informed consent is rigorously adopted in order to enable patients to make autonomous choices and assert personal preferences for the treatment on offer. This supports the Kantian view of a patient's right to autonomy and the view that respecting a patient's autonomy acts as an expression of valuing that patient's ability to make a decision. By respecting patients' esteem as individuals, this allows them the dignity of being 'in charge' of their own lives and allows them to be 'masters' of their own well-being (Hendrick 2000). In prescribing practice, patient participation is high on the agenda. Concordance is more readily achieved if the patient has had the opportunity to participate in treatment decisions by exercising autonomy and giving consent freely. Furthermore, the accuracy of the information that the patient receives impacts greatly on the legality of consent giving, and, should the prescriber fail to provide the patient with correct and evidence-based information, it is suggested that consent could be deemed 'misinformed'.

Activity box 2.8

Look at the patient in case study 2.

What factors would you consider when gaining consent from this patient? How could you guarantee that the patient consented willingly?

As a prescriber what elements of the consenting process may lead you to consider that the patient is:

- 'uninformed'
- 'misinformed'
- 'informed'.

Consent in adults lacking capacity

As prescribers we interact with many different types of patients, who, as has already been discussed, may be temporarily incapacitated due, for example, to illness, shock or reduced consciousness, or under the influence of drugs or alcohol. More complex cases involve those patients we wrongly assume to lack capacity as in the case of *Ms B v An NHS Trust* 2002 who was ventilated but communicated her wishes to refuse treatment. The court held that the patient *did* have capacity and that the continued artificial ventilation of *Ms B* against her wishes amounted to unlawful trespass. As prescribers, in order to avoid similar situations, we need to be able to establish capacity and assess our patients according to the relevant guidelines. Chapter 4 of the Mental Capacity Act (2005) Code of Practice provides detailed guidance on the assessment of capacity and prescribers should familiarise themselves with the direction contained within it.

The Department of Health (2009b, p. 9) clearly states in its guidance that:

For consent to be valid, it must be given voluntarily by an appropriately informed person who has the capacity to consent to the intervention in question (this will be the patient or someone with parental responsibility for a patient under the age of 18, someone authorised to do so under a Lasting Power of Attorney (LPA) or someone who has the authority to make treatment decisions as a court appointed deputy). Acquiescence where the person does not know what the intervention entails is not 'consent'.

However, under the Mental Capacity Act 2005 (Section 1(2)), it is stated that a person must be assumed to have capacity unless it is established that he lacks capacity. Furthermore, the Mental Capacity Act 2005 defines a person who lacks capacity as:

... a person who is unable to make a decision for themselves because of an impairment or disturbance in the functioning of their mind or brain. It does not matter if the impairment or disturbance is permanent or temporary.

The Department of Health guidance (2009b, p. 9) and the Mental Capacity Act 2005 also advise that a:

... person lacks capacity if:

- they have an impairment or disturbance (for example a disability, condition or trauma or the effect of drugs or alcohol) that affects the way their mind or brain works, and
- that impairment or disturbance means that they are unable to make a specific decision at the time it needs to be made ...

The prescriber's responsibility lies with their skill and competence to assess whether or not the patient meets the criteria contained within the Mental Capacity Act and the Department of Health guidance. To further channel our assessment of patients in our care, we should consider the Department of Health (2009b, p. 9) guidance that:

An assessment of a person's capacity must be based on their ability to make a specific decision at the time it needs to be made, and not their ability to make decisions in general. A person is unable to make a decision if they cannot do one or more of the following things:

- understand the information given to them that is relevant to the decision
- retain that information long enough to be able to make the decision
- use or weigh up the information as part of the decision-making process
- communicate their decision – this could be by talking or using sign language and includes simple muscle movements such as blinking an eye or squeezing a hand.

Chapter 4 of the Mental Capacity Act 2005 explains what is meant by the terms 'capacity' and 'lack of capacity' (Dimond 2008) and lists the following as examples of an impairment to the functioning of the mind or brain:

- conditions associated with some forms of mental illness
- dementia
- significant learning disabilities
- the long-term effects of brain damage
- physical or medical conditions that cause confusion, drowsiness or loss of consciousness
- delirium
- concussion after head injury
- the symptoms of alcohol or drug use.

As can be seen from the examples in this list, some conditions may cause permanent impairment, yet others may cause a transient or temporary lack of capacity that warrants the prescriber to act in the person's best interest. Similarly, some patients may have the ability to decide what clothes to wear or what food to eat, but lack the ability to make more major decisions such as whether or not to accept or refuse treatment (Dimond 2009).

It could be argued. thus far, that the assessment of a person's capacity to consent or refuse treatment is time-consuming and complex. Do we, as prescribers. always allow sufficient time for such assessment? Is sufficient time always available to us? It is suggested here that often our assessment of capacity is based almost subconsciously on the presenting demeanour of the patient before us. Often, we as prescribers know our patients well and a prior judgement has been made regarding the patient's mental ability. However, in some situations, e.g. in a walk-in centre, an accident and emergency department or a pharmacy, the patient is quite likely to be unknown to us and this is where an assessment needs to be made. Frequently, as experienced practitioners, a formal evaluation of mental capacity is unnecessary, but, where there is doubt or uncertainty, the prescriber should use the available published directions. It should be remembered that, although we strive for equality and tolerance as healthcare practitioners, we must never assume that a person lacks capacity simply because of unsociably acceptable behaviour, a person's appearance, an inability to speak the same language, or indeed by the person's age or appearance. Moreover, as stated in Principle 3 of the Mental Capacity Act 2005:

> A person is not to be treated as unable to make a decision merely because he makes an unwise decision.

There will always be cases in our prescribing careers where we do not agree with a patient's decision. If the person is fully autonomous and has sound mental capacity, it is our duty to respect and support that decision while truthfully guiding and informing the patient of the consequences of his or her decisions. No other adult can consent on behalf of a fully competent adult with intact mental capacity.

Having looked at consent in adults with or without mental capacity, we turn our attention to the nuances and complexities of gaining consent in children and young people. All prescribers who work with such patients need to gain a comprehensive knowledge of the legalities of consent, parental rights, and the rights of healthcare practitioners, medics and courts in order to prescribe with appropriate insight and safety. It is suggested that prescribers working with children, as with adults, do not always place sufficient emphasis on the importance of safeguarding the interests and rights of children or indeed protecting them and their interests in clinical situations. To this end, this section directs the reader to certain texts, cases and guidelines that should be read as an adjunct to the chapter.

Consent in young people aged 16 or 17 years

The BMA (2001) advocated that more autonomy should be given to children and young people and that they should be granted more influence and be given the right to be heard in respect of their own decision-making. It was suggested that less credence should be bestowed on paternalism in favour of more participation and involvement, yet, although this appears to be the ideal, the concept can and should be applied only on an individual basis. Furthermore, in prescribing practice, there appears to be significant limitations to this model, particularly in view of the knowledge that children and young people mature emotionally, developmentally, psychologically and cognitively at dissimilar rates. Under the Family Law Reform Act 1969 Section 8(1), a young person aged 16 or 17 years has a statutory right to give consent to any surgical, medical or dental treatment. There is an assumption, however, that the young person has the capacity to do so and where a young person may have learning disabilities, for example, this right can be invalidated. There are circumstances where the consent of a 16- or 17-year-old young person can be overruled, e.g. if the decision that the young person makes is not in his or her 'best interests', parents can seek to make the child a ward of court, yet the courts would always endeavour to take account of the young person's opinion and wishes.

Consent in children aged under 16

The BMA (2009) acknowledge that, in law, there is no presumption of competence for young people aged under 16 and those under this age must demonstrate their competence by meeting certain standards set by the courts. In England, Wales and Northern Ireland, the central test is whether the young person has 'sufficient understanding and intelligence to understand fully what is proposed'. In Scotland, a young person is considered competent to make treatment decisions if he or she is 'capable of understanding the nature and possible consequences of the procedure or treatment' (BMA 2009).

The Family Law Reform Act 1969 states that a parent has a right to give consent to treatment and examination on behalf of a child or young person aged under 16 years. Furthermore, although the parent may have both the right and the duty to act in the child's best interests, the parent may be prosecuted for failure to do so, particularly if the child is harmed as a consequence. Despite this parental right, the law states that the parents' decisions can be overridden in certain circumstances in order to save the life of a child. It is argued that parents' rights to act in their child's best interests was entrenched in law 'long before autonomy and privacy were pervasively applied to incompetents and minors' (Beauchamp and Childress 2001) and it was assumed that parents would always act responsibly as advocates for their child. The law established that no intervention in these parental rights would arise, unless there were extreme circumstances whereby the state and the parents disagreed about a treatment or non-treatment that may have devastating consequences for the child. Under the Children Act 1989 the court has the power to override any lack of consent from parents with a paramount consideration being stated as the overall welfare of the child (Alderson and Goodey 1998).

The Children Act 1989 is the main source of law for the care of children and young people under the age of 18 years and they ultimately come under the inherent jurisdiction of the High Court (Dimond 2008). Although there is no statutory right for a child under the age of 16 to give consent to treatment, the Children Act focuses on the principle that the child's welfare is paramount and stipulates that, provided that the child possesses the necessary understanding to consent to medical examination or treatment, the court should take account of 'the ascertainable wishes and feelings of the child concerned, considered in light of their age and understanding'.

It is important therefore to establish that when making treatment decisions for the under 16s that the child's capacity to consent has been considered. As a consequence of the *Gillick v West Norfolk and Wisbech Area Health Authority* 1985, the House of Lord's ruling was that a child under 16 years of age *is* able to give valid consent to examination or treatment if he or she is deemed to possess the requisite mental capacity to make the specific decision. This is known as 'Gillick competent', yet, in recent years, the term has been replaced (at the request of Mrs Gillick) by the term 'a child competent according to Lord Fraser guidelines'. In clinical practice, the term 'Fraser competent' is widely used, particularly in the provision of contraceptive services to the under 16s without parental consent. The criteria for a child to be deemed Fraser competent are the following:

- The girl would, although under 16, understand the doctor's advice.
- The doctor could not persuade her to inform her parents or allow them to inform the parents that she was seeking contraceptive advice.
- She was very likely to have sexual intercourse with or without contraceptive treatment.
- Unless she received contraceptive advice or treatment her physical and/or mental health were likely to suffer.
- Her best interests required the doctor to give her contraceptive advice, treatment or both, without parental consent.

In a non-medical prescribing context, the use of Fraser guidelines are particularly useful in determining 'what strategy' to adopt when using the NPC (1999) prescribing pyramid as a model. Although the criteria refer to 'the doctor' throughout, the terms 'pharmacist', 'nurse' or 'allied health professional' can be transcribed to take account of the non-medical prescribers' role in treating the under 16s. It should be remembered, however, that even if a child argues that he or she is 'Fraser competent' the courts would still insist on administering life-saving treatment if necessary. Even though a child may be considered 'Fraser competent', e.g. in *Re E* 1993, this allows only for children to opt *in* to treatment and not *out* of treatment. This case involved a 15-year-old boy whose refusal to give consent to a blood transfusion on religious grounds was overruled by the courts in that the judge gave the hospital the authority to administer treatment against both the boy's and the parents' wishes as Jehovah's Witnesses. It was held that, despite the boy's apparent intelligence and ability to make decisions, the courts felt that he lacked the capacity to understand what the transfusion would involve. The decision was therefore made on the grounds that the welfare of the child was the paramount decision. Moreover, under Section 8 (3) of the Family Law Reform Act 1969 the statutory powers that exist to allow a child aged 16 or 17 years to give valid consent do not eliminate the ability of those under 16, with adequate maturity, to give legally valid consent to treatment (Wilson 2005).

It is clear from the extensive literature and the arguments presented that truly informed consent, autonomy and mental capacity are difficult to quantify, not only in the child and incapacitated person, but in *all* individuals. It is evident from our examination of the complexities of the issues at stake that we, as prescribers, need to adopt reliable procedures to gain consent, protect autonomy and assess capacity when undertaking prescribing decisions and clinical interventions. Obtaining a comprehensive understanding of the statutory definitions and the guidelines available to us is of utmost importance.

 Activity box 2.9

To assess your learning, look at each of the case studies at the back of the book in turn, and consider what factors you would need to take into account in order to guarantee that you obtained legal consent from the patients presented.

Lasting power of attorney

HM Government (2010) identify a lasting power of attorney (LPA) as a legal document that appoints a deputy to act on a person's behalf should he or she lose capacity. The BMA (2009) highlight in their guidance that under the Mental Capacity Act in England and Wales, those aged over 18 years can make an LPA by appointing a 'welfare attorney' to make health and personal welfare decisions on their behalf if capacity is lost. They state that the Court of Protection may also appoint a deputy to make these decisions, yet neither welfare attorneys nor deputies are at liberty to demand treatment that is clinically unsuitable. The Mental Capacity Act also requires doctors to consider, as far as is reasonable and practicable, the views of the patient's primary carer. Similarly, in Scotland, the Adults with Incapacity (Scotland) Act 2000 allows people aged over 16 years to appoint a welfare attorney who has the power to give consent to medical treatment when the patient loses capacity. The Court of Session can also appoint a 'welfare guardian' on behalf of an incapacitated adult. Northern Ireland law differs somewhat, in that no person can give consent to medical treatment on behalf of another adult. Interestingly, the views of primary carers or nearest relatives have no legal status in terms of actual decision-making. Therefore, as the law currently stands, doctors may treat an incapacitated person without consent, provided that the treatment is necessary and in the patient's best interests. However, it is identified in law to be good practice for healthcare practitioners to attempt to consult with relatives in order to reach a 'best interest' decision. It is clear that, in prescribing, it is necessary to abide by the laws of the country in which you practise and be aware of the dissimilarities that exist between the countries of the UK.

Advance directives

Advance directives or 'living wills' are written decisions made in advance of the autonomous person becoming non-autonomous. They exist to express the wishes of the individual in the event of serious decisions having to be made about treatment or end-of-life choices in the event of them losing the ability to be autonomous. Although, in law, the content of advance directives is not legally binding, but is considered by medics and lawyers, the BMA and Law Society (2004) discourage patients from making such directives. There are some legitimate arguments against the use of advance directives such as the claim put forward by Robertson (1991, cited in Herring 2008, p. 182), in which it is suggested that:

> The values and interests of the competent person no longer are relevant to someone who has lost the rational structure on which those values and interests rested.

Here it is implied that people with dementia who prepared advance directives could not have predicted how they may feel once their situation changes. Some theorists have gone so far as to suggest that a person with Alzheimer's disease, for example, who prepared an advance directive with his or her critical interests at stake, no longer has the capacity to understand and his or her critical interests should not 'be given any weight' (Dresser 2003). Controversial as it seems, prescribers may potentially be presented with an advance directive dilemma. It is suggested that legal guidance be sought in order to proceed with or without treatment.

Prescribers as advocates

When patients have not yet developed, cannot develop or lose their ability to make treatment decisions for themselves, advocates can be called upon to make substituted judgements on their behalf (Vig et al 2006).

Advocacy can be described as:

> The process of identifying with and representing a person's views and concerns, in order to secure enhanced rights and entitlements, undertaken by someone who has little or no conflict of interest.

> Henderson and Pochin (2001)

In examining this definition of advocacy, it is suggested that as prescribers, we are in a unique position to represent patients in respect of 'securing enhanced rights and entitlements'. All patients are entitled to receive fair, equitable and timely treatment for conditions affecting them and our ability to prescribe goes some way to ensure that this fundamental right is attainable. In children, advocacy is usually entrusted to an adult with parental rights and, in most cases, this allegiance proceeds without conflict. In adults, however, although it has been suggested that the optimal standard for advocacy-based decisions is those decisions made by family members, 'best interest' decisions can, and are, made effectively by others including medical practitioners, nurses and the courts. In clinical practice, there are countless situations where the non-medical prescriber will be called upon to make treatment and management choices for their patients and a significant component of working in a prescribing role is to develop the competence and confidence to recognise when advocacy is required, and perform that task responsibly. Advocacy-based decisions are usually made in prescribing practice by means of consultation between families and clinicians, yet the courts will intervene if any disagreements arise.

It should be recognised that, although family members are seen as the ideal advocates, there are significant limitations in this assumption, in that family surrogates are not always ideal representatives for patient preferences (Kirschner KL 2005, cited in Vig et al 2006). Empirical studies in relation to end-of-life care, for example, have shown that the ability of family members to accurately predict patients' treatment choices is markedly flawed, not least because the decisions made are a more precise representation of their own preferences rather than the patients' (Hardwig 1993). However, Hardwig (1993) further identified that many patients still want family members to make decisions on their behalf, even though they realise that the responsibility for decision-making may be a burden and any resulting outcomes will have to be lived with thereafter.

Vig et al (2006) identified a number of ways that family surrogates plan for and make decisions on another's behalf. They highlighted that two-thirds made judgements based on conversations around future care preferences that they had had with their loved ones, yet decisions were often made without the benefit of substantial discussion. This research indicates that the family surrogates do not intentionally disregard the wishes of their family members, and moreover find it difficult to isolate their own perspectives when making decisions for others. Interestingly, some family advocates have relied heavily on previously written advance directives, without much regard for the content, until such time as they are required. As a result, the content has not been explicit and the surrogate has been unprepared for the decisions to be made. A further dilemma can arise where the decision-making process is further complicated by family members' disagreement and this may create a predicament for the prescriber.

Activity box 2.10

Read the following scenario and consider the following:

As a prescriber acting as the patient's advocate, what factors do you need to consider in order to ensure that you are acting legally?

Mr Jones is terminally ill with cancer of the lung and brain metastases. He is widowed and his daughter lives in Australia. However, she intends to travel home in the next few days. Mr Jones is being nursed at home with the help of the district nurses, his son and a very capable family friend. Mr Jones lacks capacity and has increasing pain in his back. You have been asked to review his pain relief but his son and daughter disagree about how Mr Jones should be managed.

Consent is a continuous process and should be sought with each consultation. In supplementary prescribing, for example, it is necessary to confirm that the patient is still in agreement with the devised clinical management plan and that there have been no changes in consent or that any new clinical developments have occurred (BMA 2009).

Confidentiality, sharing information and data protection

For a more comprehensive understanding, this section should be read together with the Department of Health publication *Confidentiality: NHS code of practice* (DH 2003c). In this document it is stated that:

A duty of confidence arises when one person discloses information to another (e.g. patient to clinician) in circumstances where it is reasonable to expect that the information will be held in confidence. It:

(a) is a legal obligation that is derived from case law
(b) is a requirement established within professional codes of conduct
(c) must be included within NHS employment contracts as a specific requirement linked to disciplinary procedures.

As healthcare practitioners we are accustomed to maintaining patient confidentiality. It is a fundamental aspect of healthcare, the principles of which are no less important in prescribing practice. Confidentiality of patient information is of utmost importance for trust to be achieved. The Department of Health (2003c) further identify that 'the patient information we obtain in practice is generally held under legal and ethical obligations of confidentiality and any information provided in confidence should not be used or disclosed in a form that might identify a patient without his or her consent'. Disclosure of confidential information may, in certain circumstances however, be beneficial to patients, e.g. it is often necessary for a prescriber to inform other healthcare professionals, such as the patient's GP, of the treatments prescribed, stopped or dose amended, in order to avoid inadvertent duplication of medicines or the subsequent prescribing of drugs that may interact. Patients should be informed that disclosure of information is necessary for their care to remain safe and anecdotally most patients are satisfied with this requirement. Certain prescribing situations may be more difficult to manage in respect of confidentiality and prescribers working within these areas should ensure that local confidentiality guidelines are adhered to. It is an expectation in prescribing situations that patients divulge personal and often sensitive information in order to be treated effectively. The Department of Health (2003c) recognises that patients entrust and allow NHS personnel to gather information relating to their health and personal matters as part of seeking treatment, yet they hold a legitimate expectation that staff will respect this trust. Furthermore, even if a patient is unconscious or incapacitated for any other reason, this does not diminish the duty of confidence that we have as professionals. It is essential, if the legal requirements are to be met and the trust of patients is to be retained, that the NHS provides, and is seen to provide, a confidential service (DH 2003c).

Following the Caldicott Report 1997, the Department of Health appointed Caldicott guardians to protect patient information (DH 1998). These are senior staff within health and social care who have responsibility for ensuring that patient information and records remain confidential. The Department of Health has produced a manual detailing the methods and responsibilities of Caldicott guardians (DH 2010) in their remit of protecting the sharing of patient-identifiable information between NHS organisations and non-NHS bodies. Prescribers should have an awareness of strategic information protection alongside relevant legislation that is necessary to attain comprehensive knowledge of the principles of confidentiality (Table 2.8).

Activity box 2.11

How would you manage confidential information in the following situations? When would it be legally and ethically acceptable to share information?

A 15-year-old girl requests 'emergency contraception' over the counter after unprotected intercourse the previous evening. During the consultation it transpires that she was sexually assaulted a month ago and contracted gonorrhoea.

Jean is 49 and has just been diagnosed with a genetically inherited degenerative condition. You are her physiotherapist and are discussing the rapid progression of the disease. She does not want her estranged children to be told of her diagnosis, but this would mean that they would not have the opportunity to be screened.

A 59-year-old man with diabetes receives treatment from you for erectile dysfunction and a titration of his metformin was also necessary to improve his glycaemic control. He is adamant that he does not want his GP to be informed because he is a family friend.

You have been asked to treat a 24-year-old man for a laceration that he sustained to his hand 20 minutes ago. It becomes apparent that a member of staff has had her purse stolen from the office where the window was smashed.

The daughter of one of your deceased patients has requested a copy of her mother's hospital records.

Gary is 21 and taking methadone prescribed by his GP for a heroin addiction. He attends the pharmacy on a daily basis where the dose is given and ingested at the counter in full view of the general public.

Consider what is the relevance of the Freedom of Information Act 2000 to prescribing practice?

Reducing harm, risk assessment and avoiding litigation

As a prescriber, failure to provide sufficient relevant information to patients, prescribing without due consideration being given to guidelines and evidence bases and failing to obtain valid consent could all be challenged in law. It is suggested in Figure 2.3 that, by

Table 2.8 Current legislation related to the confidentiality and accessibility of patient information

Data Protection Act 1998	The Data Protection Act governs the processing of personal data about all living people in the UK. It sets out principles for information handling with which all data controllers must comply. Its remit includes access to health records of living people, and patients' rights to have inaccurate information corrected
Access to Health Records Act 1990	This Act has mostly been superseded by the Data Protection Act 1998, and now governs only access to the health records of deceased people
Access to Medical Reports Act 1988	This Act governs access to medical reports produced about patients by a clinician
Human Rights Act 1998	Article 8 establishes a right to 'respect for private and family life'. This underpins the duty to protect the privacy of individuals and preserve the confidentiality of their health records. Current understanding is that compliance with the Data Protection Act 1998 and the common law of confidentiality should satisfy Human Rights requirements
Freedom of Information Act 2000	The Act creates a general right of access, on request, to information held by public authorities and creates exemptions from the duty to disclose information. The Act also establishes the arrangements for enforcement and appeal

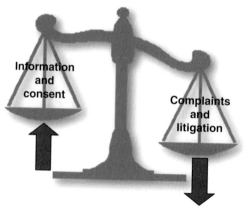

Figure 2.3 Reducing the risk of litigation.

increasing the information we impart to our patients and obtaining consent, we may reduce the probability of potential complaints and litigious proceedings being brought against us.

It is therefore suggested that, in order for the prescriber to minimise harm to their patients and avoid litigious proceedings, careful risk assessment should become a fundamental component of expert practice. Information giving and gaining consent, regular auditing of prescribing practice and accurate, detailed documentation and record keeping are all factors that should be incorporated as standard practice in prescribing. Effective risk assessment also includes personal professional development, evidence-based practice and ensuring that the patient is aware of your prescribing status. It is suggested that, if patients are not aware of the limitations of your prescribing position and harm results, they are more likely to complain than had they known and agreed to be treated by you.

The Medical Defence Union (MDU 2007) identify that drug prescription errors, dispensing errors and the incorrect administration of medication are common causes of adverse incidents and death of patients. They suggest a checklist for reducing risk for anyone involved in prescribing, dispensing or administering medication. It is with this knowledge that we propose that prescribers should be aware that common errors are easily avoided and due care and attention throughout the prescribing process will reduce the incidence. Furthermore, experiential testimony suggests that a degree of complacency can often accompany the increasing expertise of the practitioner. Common errors include wrong drug, dose, strength, quantity, duration and frequency, all of which are avoidable with careful prescribing and vigilance. Further errors include prescribing for the wrong patient, incorrect administration, failing to consider drug interactions or contraindications, and replicating mistakes on repeat prescriptions. The MDU (2007) advise that the following checklist be used for risk management:

- Patients must be told about the nature, purpose and risks of any treatment and any alternatives, and be provided with information about side effects.
- Check for known allergies or hypersensitivities, particularly when prescribing antibiotics, and ensure that these are documented consistently, on paper and computerised records.
- Have robust systems in place to review and monitor repeat medication regularly.
- It is advisable to check the correct identity of patients during each consultation and, if possible, before issuing repeat prescriptions.
- If prescribing unfamiliar drugs, check contraindications and side effects.
- When administering vaccines to young children, appropriate authority from someone with parental responsibility should be obtained and documented.
- Ensure that there are appropriate and up-to-date patient group directions or protocols in place, e.g. for child immunisations.
- All drugs should be checked before administration.
- Consider storing drugs with similar names (e.g. Depo-Provera and Depo-Medrone) or of different doses (e.g. 30 mg and 10 mg ampoules of diamorphine) separately.
- Ensure that there is a system to rotate stocks and dispose of date-expired items.
- Have an adverse incident reporting system in place so that the practice can learn from any mistakes or near misses that do occur.
- Ensure robust record keeping.

As non-medical prescribers, we have gained an insight into the professional and legal aspects of prescribing practice. The final part of this chapter looks at some of the ethical and moral concepts that may impact on your clinical decision-making and subsequent prescribing practice.

PART 3: ETHICAL ISSUES

The study of ethics is essential to healthcare practice, yet the term is not always easy to define. In addition there are numerous associated terms including morals, rights, duties and obligations that may be confusing to the reader. However, it is suggested that, although some healthcare professionals withdraw from the study of ethics, the subject is captivating once the theories become apparent and are practically applied by the practitioner. The purpose of this section is therefore to highlight some of the more established principles of healthcare ethics and relate theory to practice for the prescriber.

The BMA (2004) offers a definition of medical ethics as:

The application of ethical reasoning to medical decision-making.

Herring (2008) highlights that this definition is vague and suggests that the question remains unanswered as to *what* medical ethics is about. Edwards and Elwyn (2009), however, offer a more straightforward meaning and suggests that 'morals' and 'ethics' be classed as synonyms in the first instance and then divide the term into three components:

1 Personal ethics
2 Group ethics
3 Philosophical ethics

Personal ethics is perhaps what we all, as individuals, think of initially when asked about morals. It is concerned with the moral values that we have developed from sources such as parents, school, media and religious leaders. It encompasses our opinions on ethical issues and our understanding of what is right and what is wrong. From a prescribing perspective, we know that it is morally right to prescribe pain relief to the patient with a fractured femur, just as we also know that it is morally wrong to withhold pain relief if it is within our power to prescribe and administer it. Edwards and Elwyn (2009) suggest that all people who are able to express a view can articulate an opinion based on personal ethics. Group ethics is different in that it relates to groups of people with a similar set of standards as the term suggests. Looking back at the first part of this chapter, it is clearly evident that groups of healthcare professionals such as nurses, pharmacists and allied health professionals hold similar professional standards to each other and these are regarded as codes of 'professional ethics'. Further to Edwards and Elwyn's (2009) classification, the last sense of the term pertains to philosophical ethics. This component of ethics is concerned with a more academic approach to moral theory, language and analysis, knowledge of which is necessary to solve ethical dilemmas.

As prescribers, ethical dilemmas may occur on a daily basis and it is suggested that we draw upon a combination of personal, group and philosophical ethics to assist us in our decision-making, e.g. if a patient refuses to take the life-saving medication that you have prescribed, you may be guided by your own personal beliefs and values (such as your belief in the sanctity of life), your professional code of conduct and your knowledge and analysis of ethical theory (such as consequentialism or deontology).

Consequentialism

This ethical theory is based on making decisions from a 'common-sense' perspective by looking at the consequences of the action (Edwards 2009). Consequentialists believe that, when faced with two courses of action, the morally right action to take is the one that has the more favourable consequence. Consequentialism can be viewed as 'goal based' in that the rightness or wrongness of actions depends on their consequences and this means that the 'right' or 'moral' thing to do is the one that produces the best possible outcome and the greatest pleasure. The best-known form of consequentialism is utilitarianism (Edwards 2009). Utilitarians, perhaps the most famous being John Stuart Mill (1806-73), advocate that the most important outcome when choosing two opposing pathways is that which results in people being happy. They would also champion the philosophy of 'the greatest good for the greatest number'. In other words, to kill one person to save 100 others can be justified by utilitarians because the greater number of people experienced pleasure as a result. Furthermore, a utilitarian would consider that the action of telling the truth to a patient would be very dependent on the consequence of that truth.

Deontology

Kuhse and Singer (2001) identified that deontology originates from the Latin *'deon'* meaning 'duty'. The deontologist believes that there are fundamental rules that should be followed *whatever* the consequences and that duty and obligation are central, rather than what the effect will be. In contrast to utilitarians, it is a fundamental rule that deontologists tell the truth because it is the right thing to do and not because it will result in happiness. Immanuel Kant is thought to be the leading exponent of deontology.

Virtue ethics

Healthcare practice, including prescribing, involves certain 'virtues' such as kindness, honesty, care, benevolence, compassion, courage, temperance and loyalty as described by Edwards (2009). It is these virtues that enable us as practitioners to perform with compassion and understanding in all interactions with patients, and it is suggested here that it would be difficult to prescribe safely and effectively if a prescriber did not possess experience and virtuous characteristics.

The most influential approach to ethics is known as 'principlism'. Beauchamp and Childress (2001) are perhaps regarded as the most eminent authors on principlism and they argue that there are four equal principles that represent a common morality. These are:

1 Autonomy (respect for)
2 Beneficence
3 Non-maleficence
4 Justice.

Respect for autonomy

As discussed in Part 2, respect for autonomy means recognising and respecting people who are entitled to such basic human rights as the right to know, the right to privacy and the right to receive care and treatment. Autonomy refers to a person's ability to come to his or her own decisions and to respect those incapable of autonomy because of illness, injury, mental illness or age. This principle is often regarded as the premier principle in medical ethics due to its overarching association with consent. However, some would argue that there are some legitimate flaws in this principle. Although it is commonly agreed that respect for patient autonomy is fundamentally right and that patient choice is of the essence, sometimes 'choices' cannot be honoured, yet this does not mean that autonomy is not being respected, e.g. as prescribers, we welcome and encourage patient participation in treatment choices. However, if, by respecting a patient's autonomy it becomes evident that their autonomous choice is unacceptable (such as demanding inappropriate treatment), it is well within the realms of the practitioner's judgement to not honour that choice.

Beneficence

This principle is concerned with the duty to 'do good' and maximise good, e.g. becoming the patient's advocate. It refers to the obligation to act in a way that promotes the well-being of others – in other words, act beneficently or with beneficence. From a prescriber's perspective, our aim is always to act in a way that will optimise good for our patients, yet in doing so we may also cause them harm. A good example of this is the administration of chemotherapy. Our aim or obligation with this treatment is to do good for the patient with regard to their recovery and prognosis, yet in doing so we actually harm the patient by exposing them to immunosuppression with the associated risks. However, we act with beneficence as our intentions are honourable.

Non-maleficence

Non-maleficence is closely related to beneficence as seen in the example above. Beauchamp and Childress (2001) assert that the principle refers to the obligation to 'do no harm' or to 'minimise harm'. In the chemotherapy scenario, we can minimise harm in a number of ways, such as prescribing antiemetics to counteract the side effect of nausea and vomiting or by ensuring that the dose of chemotherapy is carefully calculated in order to reduce toxicity.

Justice

The principle of justice is a complex principle closely associated with the law. Justice requires equal treatment of equal cases and equitable distribution of benefits. In other words, there should be no discrimination on the basis of sex, race, religion or age, for example, nor should there be any inequity in the distribution of resources. In healthcare, patients should, when applying this principle, be treated fairly and equally by practitioners, using a comparable degree of means, funds and assets. Another facet of the principle of justice concerns the 'just' manner in which we are held to account for our misconduct. From a prescribing perspective, should we be seen to intentionally harm our patients, or indeed act outside of our competence, justice will be served within the parameters of UK law.

Campbell et al (2005) suggest that 'professional integrity' be added as another principle here, whereas Edwards (2009) suggests a fifth principle of 'respect for persons'. These will be explained briefly as an adjunct to this section.

Professional integrity

It is suggested that healthcare is 'a growing body of expertise and shared skills' (Campbell et al 2005, p. 13). The expansion of expert practice is dependent on respect for different disciplines but also good collaborative relationships between professions in order that high standards are maintained and competences are shared. What this means for the prescriber is that both expert and novice prescribers are obligated to cooperate with each other for the benefit of the patient and the progression of the skill.

Respect for persons

Edwards (2009, p. 28) reminds us that 'all human beings are persons' and that, when considering the first principle of respect for autonomy identified by Beauchamp and Childress (2001), we are obliged to consider that we cannot respect the autonomy of a non-autonomous person. Personhood has been discussed at great length over the years and Harris (1985) controversially suggested that non-autonomous human beings such as babies, those with dementia and people in persistent vegetative states (PVS), for example, are human beings but not persons. Whatever the view of the prescriber, it reminds us to act as that individual's advocate and in their best interests.

Best interests

The 'best interest' principle has been referred to throughout this chapter, yet we need to ascertain what actually constitutes 'best interests'. The 'best interests standard' is widely used in healthcare where patient autonomy is absent. The risks and benefits are weighed against each other in order to conclude a definitive way forward for that individual. Judgements are often based on a 'quality-of-life' criterion in that decision-makers take account of formerly autonomous patients' preferences and values. In other words, previously drawn-up express wishes of the patient are respected and the opinions of others are sought. Advance directives, legal advocates and LPA orders are all considered in best interest and 'quality-of-life' determination. Prescribers who find themselves in the position of having to make such decisions on behalf of their patients should be aware that, according to the Mental Capacity Act Code of Practice (2005), the Act does not actually define the term 'best interests', but instead provides a checklist of factors that must always be taken into account in a situation where a decision is being made for a person lacking capacity. These factors have been broadly summarised as follows:

- Equal consideration and non-discrimination
- Consider all relevant circumstances
- Consider if the person may regain capacity
- Permit and encourage the person's involvement
- Special considerations for life-sustaining treatment
- The views of other people (where practicable and appropriate)
- The person's wishes and feelings, beliefs and values, particularly where these are written down.

It is important to remember that this checklist does not define best interests as such, is not exhaustive and should be used as a guide only.

As prescribers, in addition to treating acute conditions in the normally well patient, we may be called upon to care for patients who are vulnerable, such as very old or very young people, those living with long-term conditions, terminally ill individuals and those in the last stages of life. Although some practitioners may never prescribe for such patients, it is important to highlight certain ethical concepts that are relevant to all prescribing situations. Those concepts include acting beneficently, within the law, in the person's best interests and with compassion. One of the interesting concepts that we should consider as prescribers is the doctrine of double effect and this is discussed here in the context of end-of-life care as an example.

Doctrine of double effect

Spiritual opinion aside, death is generally viewed as a normal and natural progression to the end of life, yet we are aware that death can be premature, hastened or forced through illness, accident, personal choice or unlawful acts. Within the healthcare professions, death that is anything *other* than an inherent physiological process can be subject to validation, certification and scrutiny for the protection of the public and the professional alike (Royal College of General Practitioners 2003) (covered in the Coroners Act 1988). In healthcare, the death of a patient, even when expected or inevitable, is rarely unremarkable and, rightly or wrongly, a combination of professional, moral, ethical and legal rules applies. It is the application of these rules that sometimes generates indistinct and confusing arguments, often resulting in conflict among medics, ethicists and lawyers. Combining law and ethics can be contradictory and confusing, because legal rules and philosophy do not always sit comfortably together. So what does this mean for the prescriber? Put simply, this means that, as prescribers, our choice to prescribe, what we prescribe, our mode of delivery and our prescribing intentions are all open to scrutiny, e.g. some may view our action to prescribe opiates for our patients as nothing more than a means of shortening or abruptly ending that person's life. Furthermore, this could be applied to everything that we prescribe for our patients: Are we acting beneficently or with maleficence? Can we always justify our decisions? Are we acting with criminal intentions?

Emotive terms such as 'killing someone' or 'allowing someone to die' are fraught with ambiguity and also attract moral, ethical and legal questions that warrant clarification and explicit examination in the prescribing context. It is essential to the discussion that individual determinants and variables such as religious beliefs, moral values, ethical stance, professional obligation and personal position are recognised as being integral to the interpretation of such contentious terms as these. However, in the UK, 'the law is the law' – it exists to guide us, and its foundations are enshrined in ancient Christian tradition, despite our contemporary multi-religious society. Should a prescriber be called to account in a court of law, it is with these Christian principles that the law decides whether their actions were lawful, illegal or otherwise. The doctrine of double effect (DDE), which is also referred to as the principle of double effect (PDE), the rule of double effect (RDE) or 'the doctrine', has its historical roots in mediaeval Catholic moral theology, first developed and articulated by Saint Thomas Aquinas (1225-1274) and later adapted for use in secular discussions in moral philosophy and applied ethics (Rovie 2006). Today, the application of the DDE in modern medicine is distinctly evident. In simple terms, the DDE states that (Kennedy and Grubb 2000, Beauchamp and Childress 2001, Montgomery 2003, Mason and Laurie 2006, Bass 2006):

> ... if by doing something morally good (such as giving high doses of opiates to relieve pain) has a morally bad side effect (the person's death is hastened), it is ethically acceptable to do so, providing the bad side effect (death) was not the primary intention, even if the practitioner foresaw that the bad effect would probably happen ...

However, it is sometimes impossible to act beneficently to patients without also causing them some harm, because almost all treatments have side effects. It may also be necessary to do something to a patient that would be harmful and wrong outside of a medical context, such as injecting large doses of opiates, yet it is allowed in healthcare because it will ultimately benefit the patient, despite causing harmful effects. To this end, in prescribing practice, the DDE is accepted and applied by many practitioners when undertaking medical decision-making. However, the use of the doctrine may be called into question in English law. Its legitimacy may be called upon to support or oppose a practitioner's defence, particularly where discrepancies in the intentions of that healthcare practitioner are questioned, or where justification and endorsement of an action or omission is required.

Examples of such situations have included caring for patients in the terminal phase of life in *Airedale NHS Trust v Bland* 1993. Williams (1957), in his text on the subject of the sanctity of life, criticised the DDE and argued that the basis for this statement of the law should be challenged and condemned. However, in modern healthcare practice, despite reasonable criticism from some ethicists, the DDE is still considered to be an established rule of law that is frequently applied in the courts (*Airedale NHS Trust v Bland* 1993; *R v Moor* 2000; *R v Cox* 1957). However, Williams' argument is feasible in the context of prescribing in that, as nurses, pharmacists and AHPs, it is well within our remit to kill the pain without killing the patient. As prescribers, it is paramount, therefore, that we always endeavour to prescribe treatments that are morally, ethically and legally permissible, in order to safeguard our patients, with the primary objective of acting with the best of intentions.

Conclusion

The aim of this chapter was to enlighten the prescriber of the significant importance of professional, legal and ethical concepts that are essential to prescribing practice. Some of the theoretical material incorporated within the chapter may be new to the reader, yet, I would suggest, of fundamental importance in the cognitive development of pre-scribers. The first part of the chapter has allowed prescribers to consider the relevance of working within their respective codes of conduct and reflect on professional respon-sibility and accountability. Secondly, prescribers have been given the opportunity to identify with and amalgamate legal theory and practice in order to enlighten them to the safety mechanisms and potential pitfalls of being a prescriber. It is anticipated that the prescriber armed with legal knowledge will progress into a cautious yet prophetic practitioner with advanced proficiency and skill. The final part of this chapter looked at providing the prescriber with moral and ethical theory that is pertinent to their practice. It is anticipated that the reader will use critical reflection as a means to analyse medical ethics in the context of prescribing and ultimately apply the theories to the care of their patients.

Key themes: conclusions and considerations

Public health	The legal, professional and ethical implications of non-medical prescribing must be acknowledged and understood by the non-medical prescriber
	Consider how legal, professional and ethical issues might affect your ability, or willingness, to incorporate public health targets in to your consultations
Social and cultural issues	Ethical and moral codes originate, in part, from social and cultural norms and expectations
	Consider the possible cultural and social issues that might impact on the patient's autonomy
Prescribing principles	Numerous legal, professional and ethical issues impact on every stage of the prescribing pyramid. This can range from gaining patient consent to assessment through to accurate prescription writing
	Consider the legal, professional and ethical issues relevant to negotiating a contract with your patients

Table of cases

Airedale NHS Trust v Bland [1993] AC 789, HL
Bolam v Friern Hospital Management Committee [1957] 2 All ER 118
Chatterton v Gerson [1981] 1 All ER 257
Chester v Afshar [2005] 1 AC 134

Donoghue v Stevensen [1932] AC 562
Gillick v West Norfolk and Wisbech Area Health Authority [1985] 3 All ER 402
Lister and ors v Hesley Hall Ltd [2001] ICR 665, *House of Lords* [2001] UKHL 22
Ms B v An NHS Trust [2002] 2 All ER 449
Re E (A minor: wardship: medical treatment) [1993] 1 FLR 386 FD.
R v Cox [1957] Crim LR 365
R v Moor [2000] cited in Smith (2000)
Sidaway v Bethlem Royal Hospital Governors [1985] 1 All ER 643

References

Alderson P, Goodey C (1998) Theories of consent. *BMJ* **317**: 1313-15.

Avery AJ, Pringle J (2005) Extended prescribing by UK nurses and pharmacists (Editorial). *BMJ* **331**: 1154-5.

Bass M (2006) *Palliative Care Resuscitation*. Chichester: John Wiley & Sons.

Beauchamp TL, Childress JF (2001) *Principles of Biomedical Ethics*, 5th edn. Oxford: Oxford University Press.

British Employment Law (Emplaw) (2010) *Vicarious Liability* (online). Available at: www.emplaw.co.uk (accessed 26 April 2010).

British Medical Association (2001) *Consent, Rights and Choices in Healthcare for Children and Young People*. London: BMJ Books.

British Medical Association (2004) *Medical Ethics Today*. London: BMJ Books.

British Medical Association (2005) BMA Calls for urgent meeting with Patricia Hewitt on plans to extend prescribing powers. Press release, 10 November 2005. London: BMA.

British Medical Association (2009) *Consent Toolkit*, 5th edn. London: BMA.

British Medical Association and Law Society (2004) *Assessment of Mental Capacity*. London: BMJ Books.

British Medical Association and Royal Pharmaceutical Society of Great Britain (2010). *British National Formulary* (latest version). Available at: http://bnf.org/bnf.

Campbell A, Gillett G, Jones G (2005) *Medical Ethics*. Oxford: Oxford University Press.

Care Quality Commission (2010) 'Management of Controlled Drugs in Care Homes' (online). Available at www.cqc.org.uk (accessed 21 May 2010).

Department of Health (1998) *Implementing the Caldicott Report: Consultation document*, London: DH.

Department of Health (1999) *HSC 1999/198 The Public Disclosure Act 1998 Whistleblowing in the NHS*. London: DH.

Department of Health (2003a) *Whistleblowing in the NHS Policy Pack*. London: The Stationery Office.

Department of Health (2003b) *Making Amends: A consultation paper setting out proposals for reforming the approach to clinical negligence in the NHS. A Report by the Chief Medical Officer*. London: DH.

Department of Health (2003c) *Confidentiality: NHS code of practice*. London: DH.

Department of Health (2005a) *NHS Redress Bill* (online). Available at www.dh.gov.uk/actsandbills (accessed 17 April 2010).

Department of Health (2005b) *NHS Redress: Statement of policy*, London: DH.

Department of Health (2007) *Safer Management of Controlled Drugs: A guide to good practice in secondary care (England)*, London: The Stationery Office.

Department of Health (2009a) *High Quality Care for All: Our journey so far*. London: The Stationery Office.

Department of Health (2009b) *Reference Guide to Consent for Examination or Treatment*. 2nd edn. London: The Stationery Office.

Department of Health (2010) *The Caldicott Guardian Manual*. London: DH.

Dimond B (2008) *Legal Aspects of Mental Capacity*. Oxford: Blackwell Publishing.

Dimond B (2009) *Legal Aspects of Consent*. 2nd edn. London: Quay Books.

Doormaal JE van, van den Bemt PMLA, Mol PGM et al (2009) Medication errors: the impact of prescribing and transcribing errors on preventable harm in hospitalised patients. *Quality Safety Healthcare* **18**: 22-7.

Dresser R (2003) Precommitment: A misguided strategy for securing death with dignity. *Texas Law Rev* **81**: 1823.

Dworkin G (1989) *The Theory and Practice of Autonomy*. Cambridge: Cambridge University Press.

Edwards S (2009) *Nursing Ethics: A principle-based approach*. London: Palgrave.

Edwards A, Elwyn G, eds (2009) *Shared Decision-Making in Health Care: Achieving evidence-based patient choice*, 2nd edn. Oxford: Oxford University Press.

East Riding of Yorkshire Primary Care Trust (2007) *Transcribing Protocol* (online). Available at: www.ery.pct.uk (accessed 4 May 2010).

Fallowfield L, Ford S, Lewis S (1994) Information preferences of patients with cancer. *Lancet* **344**: 1576.

Farrell AM, Devaney S (2007) Making amends or making things worse? Clinical negligence reform and patient redress in England. *Legal Studies* **27**: 630-48.

Fulford K, Howse K (1993) Ethics of research with psychiatric patients: principles, problems and the primary responsibility of researchers. *J Med Ethics* **19**: 85-91.

Garwood-Gowers A, Tingle J, Lewis T (2001) *Healthcare Law: The impact of the Human Rights Act 1998*. London: Cavendish Publishing Ltd.

General Medical Council (1998) *Seeking Patients' Consent: Ethical considerations*. London: GMC.

General Medical Council (2002) *Research: The role and responsibilities of doctors*. London: GMC.

General Medical Council (2008a) *Seeking Patients' Consent: The ethical considerations*. London: GMC.

General Medical Council (2008b) *Good Practice in Prescribing Medicines: Guidance for doctors*. London: GMC.

General Pharmaceutical Council (GPhC) (2010) *Governance* (online) Available at www. pharmacyregulation.org (accessed 04.11.2010)

General Pharmaceutical Council (GPhC) (2010) *Standards of Conduct, Ethics and Performance*. London. GPhC.

Gillon R (1985) *Philosophical Medical Ethics*. Chichester: John Wiley.

Glare J (2009) Prescribing or transcribing errors are common in hospitalised patients though few lead to harm. *Quality Safety Healthcare* **18**: 22-27.

Gulliver A (2006) How New prescribers can limit liability. *Prescribing Med Manag* 2006: PM3.

Hardwig J (1993) The problem of proxies with interests of their own: Toward a better theory of proxy decisions. *J Clin Ethics* **4**: 20-27

Harris J (1985) *The Value of Life*. London: Routledge.

Hawley G, ed. (2007) *Ethics in Clinical Practice: An interprofessional approach*. London: Pearson Education Ltd.

Health Professions Council (2008) *Standards of Conduct. Performance and Ethics*. London: HPC.

Henderson R, Pochin M (2001) *A Right Result? Advocacy, justice and empowerment*. Bristol: Policy Press.

Hendrick J (2000) *Law and Ethics in Nursing and Healthcare*. Cheltenham: Stanley Thornes Ltd, 30.

Herring J (2008) *Medical Law and Ethics*. Oxford: Oxford University Press.

HM Government (2010) What is a Lasting Power of Attorney? (online). Available at: www.direct.gov.uk (accessed 28 April 2010.)

Jefford M, Tattersall MH (2002) Informing and involving cancer patients in their own care. *Lancet Oncol* **3**: 629-37.

Jefford M, Savulescu J, Thomson J et al (2005) Medical paternalism and expensive unsubsidised drugs. *BMJ* **331**: 1075-7.

Jones MA (1999) Informed consent and other fairy stories. *Med Law Rev* **7**: 103.

Jones S, Davies K, Jones B (2005) The adult patient, informed consent and the emergency care setting. *Accid Emerg Nurs* **13**: 167-70.

Kennedy I, Grubb, A (2000) *Medical Law*. 3rd edn. London: Butterworths.

Kessel A (1994) On failing to understand informed consent. *Br J Hosp Med* **52**: 235-8.

Kottow M (2003) The battering of informed consent. *J Med Ethics* **30**: 565-9.

Kuhse H, Singer P, eds (2001) *A Companion to Bioethics*. Oxford: Blackwell Publishing.

Kular M (2010) Providing effective telephone consultations. *Independent Nurse* 19 April: 42.

Lavelle-Jones C, Byrne D, Rice P, Cuschieri A (1993) Factors affecting quality of informed consent. *BMJ* **306**: 885-90.

Mason JK, Laurie GT (2006) *Law and Medical Ethics*, 7th edn. Oxford: Oxford University Press.

Medical Defence Union (2007) *Wrong Drug Errors Top List of GP Medication Incidents* (online). Available at: www.the-mdu.com (accessed 24 April 2010).

Medicines and Healthcare products Regulatory Agency (2008) *Supply and Administration of Botox®, Vistabel®, Dysport® and Other Injectable Medicines Used in Cosmetic Procedures* (online). Available at: www.mhra.gov.uk (accessed 22 April 2010).

Medicines and Healthcare products Regulatory Agency (2010) *Exemptions from Medicines Act Restrictions* Available at: www.mhra.gov.uk (accessed 22 April 2010).

Montgomery J (2003) *Health Care Law*, 2nd edn. Oxford: Oxford University Press.

National Prescribing Centre (1999) Signposts for prescribing nurses – general principles of good prescribing, *Prescribing Nurse Bulletin* **1**, No. 1.

National Prescribing Centre (2009) *A Guide to Good Practice in the Management of Controlled Drugs in Primary Care (England)*, 3rd edn (online). Available at: www.npc.co.uk (accessed 21 May 2010).

National Prescribing Centre (2010) *Frequently Asked Questions* (online). Available at: www.npc.co.uk (accessed 21 May 2010).

NHS Business Services Authority (2009) *NHS Security Management Service Security of Prescription Forms Guidance*. London: NHS Business Services Authority.

NHS Education for Scotland (2010) Glossary (online). Available at: www.nes.scot.nhs.uk/initiatives/patient-group-directions/glossary (accessed 15 September 2010).

NHS Employers (2010) *Whistleblowing* (online). Available at: www.nhsemployers.org (accessed 20 May 2010).

NHS Purchasing and Supply Agency (2010) *Borderline Substances* (online). Available at: www.pasa.nhs.uk (accessed 21 May 2010).

Nursing and Midwifery Council (2006) *Standards of Proficiency for Nurse and Midwife Prescribers*. London: NMC.

Nursing and Midwifery Council (2008a) *The Code: Standards of conduct, performance and ethics for nurses and midwives*. London: NMC.

Nursing and Midwifery Council (2008b) *Position Statement: Remote assessment and prescribing*. London: NMC.

Nursing and Midwifery Council (2010a) *Standards for Medicines Management*. London: NMC.

Nursing and Midwifery Council (2010b) *Nurse and Midwife Independent Prescribing of Unlicensed Medicines*. London: NMC.

O'Neill O (2003) Some limits of informed consent. *J Med Ethics* **29**: 4-7.

Pharmaceutical Services Negotiating Committee (2010) *Independent Prescribing of Unlicensed Medicines* (online). Available at: www.psnc.org.uk (accessed 21 May 2010).

Rovie E (2006) Re-evaluating the historical doctrine of double effect: Anscombe, Aquinas and the principle of side effects. *Studies in the History of Ethics* February 2006.

Royal College of General Practitioners (2003) *Death Certification and the Investigation of Deaths by Coroners*. London: RCGP.

Royal College of Nursing (2005) *Informed Consent in Health and Social Care Research*. London: RCN.

Royal Pharmaceutical Society of Great Britain (2007) *Professional Standards and Guidance for Pharmacist Prescribers*. London: RPSGB.

Royal Pharmaceutical Society of Great Britain (2007c) *Professional Standards and Guidance for Patient Consent*. London: RPSGB.

Royal Pharmaceutical Society of Great Britain (2009) The wholesale of medicines to registered chiropodists. In: *Law and Ethics Bulletin*. London: RPSGB.

Royal Pharmaceutical Society of Great Britain (2010) *Clinical Governance* (online). Available at: www.rpsgb.org/registrationandsupport/clinicalgovernance (accessed 12 April 2010).

Savage J, Moore L (2004) *Interpreting Accountability*. London: Royal College of Nursing Institute.

Shipman Inquiry (2004a) *Fourth Report: The Regulation of Controlled Drugs in the Community* (online). Available at: www.the-shipman-inquiry.org.uk (accessed 14 April 2010).

Shipman Inquiry (2004b) *Safeguarding Patients: Lessons from the Past – Proposals for the Future* (online). Available at: www.the-shipman-inquiry.org.uk (accessed 14 April 2010).

Shipman Inquiry (2010) *Independent Public Inquiry into the Issues Arising from the Case of Harold Fredrick Shipman* (online). Available at: www.the-shipman-inquiry.org (accessed 14 April 2010).

Silverman W (1989) The myth of informed consent: in daily practice and in clinical trials. *J Med Ethics* **15**: 6-11.

Smith JC (2000) A comment on Moor's case. *Criminal Law Review* **41**.

Staines, R (2009) NMC defends decision to strike off undercover nurse Margaret Haywood (online). Available at: www.nursingtimes.net (accessed 20 May 2010).

Tingle J, Cribb A (2002) *Nursing Law and Ethics*, 2nd edn. Oxford: Blackwell Publishing, 125.

Vig EK, Taylor JS, Starks H, Hopley EK, Fryer-Edward K (2006) Beyond substituted judgment: how surrogates navigate end-of-life decision-making. *J Am Geriatr Soc* **54**: 1688-93.

Wager E, Tooley PJH, Emanuel MB, Wood SF (1995) How to do it: get patients' consent to enter clinical trials. *BMJ* **311**: 734-7.

Weaver JM (2006) It's time to throw out old-fashioned Latin abbreviations. *Anesth Progr* **53**: 1-2.

Williams G (1957) *The Sanctity of Life and the Criminal Law*. London: Faber and Faber.

Wilson P (2005) Jehovah's Witness children: when religion and the law Collide. *Paediatr Nurs* **17**: 34-9.

Acts

Adults with Incapacity (Scotland) Act 2000

Children Act 1989

Coroners' Act 1988

European Convention on Human Rights and Biomedicine of 1997

Family Law Reform Act 1969

Human Rights Act 1998

Medicines Act 1968

Mental Capacity Act (2005) Code of Practice

Misuse of Drugs Act 1971

Prescription Only Medicines (Human Use) Order 1997 SI 1997/1830 Medicines (Sale or Supply) (Miscellaneous Provisions) Amendment.

Public Interest Disclosure Act 1998

Chapter 3
Factors Influencing Prescribing

Val Lawrenson

Learning objectives

After reading this chapter and completing the activities within it, the reader will be able to:

1 identify the influences upon non-medical prescribing practice
2 critically analyse the impact of the influences on non-medical prescribing in relation to practice
3 identify and evaluate strategies to address the influences on non-medical prescribing in order to support safe and effective prescribing

Prescribing is a complex activity and each consultation is unique, although common themes may emerge. To ensure patient safety and cost-effective prescribing, the practitioner has to be aware of the many factors that might influence practice. In addition to ethical, professional and legal issues, non-medical prescribing is subject to a variety of other influences that impact on the non-medical prescriber's ability to prescribe safely and effectively. For the purpose of this chapter, consideration of these influences is undertaken in the context of the prescriber, the patient, the product and other professionals. This chapter briefly explores some of the issues related to each of these influences and proposes strategies to overcome related difficulties in order to promote concordance.

The prescriber

Julia Cumberledge clearly recognised the benefits of non-medical prescribing (Department of Health and Social Security (DHSS) 1986) however this appreciation is not always shared. Indeed, despite claims of benefits to prescribers, patients and the organisation (While and Biggs 2004, Jones and Jones 2005), many non-medical

The Textbook of Non-medical Prescribing, edited by Dilyse Nuttall and Jane Rutt-Howard.
© 2011 Blackwell Publishing Ltd

prescribers who are eligible to prescribe still do not do so (Hall et al 2006, Hobson and Sewell 2006, George et al 2007). Hall et al (2006) found that community nurses were not prescribing consistently, with 50% more health visitors than district nurses being described as infrequent or reluctant prescribers. Similarly, Hobson and Sewell (2006) found that, whilst pharmacist non-medical prescribers working in primary and secondary care settings were clearly able to articulate the benefits of supplementary prescribing, not all of the 532 pharmacists registered as supplementary prescribers were using their prescribing skills. The implementation of non-medical prescribing, to allow pharmacists and other allied professionals to prescribe, has been heralded as a positive innovation. However, according to Avery et al (2007), despite the UK having invested in non-medical prescribing, the infrastructure required to support non-medical prescribers remains fragile. They argue that this is particularly evident within the acute settings where non-medical prescribing has not achieved priority status. Although there is limited evidence on the impact of the extension of non-medical prescribing to include pharmacists and other allied professionals, it is envisaged that many of the strategic barriers to its success are shared with nurses (Avery et al 2007).

Whilst welcomed as a logical extension to practice not everyone is ready to accept the increased responsibility that accompanies the autonomy associated with implementation of non-medical prescribing (Lewis-Evans and Jester 2004). Although for the most part practitioners are able to manage the tension between nursing and medical approaches to consultation (Bradley and Nolan 2007), Wells et al (2009) propose that the success of non-medical prescribing is influenced by ambivalence. This argument gains some support from Young et al (2009) who found that, where the benefits of non-medical prescribing are considered obvious, implementation appears to be more successful. According to Stenner et al (2010) ambivalence, arising from the role change as a result of implementation of prescribing could be one of the factors that influence practitioners' responses to prescribing. However, we must be mindful not to dismiss the challenges that non-medical prescribers in both the primary and secondary care environments face as an indication of misgivings related to the benefits of role expansion. To ensure successful implementation of prescribing within your clinical role, you will need to perceive the benefits and be willing to take on the responsibilities associated with this role expansion.

Activity box 3.1

Consider the impact of the expansion of your role to include non-medical prescribing on the following:

- The patient
- Yourself
- Your colleagues
- The organisation
- The profession

Personal characteristics

As individual practitioners, we each have personal beliefs, based on the optimum method of treatment and the perceptions of the effectiveness of particular treatment regimens. Hughes et al (2007) refer to these particular influences on prescribing as prescriber characteristics. Personal characteristics, combined with a lack of specialist knowledge and graduate level academic ability, are said to have an influence on the quality of prescribing practice (Hughes et al 2007). Their study suggested that prescribers without additional qualifications in their field of expertise lacked confidence and, subsequently, were reluctant to prescribe. Similar findings have been presented by Cooper et al (2008) who also made reference to expert knowledge when they expressed concerns that pharmacist prescribers might be unaware of current clinical knowledge, which clearly would be to the detriment of patients in their care. It is important that non-medical prescribers use their appraisal to identify learning opportunities to ensure that they are able to access appropriate courses and receive formal feedback on practice (see Chapter 9).

Prescriber Confidence, and its impact on practice, has also been highlighted by While and Biggs (2004). They found that non-medical prescribers who generated more than three prescriptions a week were more confident than those who prescribed less. The number of prescribing situations was also linked to familiarity with the product and increased prescriber confidence (While and Biggs 2004).

Activity box 3.2

Consider the number of times that you are likely to generate a prescription in a week.

Do you consider this to be sufficient to ensure familiarity with the products in your personal formulary?

What strategies could you implement in order to ensure familiarity and maintain your confidence? (See Chapter 9 for more about continuing personal development.)

Contact your trust prescribing lead to find out more about the support available to you while you gain confidence in your prescribing role.

The length of time from qualifying to receipt of a prescription pad and being able to prescribe was found to contribute to a lack of practitioner confidence (Hall et al 2006). Non-medical prescribers suggested that this delay contributed to a loss of confidence which, in some cases, led to prescribers reverting to their traditional prescribing practice. George et al (2007) also commented on the delay in getting prescriptions booklets although they indicated that, for pharmacists, this delay was more of a cause of frustration than a factor that impacted on confidence.

Prescriber feelings of vulnerability

Within secondary care prescriptions are commonly documented on hospital drug charts which accommodate multiple prescriptions by multiple prescribers (Morran 2007). In contrast, even though increasingly prescribers in primary care are able to use computer-generated prescriptions, many still use individual prescriptions from their own prescription pad. The location of the prescribing episode is also recognised as having impact on the prescribing process as a result of prescriber vulnerability (Hall et al 2006). Unlike in the hospital setting, non-medical prescribers working in the community are likely to undertake most of their consultations in client's homes, clinics, pharmacist premises or other community environments. For the most part the prescriber will be familiar with these environments. However, there may be situations when the prescriber feels vulnerable, e.g. when entering areas of high crime or deprivation. In this scenario prescribers will need to exercise particular vigilance about the safety and security of both themselves and the prescription pad. Hall et al (2006) described how the practitioners' feelings of vulnerability influenced prescribing because, in these scenarios, where a prescription was necessary, the patient was referred to the GP.

Activity box 3.3

Find out how prescribers working in secondary care environments ensure safety of the prescriptions.

Institutional and resource factors

Changes in role, responsibilities and funding

It could be argued that, although changes in healthcare provision have acted as the driver for non-medical prescribing, they also exert a negative influence on prescribing practice. In addition to insufficient knowledge of the clinical condition insufficient clinical opportunity is said to influence prescribing, particularly where those previously active as prescribers have taken on managerial roles (Wells et al 2009). The lack of financial remuneration for the additional responsibilities has also been highlighted as a factor influencing prescribing practice (Thurtle 2007, Cooper et al 2008). Although experienced clinical pharmacist and community pharmacist salaries are higher than those of nurses the type of prescribing undertaken by nurses and pharmacists is identical. According to Hobson and Sewell (2006) this might be one factor that contributes to the lack of pharmacist prescribers, particularly in primary care where funding could be an issue. Avery et al (2007) and Cooper et al (2008) discussed funding in relation to remuneration for those providing clinical support for non-medical prescribers. This did not seem to be problematic in secondary care environments where medical staff were salaried; however, in primary care a lack of sufficient designated medical practitioners was considered to be influenced by remuneration.

Organisational culture

Hughes et al (2007) refer to the socially constructed nature of the phenomenon. This is the way in which norms, beliefs and values, having been accepted by all group members, are integrated into practice. According to Hughes et al (2007), organisational culture and the values of professionals can have a major influence on the decision not to prescribe. Indeed Thurtle (2006) found this to be the case for some health visitors, where a culture of not prescribing had been established. Organisational culture has also been highlighted as having an impact on prescribing for pharmacists working in primary and secondary care. Here different approaches to the implementation of non-medical prescribing have contributed to confusion about the role and responsibilities of sup-plementary prescribers which, according to Hobson and Sewell (2006), is a factor influencing prescribing practice. As the way in which the organisation responds to the challenges associated with implementation of non-medical prescribing clearly impacts on its success, newly qualified prescribers are advised to consider the culture of the organisation in which they are to practise. If practice needs to be challenged, the new prescriber will require skills in communication and assertiveness. Indeed, in the areas where clear barriers to implementation exist, a degree of courage may also be necessary.

Whilst there will be some similarities not all non-medical prescribers will face the same challenges to implementation of prescribing. Indeed local variations are known to impact on the success of the intervention. Therefore, identification of local barriers to prescrib-ing is one strategy that will ensure that trusts are able to provide appropriate organi-sational support mechanisms. Discussions with practitioners, who are not actively prescribing despite their eligibility, would be one way forward. In addition to this, during the early stages of prescribing, the provision of preceptorship or mentoring by an expe-rienced prescriber would also provide the support required until confidence is estab-lished. Cooper et al (2008) suggested that implementation of a buddying system was one way in which newly qualified supplementary pharmacist prescribers were able to gain confidence in their new role. This strategy is equally relevant to other non-medical prescribers, particularly perhaps those who find themselves working in isolation.

Activity box 3.4

Find out how many non-medical prescribers there are in your local trust.
What percentage of those eligible to prescribe do not regularly prescribe?
Consider what factors might influence their decision not to prescribe.

Organisational issues associated with the prescribing process

Time

According to Hall et al (2006), although community practitioner prescribing has been welcomed by patients, there are conflicting reports as to its associated benefits. It was initially envisaged that not having to wait around GP offices for prescriptions would save nurses time. In the event, French (2002) demonstrated how time-consuming the administrative processes associated with prescribing were and argued that it was this that often influenced practitioners' decisions to refer patients to their general practitioner (GP). As many community practitioners refer to the time-consuming nature of the prescribing process, Hall et al (2003a) suggest that time is perhaps used differently rather than saved. The length of time that consultations take has been considered to influence prescribing in a variety of ways. Kimmer and Christian (2005) found that the pressure of timed appointments often resulted in generation of a prescription that they argued could be counterproductive in the case of self-limiting conditions. Lado et al (2008) similarly argued that prescriptions might be generated in order to compensate for restrictions on consultation time. Undertaking a thorough holistic assessment takes time; concerns related to the need for longer consultation times as well as the time required to devise and implement clinical management plans have also been identified as barriers to implementation by other non-medical prescribers (Cooper et al 2008).

Not all references to time relate to insufficiencies and in some areas non-medical prescribers describe having sufficient time to undertake their assessment, which consequently facilitates safe and effective prescribing (Hall et al 2003a, Jones and Jones 2005). In addition to this, those working in isolated areas indicate that implementation of non-medial prescribing has reduced the time patients wait for appropriate interventions – thus achieving one of the aims of outlined by Department of Health (DH 2006) as quicker access to healthcare.

Activity box 3.5

Consider how expansion of your role to include non-medical prescribing might impact on the time available for your consultations.

Devise a way to ensure that prescribing is safe and effective within the constraints that you have identified.

The need for accurate documentation is fundamental and the importance of good communication within prescribing is evident. However, as has previously been noted non-medical prescribers have found procedures accompanying generation of a prescription to be time-consuming and involve much duplication (Lewis-Evans and Jester 2004). These two factors have been found to influence prescribing and contributed to individual practitioners' decision to refer patients rather than prescribe for them (Lewis-Evans and Jester 2004, While and Biggs 2007). By way of an example, generation of a prescription by a non-medical prescriber could impact on continuity of care as a consequence of the patient or representative having to visit the pharmacy to have the prescription dispensed. In situations like this the prescribing decision may be influenced by the knowledge that the patient is already receiving items from another source, such as their GP. Repeat prescriptions might be viewed in a similar way, e.g. if the patient is already in receipt of non-Community Practitioners formulary items from the GP, the products that the non-medical prescriber might prescribe could be added to the existing prescription (Hall et al 2006). This might be a strategy that some community matrons choose to employ because patients on their caseloads are likely to have repeat medication arrangements already established.

To ensure patient safety, it is important that the prescriber has access to information related to previous diagnoses or concurrent medication. Obviously the inability to access information held in electronic patient medical notes impacts on prescribing decisions for all non-medical prescribers, as does access to the technology to print prescriptions (Hall et al 2006, Guillaume et al 2008). For those working in primary care, an additional barrier to prescribing is the need to generate handwritten prescriptions, particularly as many GP practices now operate electronic paperless systems (Hall et al 2006, George et al 2007).

As it is some time since the initial implementation of nurse prescribing, it is perhaps not surprising that strategies have been found to circumvent the increased workload and repetition involved. Evidence of these strategies can be seen in the literature, including the use of carbonised prescription pads, photocopies being filed in patient's notes or prescriptions being faxed to GP surgeries for their records. While et al (2005) found that some prescribers reverted to their traditional practice of indicating the products required and then having the prescription generated electronically, before being signed by the doctor. Reverting to ordering products using a computerised system should be avoided because ultimately it will lead to prescribers being deskilled (Fisher 2005a, 2005b). However, it appears as if the strategy might be commonly employed, because the inability to computer generate prescriptions was also found to influence prescribing in studies undertaken by Thurtle (2006) and Courtney (2007). Although not all non-medical prescribers can relate to this particular scenario, it must be recognised that, for others, the influence of time pressures could result in this becoming the practice of choice.

An alternative strategy to reduce the amount of time that non-medical prescribers engage in administrative processes has been to notify GPs only when new items were prescribed or if there had been a change to the item prescribed (Fisher 2005a, 2005b). These findings were reinforced by Hall et al (2006) who indicated that, although the prescriber kept their own record of each prescription, the GP was informed only if the item prescribed was a medicine. At their request GPs were not informed of prescriptions for dressings unless, as stated earlier, there had been a change to the initial treatment plan (Hall et al 2006).

 Activity box 3.6

What does your local policy say about how and when you must communicate details of your prescribing decisions?

Speak to two members of the healthcare team whom you will need to keep informed about your prescribing practice. Find out what they require from you in relation to communication about your prescribing decisions.

Professional issues

Codes of professional conduct protect both the public and the practitioner and, as professionals, we have a duty to comply with these codes (for further information see Chapter 2). Government guidelines (DH 2006) indicate the need for employers to ensure that the practitioner has access to relevant ongoing education and training. In addition to this, all professional codes (Health Professionals Council (HPC) 2006, Nursing Midwifery Council (NMC) 2006, General Pharmaceutical Council (GPhC) 2010 make reference to the need for practitioners to maintain their knowledge and competence. Nevertheless, the availability of funding sources remains an issue (Hall et al 2004) and support for continuing professional development (CPD) for the prescribing role remains inconsistent (Carey et al 2010). Access to CPD is viewed as necessary by non-medical prescribers. Indeed, Thurtle (2006) argued that access to personal and professional development was one factor that influenced health visitors' decisions not to prescribe. Examples from the literature demonstrate the lack of supportive infrastructures and, in particular, that funding for and access to CPD is not limited to nurses but is equally relevant to other non-medical prescribers (George et al 2007, Cooper et al 2008).

Activity box 3.7

Identify three ways in which you could maintain your knowledge and competence in relation to prescribing practice without necessarily requiring funding for formal study.

As a range of variables is likely to inform the prescribing decision, any decisions made must have a logical basis. As such, the non-medical prescriber will need to be able to provide a sound, evidence-based rationale to support his or her professional judgement in relation to the option chosen (Dimond 2005). As registered practitioners, non-medical prescribers have a responsibility to ensure that they are knowledgeable and competent and prescribe only within their competency (HPC 2006, NMC 2006, GPhC 2010). Non-medical prescribers not only have to be aware of the nuances of their own clinical field but also have to be able to use a range of different strategies in order to collect the evidence needed to underpin the holistic assessment. It is therefore important that they have a sound knowledge of their clinical area as well as an understanding of consultation and history-taking models. If there are areas in which the non-medical prescriber feels less confident, these need to be highlighted in his or her personal development plan or individual performance review, guidance on which can be found in Chapter 9.

Activity box 3.8

Identify three conditions for which you will be expected to prescribe. Reflect on your knowledge of the investigations that will be necessary in order to ensure an accurate diagnosis. If you discover any gaps in your knowledge/experience, devise an action plan to address this deficit.

The patient

The consultation

As indicated in Chapter 4, a structured approach to history taking and well-developed history-taking skills are needed to inform a diagnosis (Offredy 2002). To ensure safe and effective prescribing, it is important to be aware of any existing pathology and underlying medical conditions, because many patients present with multiple pathologies. Where possible accessing patients records as well as undertaking a comprehensive history will provide the information needed to inform the prescribing decision. Communication and the transfer of appropriate information are clearly a cornerstone of safe prescribing practice and the duty of care owed by health professionals to their clients is non the less important in the prescribing consultation (Dimond 2005). Systematic application of the principles of prescribing (NPC 1999) breaks down the complex decisions that underpin a prescribing consultation, thus making them more manageable (Thompson 2007). Adherence to these principles also ensures that decisions made during the consultation have a logical basis (Dimond 2005).

As professionals, we are aware of the impact of communication in relation to the success of care interventions (Latter 2008). The prescriber's ability to quickly and effectively build a therapeutic relationship is never more obvious than in a prescribing consultation. Many of these consultations are time limited, which means that the non-medical prescriber's ability to gather sufficient information on which to base an accurate diagnosis is crucial. To gather appropriate, relevant and accurate data to inform the prescribing decision, it is important that a relationship of trust is developed. It is also important to recognise the shift from a professionally determined compliance agenda to the integration of concordance within non-medical prescribing consultations (Latter et al 2007). To achieve concordance, the practitioner needs to embrace a non-judgemental, empowering care philosophy that will enable clients to make choices about their health (Day 2007).

The development of the therapeutic alliance required to ensure successful patient-centred services requires effective communication, which according to Mead and Bower (2000) is built on the practitioner's own awareness of self. Many healthcare practitioners assume that their communication skills are good and consider themselves to be non-judgemental. However, in some situations this may not be the case.

Activity box 3.9

Reflect on a situation in which you have given advice, but the outcome had not been as you intended.

- What happened?
- What was it about the communication that could have impacted on the success of the intervention?
- What other factors may have contributed to the ineffectiveness of the communication?
- What strategies could you employ in future to ensure similar misunderstandings did not occur?

Patient expectations

To practise safely and cost-effectively, it is important that prescriptions are generated only when necessary (NPC 1999). Non-medical prescribers are required to develop an awareness of all the options available to them, which includes the generation of a prescription. The patient, however, may not be aware of the alternatives and some are likely to arrive at the consultation with an expectation that a prescription will be the ultimate outcome. Many prescribers assume that the patient attends the consultation with an expectation that a prescription will be generated. However, according to Lado et al (2008) the number of patients who actually expected a prescription was overestimated by the healthcare professional. Patients' expectations as to who will undertake the consultation are often based on their previous experiences so, even though some practitioners roles have been expanded to include non-medical prescribing, patients may still expect the consultation to be undertaken by a medical practitioner. Although not commonly highlighted, in mental health nursing, Harrison (2003) found that some patients were concerned about the non-medical prescribers' skills and knowledge to undertake the prescribing role.

Later in this chapter, factors that influence prescribing, such as culture, health beliefs and the media, are explored individually. However as patients' knowledge and understanding influences their expectations it is pertinent to include reference to it here. As a consequence of increased access to information sources, healthcare professionals are now dealing with an informed public who are more aware of health issues. It is acknowledged that not all the information that patients acquire is evidence based or even in some cases rational. Nevertheless the information that the patient has impacts on expectations. McKinley and Middleton (1999) found that 60% of patients had already formed a view about the cause of their presenting problems and 38% had an explanation for their symptoms. These patients attended the consultation with an expectation that the specific questions that they had would be answered (McKinley and Middleton 1999).

Emotions, such as anger, distress or anxiety, can influence the prescribing consultation in a variety of different ways. Each has the ability to influence communication and could impact on the patient's ability to assimilate the information that he or she is given. Some patients request a consultation only when they have exhausted alternative approaches to managing their conditions. In fact McKinley and Middleton (1999) found that nearly a quarter of the patients who attended the clinic reported that they had reached the height of their anxiety. The non-medical prescriber is advised to remain cognisant of this because anxiety can influence not only patient expectation but also the effectiveness of the consultation in relation to the patient's involvement in the treatment plan (Granby 2005).

In many consultations, although by no means all, a previous relationship has already been established. In these cases it considered easier for the prescriber to collect information relevant to the presenting consultation (Cioffi 2003). On the other hand, a consultation in which there is no prior relationship is considered more complex. Each consultation is unique, as is the patient with whom it takes place, and the influence of an existing relationship between the prescriber and patient should not be underestimated (Granby 2005). Existing relationships can influence prescribing either positively or negatively. Patients may have an expectation that a prescription will be provided based on their interpretation of the interactions with the non-medical prescriber. Too friendly a relationship may contribute to a mismatch in expectations whereas a distant or aloof approach might impact on clients' willingness to divulge their information. The presentation of a friendly, approachable, yet professional manner will go some way to ensuring that the relationship between the prescriber and patient remains firmly based on one of respect and trust.

Leyshon (2007) indicates that, although the health professional may have expert disease-related knowledge, the patient is the expert in his or her own preferences and experiences of the condition. Historically, the relationship between the patient and healthcare professional has been paternalistic. The patient had a passive role within the consultation, with the healthcare professional taking the lead in assessment, diagnosis and decision-making about the treatment regimen. Changes in this relationship now mean that the patient expects to have a more active role which, according to Leyshon (2007), goes some way to enhancing the success of care interventions. Lewis-Evans and Jester (2004) describe the outcomes of this more egalitarian relationship between prescriber and patient as concordance. They suggest that, in situations where the patient respects the practitioner and is confident in his or her ability to prescribe, concordance is enhanced. It is therefore important that the non-medical prescriber presents him- or herself confidently to the patient. One way to ensure confidence is for the non-medical prescriber to be knowledgeable about his or her specialist field of practice. Keeping abreast of the latest developments and being able to explain these to patients will go some way to enhancing credibility (Creedon et al 2009).

Activity box 3.10

Identify three resources that will help you deliver evidence-based practice.

Patient as consumer

As a consequence of changes to the categorisations of some medicines, the ability to self medicate has greatly increased. This can be viewed as a positive development as patients take responsibility for the management of their disorders and become self-sufficient (Aronson 2004). The increased availability of products on the shelves in pharmacists, supermarkets and stores contributes to a sense of empowerment. However, as most people have little understanding of the physiological systems of the body, one disadvantage of the consumer ideology is an increased risk of potentially serious conditions going undiagnosed (Hughes et al 2002). To ensure safety, non-medical prescribers need to stay increasingly alert to the concept of self-medication. They will need to remain mindful that patients regularly omit to tell health professionals that they are taking over-the-counter medications because they perceive being able to purchase them as an indication of their safety (Bond and Hannaford 2003). Non-medical prescribers will need to develop what Crouch and Chapelhow (2008) call pharmacovigilance. Skills required for pharmacovigilance include awareness of side effects, adverse drug reactions, potential interactions of medicines, food and drink and other medicines. While recognising that it is unrealistic for the non-medical prescriber to have an in-depth knowledge of each potential combination, there is an expectation that they will be able to recognise the potential dangers and to know how to access appropriate information in order to enhance patient safety.

 Activity box 3.11

Identify two sources of information relating to potential interactions between medicines that patients might purchase over the counter.

Identify the potential interactions between one medicine that patients might purchase over the counter with one of the medicines that you are likely to prescribe.

Culture

It is difficult to provide a finite definition for 'culture' so here the term is used to represent the concept that encompasses traditions, expected behaviour, beliefs and knowledge of a social grouping. As a consequence of globalisation, healthcare professionals are finding themselves interacting with increasingly more ethnically and culturally diverse populations. According to the 2001 census 7.9% of the population in England and Wales was from Asian or Asian British, black or black British, Chinese or other minority groups (Office for National Statistics 2003). Therefore, the need for healthcare workers to appreciate how culture influences health-seeking behaviour, the interpretation of symptoms and compliance with treatment regimens is clear (Berry-Caban and Crespo 2008).

Anthropology teaches us that disease, health and illness are culturally defined. The reasons why patients attend the consultation, how they understand the cause and treatment of their illness, and what they expect from the prescriber are all informed by their individual beliefs (Langer 2008). Although a lack of concordance could be intentional, Langer (2008) argues that it is more appropriate to view a lack of concordance as a problem related to the kind of communication relationship between the patient and practitioner, rather than as a maladaptive characteristic of the patient. Table 3.1 provides some examples to demonstrate the impact of culture on health behaviour.

Failure of the non-medical prescriber to recognise and address cultural factors may contribute to a powerful source of information being overlooked (Otway and Bowskill 2006). This could impact on the appropriateness of the information underpinning the assessment and diagnosis, and subsequently influence safety and effectiveness of the consultation. Working with patients and negotiating treatment plans that make sense in the context of their lives and cultural belief systems will enhance concordance and facilitate self management (Langer 2008). In view of the potential impact of culture on the prescribing outcomes it is important that prescribers develop what Berry-Caban and Crespo (2008) term 'cultural competency'. Cultural competency ensures an understanding, appreciation and respect of cultural differences within groups, which is clearly relevant to prescribing practice.

Otway and Bowskill (2006) highlight the importance of good communication skills in ensuring that those for whom English is not the first language obtain appropriate treatment and care. They suggest that meeting the needs of patients who do not share the same language as the health professional is a complex process, and highlight the need for the practitioner to be able and willing to understand the patient's point of view.

The awareness of the dynamics that result from cultural differences such as value preferences, perception of illness, health beliefs and communication style will help practitioners adapt treatment plans that meet culturally unique needs (Langer 2008). Therefore, to demonstrate cultural competence the non-medical prescriber needs to have some understanding of culture, traditions, values and family systems. They will need to reflect on their own values, stereotypes and biases about ethnicity and socio-

Table 3.1 Culture and health behaviour

Nula is a Muslim. She perceives Allah (God) to be the ultimate decider of health, life and death. In Islam, illness is seen as atonement for prior sins and death is part of the journey to meet God. Nula has delayed seeking healthcare intervention for her symptoms which as can now be seen has contributed to the advanced presentation of the disease

In the West African culture an individual's health status is indicated by his or her physical appearance. This display of heath includes the amount of body fat and clarity of the skin. Individuals from this particular cultural background are more receptive to health promotion strategies that include eating right, avoiding drafts and eliminating properly

In the Polish culture there is a belief that almost all illnesses can be explained as having a physical/biological cause. Treatments aimed at correcting these causes are more likely to be successful than, say, psychological or self-help interventions

economic class. To ensure safe prescribing practice, they will need to demonstrate acceptance of ethnic/racial differences, practice empathically and to reflect genuineness, as well as have the capacity to respond flexibly to individual patient needs (Berry-Caban and Crespo 2008). A holistic assessment using a recognised consultation model is one way to elicit the patient's understanding and expectations, and so ensure the safety and effectiveness of the prescribing decision.

Activity box 3.12

Identify three minority groups for whom you might have to prescribe.
    Jot down what you know about each cultural group's perception of health and illness.
    If your knowledge is limited undertake a literature search.
    Reflect upon one of your consultations in which your patient was from an ethnic minority group. Critically analyse your actions in meeting the needs of the patient in relation to the health/illness perceptions identified.

Health beliefs

In the previous section reference was made to culture and how this has the potential to influence prescribing. For the most part, the inference was that culture and country of origin were conjoined. However, it is important not to stereotype patients because, even within a homogeneous culture, there are still wide variations in subcultures. A patient-centred approach to the consultation is important to ensure that each patient has his or her needs and beliefs explored.

    According to Harvey and Lawson (2009), education and knowledge alone are often insufficient to ensure concordance and the successful outcome of care interventions. Health behaviour and the patient's motivation to participate in healthcare activities are influenced by their health beliefs, illness representations or personal models (Ogden 1996). Health psychology attempts to offer theoretical explanations for health behaviour by exploring factors that influence health behaviour, including health beliefs and practitioner–patient relationships. Numerous health belief models have arisen as a consequence of the increased interest in health psychology and health behaviour. Approaches to health belief include: the health belief model, theory of reasoned action and the locus of control theory. There is a link between how patients perceive the relevance of suggested therapies and their 'heath belief model', i.e. their belief in their susceptibility to a disease or illness. The patient-perceived relevance of the suggested therapy is also linked to their perceptions of the degree of severity of the illness and the consequences for health and daily functioning (Langer 2008). There is also a link between patients' concerns about risks, harm or addiction and health belief models and concordance (Robinson 2010). Therefore in this section a brief overview of some of the models underpinning health behaviour is presented, although it is not within the remit of this chapter to address the health belief models in any depth and therefore non-medical prescribers are reminded of the important influence that heath beliefs can have on prescribing and advised to undertake further reading in relation to health psychology.

Health belief models

The health belief model was originally devised by Rossenstock in 1966 and then further developed by Becker in 1974. It is based on the assumption that the individual behaves in a rational manner and implies that, faced with pressure to change behaviour, the individual will consider the advantages and disadvantages of a particular course of action. These two factors, combined with the individual's perception of the seriousness of the illness, are what are said to contribute to changes in behaviour (cited in Harvey and Lawson 2009). The theory of reasoned action/theory of planned behaviour was proposed by Fishbein and Ajzen in 1970. This theory suggests that changes in behaviour are influenced by individuals' attitude towards the behaviour, e.g. if they believe that the changed behaviour will bring about the effect that they desire. Subjective norms, i.e. the individual's perceptions of what others expect or would like, are an important component of the theory of reasoned action, e.g. the degree to which significant others perceive the benefits of change and how motivated the individual is to comply with this pressure. This model places the individual within their social context and demonstrates the important role of culture, family and friends in influencing health behaviour. (Harvey and Lawson 2009). Individuals' beliefs that they have the necessary skills, abilities and information to carry out the required change are also a key component of this particular theory (Ogden 1996). Past experiences, particularly if the patient has been unsuccessful in implementing a change, can influence motivation and influence success in this particular health belief model.

The locus of control theory was proposed by Sarafino in 1994. Within this model, reference is made to internal and external loci of control as well as a fatalistic perspective. Patients, who are empowered and consider their health to be determined by their own actions, are said to have an internal locus of control. They consider themselves to have both the skills, abilities and desire to make changes, and the necessary external resources to support any change, e.g. health education support networks. On the other hand, those who perceive restoration or maintenance of health as the responsibility of the healthcare professional are said to have an external locus of control. Those with a fatalistic perspective are perhaps among the most difficult to manage because they consider health to be determined by luck, fate, destiny or religious beliefs. As a non-medical prescriber you will encounter patients who hold each of these different health beliefs.

The patient's awareness of the need to take medication, to make changes to health behaviour and his or her understanding of the consequences impact on the effectiveness of prescribing (Barber and Robertson 2009). Therefore a lack of understanding, by the non-medical prescriber, of how an individual's beliefs and culture impact on his or her behaviour will inevitably influence the prescribing consultation. To enable the correct assessment of the patient's understanding of the illness and to enhance the effectiveness of the consultation, it is important that the non-medical prescriber has an understanding of various models that attempt to explain the relationship between beliefs and behaviour in more depth. This understanding will support the development of patient-centred care programmes that will increase the chances of concordance (Langer 2008).

Activity box 3.13

Reflect on one of your consultations in which the outcome was not as you had envisaged.

Critically evaluate the outcome in relation to one of the health belief models identified.

Undertake a literature search related to health belief models.

The product

Product choice

Granby (2005) makes the point that it is no longer acceptable to base clinical decisions on personal opinions. Indeed the introduction of clinical governance and the implementation of evidence-based practice, with its emphasis on accountability, quality and efficiency, go some way to eliminating this type of care delivery (Granby and Chapman 2004). The National Institute for Health and Clinical Excellence (NICE) guidelines and evidence-based practice are often key drivers influencing prescribing. Therefore, each practitioner needs to ensure that his or her knowledge of relevant guidelines remains current. It is also important for prescribers to be aware of any local protocols related to their clinical field because these will also be expected to inform product choice.

Kimmer and Christian (2005) identify that difficulties in keeping abreast of the changes are worthy of consideration, particularly when practitioners are governed by codes of conduct that refer to working within one's competence (see Chapter 2 for more on codes of conduct). The National Prescribing Centre (1999) provide the mnemonic EASE to aid the non-medical prescriber when considering the product choice (see the introduction for a full explanation of the prescribing principles).

Effectiveness and cost are often presented concurrently; however, cost-effectiveness is not necessarily linked solely to product price and the prescriber must remain aware of the additional drivers that may influence cost. Case study 1, at the back of this book, demonstrates how the cost of the product choice also includes the number of nurses' visits, the loss of earnings and the potential barriers to concordance. Patient acceptability is a key factor in enhancing concordance so non-medical prescribers need to remain mindful of convenience, size, shape, portability and storage of products because these can all impact on patients' perceptions of product acceptability. To assess suitability of the product choice, the non-medical prescriber will need to pay particular attention to related information gathered during the holistic assessment.

Activity box 3.14

In relation to your clinical field identify two national guidelines that influence product choice.

Critically evaluate the advantages and disadvantages related to implementation of each of these guidelines in relation to product choice decisions.

Prescribing formularies

Strategies that support the implementation of evidence based practice include prescribing policies and formularies. Hughes et al (2007) refer to these strategies as external influences on prescribing practice. The most readily recognised formulary to influence prescribing practice is the *British National Formulary* (BNF) or the *British National Formulary for Children* (BNFC) (Sains 2008). These authoritative reference sources provide information on the most up-to-date items available to UK prescribers. According to Sains (2008), although best practice is to use these formal governance frameworks to inform prescribing decisions, some prescribers refer to a mental list of tried and tested products.

To support prescribing decisions and ensure implementation of standardised care, many organisations expect prescribers to comply with a local formulary (Sains 2008). A formulary is a collection of guidelines that suggest first- and second-line treatments. In primary care, formularies may be related to continence, wound or skin care products, whereas, in acute settings, formularies for specialist clinical areas exist, e.g. skin preparations in dermatology.

The decision to include items in the formulary is based on clinical and cost-effectiveness which are often determined by a panel of local stakeholders including practitioners, pharmacists and specialist nurses. The outcome of this collaboration is a formulary that provides guidance to the non-medical prescriber in relation to the items that are available for specific situations.

Activity box 3.15

Which formularies influence prescribing in your clinical area?

What criteria are used to determine whether or not a product is available to you in the formulary?

See if you can arrange to participate on the panel responsible for revising the formulary that you are most likely to frequently prescribe from.

While and Biggs (2004) suggest that local formularies and policies can help to build prescribers' confidence, particularly in the immediate post-qualifying period, because they act as both decision-support and educational tools. It is also thought that, by removing some of the responsibility on the practitioner to be aware of the price of items at the point of use, they also enhance financial probity (Sains 2008). Prescribing is a complex interaction and it is unlikely that the products contained in local formularies will cover all eventualities. However, implementation of formularies has been found to strengthen the robustness of clinical governance with regard to prescribing (Sains 2008).

Not all authors agree that local formularies influence prescribing in a positive manner and limitations imposed as a consequence of the implementation of local formularies are said to generate frustration for many prescribers (Lewis-Evans and Jester 2004, Carey et al 2009a, 2009b). Bradley and Nolan (2007) argue that restricting prescribing decisions to items in local formularies undermines nurses' confidence and discourages them from using their prescribing authority.

Hall et al (2008) indicated that influences on prescribing decisions, in particular the decision to make changes to prescribed items, involved the weight of evidence in favour of the change, as well as the authority of the sources recommending the change. In these situations, the influence of the person providing clinical support was found to impact at least initially on the prescribing choices of newly qualified non-medical prescribers. Hall et al (2008) also discovered that those who worked as district nurses immediately before becoming a prescriber prescribed the same items that they had used as a district nurse.

Similar themes have been reported by both Sbarbaro (2001), who demonstrated how the endorsement of local opinion leaders influenced product choice, and Kisa (2006), who demonstrated how physicians' experiences in medical school contributed to prescribing practice. These studies demonstrate how those considered to be authoritative sources by the newly qualified prescriber have an influence on prescribing practice. Fortunately the studies suggest that exposure to these influences can be reversed and it is believed that, as a consequence of personal and professional development, non-medical prescribers will acquire the skills and knowledge required to critically analyse current practice and make changes where appropriate.

Activity box 3.16

Identify two products that you prescribe regularly.
  Critically evaluate the influences that have informed your decision to prescribe these items.

Hall et al (2003b) indicate that the prescriber's and/or the patient's previous experience of the product can influence the prescribing decision. Prescribers reported more confidence in their prescribing decisions if they had previous experience of the product and if the patient had no previous reactions to it. One word of caution is that reliance on previous experience may limit the prescriber's individual formulary (the development of which is promoted in Chapter 5), thus impacting on the delivery of evidence-based practice. This concern is supported by the additional finding, from the study by Hall et al (2008), that the main influence on product choice resulted from the prescriber's previous experience of it. Thereafter the favoured item was changed only if the product was not considered effective in terms of healing rates or, in the case of patient discomfort.

Schumock et al (2004) found that physicians, pharmacists and formulary committee members rated safety of the product as highly influential to prescribing. It is reasonable to argue that non-medical prescribers would not knowingly prescribe a product that was unsafe. The Medicines Safety Agency (MSA) publish alerts when products are found to be unsafe, and the non-medical prescriber has a responsibility to access the MSA reports to check if there are any safety issues associated with products that they intend to prescribe.

Activity box 3.17

Access the Medicines and Healthcare products Regulatory Agency to see the latest monthly updates on drug safety issues at www.mhra.gov.uk.

External influences on prescribing practice

Pharmaceutical companies

The UK pharmaceutical Industry has been described as the world's third largest exporter of medicines (www.dh.gov.uk/en/Healthcare/medicinespharmacyandindustry/DH_866). In 2004, 73 000 people were directly employed in the UK pharmaceutical industry, and £3.2 billion was invested in UK-based research and development. The total NHS research and development budget for 2005–6 was £650 million.

The Association of the British Pharmaceutical Industry (ABPI) is the trade association for pharmaceutical companies that produce prescription medicines in the UK. Its member companies research, develop, manufacture and supply more than 90% of the medicines prescribed through the NHS. The Pharmaceutical industry is governed by the Department of Health and members of the ABPI hold key positions on committees where they represent the views of the industry to the Government and politicians.

In recognition of the harm that inappropriate use of medicines can cause, the advertising of medicines is controlled by a combination of statutory measures (with both criminal and civil sanctions). The advertising standards are enforced by the Medicines and Healthcare products Regulatory Agency (MHRA) and self-regulation through codes of practice for the pharmaceutical industry.

The MHRA, as licensing authority, has a statutory duty on behalf of ministers to consider breaches of the Medicines Act 1968 and Regulations on the promotion of medicines. Its key function is to protect public health by promoting the safe use of medicines, ensuring that they are honestly promoted with regard to their benefits, uses and effects, in compliance with current legislation. All advertising and promotion of medicines must be responsible and of the highest standard to ensure the safe use of medicines, both in self-medication and where medical supervision is required. To this end, the MHRA has devised guidelines for the advertising and promotion of medicines in the UK. The MHRA's Advertising Standards Unit routinely scrutinises medical journals and magazines available to the general public and checks samples of advertisements before their publication in order to ensure safe and honest promotion.

 Activity box 3.18

Access the MHRA Guidance Note 23 *The blue guide: Advertising and promotion of medicines in the UK* at www.mhra.gov.uk.

Pharmaceutical companies are continually pushing the boundaries of knowledge and a greater understanding of human physiology, e.g. neurology, endocrinology and the newly defined science of proteins contribute to an increased understanding of how medicines work. However, the continued expansion of knowledge about pharmacology is accompanied by the medicalisation of lifestyle problems (Fitzpatrick 2005), which has inevitably resulted in the development and marketing of lifestyle drugs. Issues related to lifestyle, such as alcohol and drug dependency, obesity and impotence, are now being seen as diseases, with an expectation that medication can be used to treat these.

According to Komesaroff and Kerridge (2002) drug promotion and marketing consumed a quarter to a third of drug company budgets in 2000. Therefore the need for these two strategies to be effective is clear. To successfully maintain their place in the market, pharmaceutical companies spend vast amounts of money on intensive marketing campaigns. These campaigns involve a variety of strategies including advertising, sponsorship, funding for professional development and personal selling (Crock 2009). One of the most effective strategies to influence prescribing practice is dissemination of product information by company representatives. Pharmaceutical representatives are very knowledgeable about the products produced by their companies. Indeed in a healthcare environment where information is constantly updated, many non-medical prescribers rely on pharmaceutical representatives as valuable sources of information.

As many non-medical prescribers increasingly come to rely on information provided by pharmaceutical companies to inform prescribing decisions, it could be argued that the evidence base affecting prescribing practice is at risk. Hall et al (2008) proposed that this reliance could ultimately result in prescribing patterns being controlled by the pharmaceutical industry rather than local trusts or the NPC. Indeed Crock (2009) found that prescribing behaviour was altered in favour of sponsors' products and that the evidence base underpinning practice was reduced after sponsorship by drug companies. Although there is little evidence available in the literature related to the impact of the pharmaceutical industry on non-medical prescribing, there is no reason to believe that non-medical prescribers are any less likely to be influenced than doctors. To avoid this scenario, the prescriber is reminded of the need for healthy scepticism when considering the use of resources provided by pharmaceutical companies. They are also referred back to the prescribing competency frameworks: HPC (2006), NMC (2006) and RPSB (2006).

The relationship between non-medical prescribers and the pharmaceutical companies could be described as tenuous. On the one hand, they can act as valuable resources of information for both prescribers and patients, and on the other their selling strategies, including the provision of inducements, could lead to ethical and professional compromise (Crock 2009). One strategy introduced to minimise the risk of bias and unethical prescribing has been the need for presentations given by pharmaceutical company representative to be based on scientific or educational content. Indeed many trusts have introduced policies that influence the relationship between non-medical prescribers and pharmaceutical companies. In response to concerns about the relationship between the industry and healthcare providers The ABPI has devised a code of conduct that provides guidance related to the marketing of their products. The ABPI's Code of Practice is drawn up in consultation with the BMA, RPSGB and MCA. It aims to ensure that the promotion of medicines is carried out in a responsible, ethical and professional manner (ABPI 2006).

The pharmaceutical industry also employs advertising as a way to communicate and influence prescribing behaviour. Advertising is a paid form of non-personal communication that is transmitted through the mass media. It has a range of purposes which include stimulating demand, educating the market's customers, increasing the use of a product, or to remind and reinforce customers' behaviour (Dibb et al 2005).

It has been estimated to cost £433m to get a new drug on to the market (Kmietowic 2004) so the need for a financial return is clear. The effectiveness of any advertising media depends on how many people are exposed to the message (Dibb et al 2005). Strategic marketing for the pharmaceutical industry includes advertising in high impact journals. These are professional journals that are known to reach the target audience, in this case prescribers. The inclusion of promotional material and research funded by pharmaceutical companies might contradict the editorial board's obligation to maintain independence (Stokamer 2003). Nevertheless many peer-reviewed nursing and medical journals rely on the inclusion of advertisements for their fiscal survival. Scott et al (2004) found that pharmaceutical advertising in medical journals influenced doctors' prescribing behaviour through both the scientific validity of the text and the images used to convey the message. These two components may not necessarily influence non-medical prescribers; however, each advertisement is underpinned by the psychology of consumer behaviour (Dibb et al 2005).

Many readers will consider themselves unlikely to be influenced by this particular marketing approach. However, studies regularly demonstrate how prescribing patterns have been changed as a consequence of advertisement campaigns (Bradford et al 2006, Davies and Hemingway 2006, Dean and Webb 2007). According to Dibb et al (2005) the aim of advertising is to bring about changes in behaviour. In the case of pharmaceutical industry, it is to influence decisions so that the product being promoted is prescribed.

To communicate effectively an advertisement uses words, symbols and illustrations that are meaningful, familiar and attractive to the target audience. The intention is that the format will grab attention, gain interest and make the product appear desirable; the ultimate outcome is that the consumer will be encouraged to take action (Dibb et al 2005). An advertisement often contains text, artwork or illustrations, and has a specific layout. Illustrations or images are used to attract attention and to communicate an idea quickly. If they are successful, the reader is encouraged to engage with the verbal portion of the advertisement which enhances its potential for success. The aim of the advertising message is to systematically move the reader thorough a persuasive sequence. To achieve this, copywriters apply the following guidelines when devising advertisements:

- Identify a specific desire or problem
- Suggest the product as the best way to satisfy that desire or solve the problem
- State the advantages and benefits of the product
- Indicate why the product is the best for the buyer's particular situation
- Substantiate the claims and advantages
- Ask the buyer for action (Dibb et al 2005).

Activity box 3.19

Identify an advertisement in any professional journal to which you subscribe.
   Consider the strategic placement of the advertisement, e.g. in between articles of particular relevance to your field of practice.
   Critically evaluate the advertisement in relation to the five objectives outlined by Dibb et al (2005).

The media

Although reference has been made to the influence of pharmaceutical companies on prescribing, it is important that we do not overlook the impact of the media, because this is perhaps more subtle. Media communication is a complex activity based on utilisation of a range of different communication channels and communications psychology. Often when we refer to the media we envisage television and newspapers. However, a wide range of communication strategies is encompassed by the term. Electronic media, such as television and cinema, and print media, such as newspapers and magazines, are important advertisement media. The potential for advertisements to influence prescribing is evident when we consider advances in telecommunications such as email and the internet, which facilitate dissemination of information to a worldwide audience.

As the policy makers move increasingly towards the concept of patient autonomy, the distribution of health information gains momentum. Indeed the internet is gaining prominence as a source of information for patients. This is not necessarily a positive thing because some internet sources and information shared in forums can have questionable evidence bases. Nevertheless, patients do use the internet and may arrive at the consultation equipped with sufficient knowledge to influence the prescribing decision. Recognition that patient expectations may not necessarily be underpinned by relevant and accurate information is crucial. Non-medical prescribers will need to exercise a range of communication skills including active listening, discernment and tact.

Most importantly, if the success of the consultation is to be guaranteed, the prescriber will need an awareness of current health messages, an accurate knowledge base and the ability to communicate effectively (Berry et al 2008).

It is likely that you will be able to identify something in the media that has influenced prescribing practice. Perhaps one of the most influential has been the impact of the mumps, measles and rubella study (MMR) and the impact this had on the uptake of immunisation. More recently the papillomavirus immunisation has been in the spotlight. The influence that the media has on prescribing can be seen from the two examples provided: this influence can be positive, e.g. the increased uptake of screening after the death of Jade Goody or negative, e.g. in the case of a report suggesting a link between autism and the MMR immunisation (which was subsequently disproved). In the case of mass public health campaigns, e.g. influenza, it may be that an increased number of patients are requesting immunisation as a consequence of concentrated media communication strategies.

Activity box 3.20

Consider how a phenomenon recently reported in the press has impacted on your prescribing practice.

It could be that patients are more aware of the issue and are therefore asking your advice. On the other hand, it may be that you have noticed that your client group is more knowledgeable about the health topic.

Other professionals

Relationships with the wider multidisciplinary team

The emphasis on team working and collaboration within healthcare is evident within Government policy. Indeed, in prescribing it is indicated as a competency prescribers must demonstrate (NMC 2006). Professional codes of conduct also direct us towards the importance of team working (General Pharmaceutical Council 2010, HPC 2006, NMC 2009). The issues relating to multidisciplinary team working are explored at length in Chapter 6. A key message from that chapter is that non-medical prescribing can improve multiprofessional working.

While et al (2005) demonstrated how insufficient understanding of roles and the lack of a shared view compound the difficulties related to prescribing decisions. In their view the understanding of different roles is crucial to the success and safety of prescribing. Cooper et al (2008) reiterated the challenges presented by insufficient understanding of roles when referring to supplementary pharmacist prescribers. Similar to Bradley and Nolan (2007), Courtney (2008), Cooper et al (2008) examined professional relationships and the need for clarity about the practitioner's own role and the boundaries of prescribing. As support from within the immediate prescribing team is particularly helpful in the context of non-medical prescribing, it is important that members of the multidisciplinary team are made aware of the role of the non-medical prescriber (Bradley and Nolan 2007). The way that GPs work with prescribers can be variable with Fisher (2005a, 2005b), demonstrating how some are happy with the arrangement whereas others continue to have concerns. Existing relationships between the medical professionals and prescribers have been analysed by Rana et al (2009). Senior staff, such as consultants, were found to be less concerned about safety aspects of non-medical prescribing than junior doctors. According to Rana et al (2009) this is possibly because the consultants knew the non-medical prescriber better than the junior doctors did and were therefore more confident in their abilities.

Communication and the transfer of appropriate information are a cornerstone of safe prescribing practice, and keeping members of the team informed of prescribing decisions is vital to ensure safety and continuity of care. In addition to patient safety keeping others informed of prescribing decisions, either orally or in writing, is considered an effective strategy to raise their awareness of the non-medical prescribing role. It is also a way to avoid misunderstandings, share knowledge and most importantly build trust (Stenner and Courtney 2008). To appreciate the benefits that team working can generate and to enhance safety in prescribing, the practitioner needs to be aware of local policies relating to dialogue and communication with other agencies as well as other members of the care team.

Lewis-Evans and Jester (2004) referred to other members of the multidisciplinary team and their influence on prescribing practice, particularly in respect of support for the prescriber. The contribution of pharmacists' specialist knowledge and how this was used to develop nurse prescribers' practice has been highlighted (Lewis-Evans and Jester 2004). Pharmacists were seen as having greater knowledge of wound care products than GPs and were therefore more readily approached than GPs for advice about prescriptions.

The evidence demonstrates that successful implementation of non-medical prescribing is influenced by the nature of existing relationships (Wells et al 2009). Indeed Cooper et al (2008) highlighted how relationships between non-medical prescriber pharmacists and hospital managers and doctors have a major influence on implementation. Similar findings have been presented by Nolan et al (2001), Fisher (2005a, 2005b) and Stenner and Courtney (2008). The strength of this evidence suggests that new non-medical prescribers would be advised to cultivate their relationship with not only the current prescriber but also all members of the multidisciplinary care team.

 Activity box 3.21

Critically reflect on the relationships that currently exist between yourself and other members of the multidisciplinary team.

Identify areas of potential strength and weakness in relation to your role as a non-medical prescriber.

Consider how you might prepare the multidisciplinary team for the changes to practice that will result as a consequence of your developing role as a prescriber.

The aim of this chapter was to briefly explore some of the issues related to prescribing practice: prescriber, patient, product and other professionals. It is acknowledged that the content is not exhaustive. Reading the chapter and working through the suggested activities will enable readers to critically evaluate the factors that influence their own practice. They will then be able to identify strategies that can be implemented in order to minimise potential influencing factors and subsequently enhance their practice.

Key themes: conclusions and considerations

Public health	The ability for individuals to undertake a public health approach within the context of non-medical prescribing will be impacted on by influences relating to the prescriber, patient, product and other professionals
	Consider how, in relation to four key areas of influence stated above, your ability to adopt a public health approach may be aided or hindered
Social and cultural issues	Social and cultural issues have been shown to have a significant impact on health and health beliefs
	Consider your learning needs in relation to cultural issues and identify how these needs may be met
Prescribing principles	The prescribing principles not only influence prescribing but are also influenced (in terms of how they are utilised) by the influences relating to the prescriber, patient, product and other professionals
	Consider how the prescriber, patient, product and other professionals influence your ability to 'consider the appropriate strategy' (prescribing principle 2)

References

Aronson J (2004) Classifying drug interactions. *Br J Clin Pharmacol* **58**(4).

Association of the British Pharmaceutical Industry (2006) *Code of Practice for the Pharmaceutical Industry*. London: ABPI.

Avery G, Todd J, Green G, Sains K (2007) Non-medical prescribing: the doctor-nurse relationship revisited. *Nurse Prescrib* **5**: 109-13.

Barber P, Robertson D (2009) *Essentials of Pharmacology for Nurses*. Maidenhead: McGraw-Hill.

Berry-Caban C, Crespo H (2008) Cultural competency as a skill for health care providers. *Hispanic Health Care Int* **6**: 115-21.

Berry D, Bradlow A, Courtney M (2008) Patients' attitudes towards, and information needs in relation to, nurse prescribing in rheumatology. *J Clin Nurs* **17**: 266-73.

Bond C, Hannaford P (2003) Issues related to monitoring the safety of over-the-counter (OTC) medicines. *Drug Safety* **26**: 1065-77.

Bradford D, Kleit A, Nietert P, Steyer T, McIlwain T, Ornstein S (2006) How direct-to-consumer- television advertising for osteoarthritis drugs affects physicians' prescribing behaviour. *Health Affairs* **25**: 1371-6.

Bradley E, Nolan P (2007) Impact of nurse prescribing: a qualitative study. *J Adv Nurs* **59**: 120-8.

Carey N, Stenner K, Courtney M (2009a) Stakeholder views on the impact of nurse prescribing on dermatology services. *J Clin Nurs* **19**: 498-506.

Carey N, Stenner K, Courtney M (2009b) Adopting the prescribing role in practice: exploring nurses' views in a specialist children's hospital. *Paediatr Nurs* **21**: 25-9.

Carey N, Stenner K, Courtenay M (2010) Stakeholder views on the impact of nurse prescribing on dermatology services. *J Clin Nurs* **19**: 498-506.

Cioffi RNJ (2003) Communicating with culturally and linguistically diverse patients in an acute care setting: nurses' experiences. *Int J Nurs Studies* **40**: 299-306.

Cooper R, Anderson C, Avery T, et al (2008) Stakeholders' view of UK nurse and pharmacist supplementary prescribing. *J Health Service Res Policy* **13**: 215-21.

Courtney M (2007) Nurse prescribing - the benefits and the pitfalls. *J Commun Nurs* **21**: 11-14.

Courtney M (2008) Nurse prescribing, policy, practice and evidence base. *Br J Commun Nurs* **13**: 563-6.

Creedon R, O'Connell E, McCarthy G, Lehane B (2009) An evaluation of nurse prescribing. Part 1: A literature review. *Br J Nurs* **18**: 1322-7.

Crock E (2009) Ethics of pharmaceutical company relationships with the nursing profession: no free lunch .... and no more pens? *Contemp Nurse* **33**: 202-9.

Crouch S, Chapelhow C (2008) *Medicines Management, A Nursing Perspective*. Harlow: Pearson Education Ltd.

Davies J, Hemingway S (2006) Pharmaceutical influences - nurse prescribers: eyes wide open. *Nurse Prescriber* **1**(12): e224.

Day P (2007) School nurse independent prescribing in practice. *Br J School Nurs* **2**: 267-71.

Dean J, Webb J (2007) Disease mongering a challenge for everyone involved in healthcare. *Br J Clin Pharmacol* **64**: 122-4.

Department of Health (2006) *Improving Patients' Access to Medicines: A guide to implementing nurse and pharmacist independent prescribing within the NHS in England*. London: The Stationery Office.

Department of Health and Social Security (1986) *Neighbourhood Nursing: A focus for care (Cumberledge Report)*. London: HMSO.

Dibb S, Simkin L, Pride W, Ferrell O (2005) *Marketing: Concepts and strategies*, 5th European edn. New York: Houghton Mifflin.

Dimond B (2005) Explaining common deficiencies that occur in record keeping, *Br J Nurs* **14**: 568-70.

Fisher R (2005a) District nurses: relationships in nurse prescribing. *Br J Commun Nurs* **9**: 416-19.

Fisher R (2005b) Relationships in nurse prescribing in district nursing practice in England: a preliminary investigation. *Int J Nurs Pract* **11**: 102-7.

Fitzpatrick M (2005) Selling sickness: how drug companies are turning us all into patients. *BMJ* **331**: 701.

French G (2002) What is the evidence on evidence-based nursing? An epistemological concern. *J Adv Nurs* **37**: 250-257.

General Pharmaceutical Council (2010) *Standards of Conduct, Ethics and Performance*. London: GPhC.

George J, McCaig D, Bond C, Cunningham I, Diak H, Stewart D (2007) Benefits and challenges of prescribing training and implementation: perceptions and early experiences of RPSGB prescribers. *Int J Pharm Pract* March 2007: 23-30.

Granby T (2005) Evidence-based prescribing. *Nurse Prescriber* **2**(2) (online). Available at: www.nurse-presciber.co.uk (accessed 4 February 2010).

Granby T, Chapman S (2004) Evidence-based prescribing. In: Courtney M, Griffiths M (eds), *Independent and Supplementary Prescribing: An essential guide*. London: Greenwich Media, Chapter 10.

Guillame L, Cooper R, Avery A et al (2008) supplementary prescribing by community and primary care pharmacists: an analysis of PACT data, 2004-2006. *J Clin Pharm Therap* **33**: 11-16.

Hall J, Cantrill J, Noyce P (2003a) The information sources used by community nurse prescribers. *Br J Nursing* **12**: 810-18.

Hall J, Cantrell J, Noyce P (2003b) Influences on community nurse prescribing. *Nurse Prescrib* **1**: 127-32.

Hall J, Cantrill J, Noyce P (2004) Managing independent prescribing: the influence of primary care trusts on community nurse prescribing. *Int J Pharmaceut Pract* **12**: 133-9.

Hall J, Cantrill J, Noyce P (2006) Why don't trained community nurse prescribers prescribe? *J Clin Nurs* **15**: 403-12.

Hall J, Noyce P, Cantrill J (2008) Why do district nurse prescribers alter their prescribing patterns? *Br J Commun Nurs* **13**: 507-13.

Harrison A (2003) Mental health service users' views of nurse prescribing. *Nurse Prescrib* **1**: 78-85.

Harvey J, Lawson V (2009) The importance of health belief models in determining self-care behaviour in diabetes. *Diabetic Med* **26**: 5-13.

Health Professions Council (2006) *HPC In Focus*, Issue 6. London: HPC.

Hobson R, Sewell G (2006) Supplementary prescribing by pharmacists in England. *Am J Health-System Pharmacol* **63**: 244-53.

Hughes C, Lapane K, Watson K, Davies H (2007) Does organisational culture influence prescribing in care homes for older people? *Drugs Ageing* **24**: 81-93.

Hughes L, Whittlesea C, Luscomb D (2002) Patients' knowledge and perceptions of the side effects of over the counter medication. *J Clin Pharm Therap* **27**: 243-8.

Jones A, Jones M (2005) Mental health nurse prescribing: issues for the UK. *J Psychiatr Mental Health Nurs* **12**: 527-35.

Kimmer E, Christian A (2005) A review of the usefulness and efficacy of independent nurse prescribing. *Nurse Prescrib* **3**: 39-42.

Kisa S (2006) Factors that influence prescribing decisions among Turkish physicians. *Clin Res Regulat Affairs* **23**: 177-89.

Komesaroff P, Kerridge I (2002) Ethical issues concerning the relationship between medical practitioners and the pharmaceutical industry. *Med J Aust* **176**: 118-21.

Kmietowic Z (2004) Drug company influences extend to nurses, pharmacists and patient groups. *BMJ* **329**: 1206.

Lado E, Vacariza M, Fernandez-Gonzales C, Gestal-Otero J, Figueiras A (2008) Influence exerted on drug prescribing by patients' attitudes and expectations and by doctors' perception of such expectations: a cohort and nested case-control study. *J Eval Clin Pract* **14**: 453-9.

Langer N (2008) Integrating Compliance, communication, and culture: delivering health care to an ageing population. *Educ Gerontol* **34**: 385-96.

Latter S (2008) Safety and quality in independent prescribing: an evidence review. *Nurse Prescrib* **6**: 59-66.

Latter S, Maben J, Myall M, Young A (2007) Evaluating nurse prescribers' education and continuing professional development for independent prescribing practice: findings from a national survey in England. *Nurse Educ Today* **27**: 685-96.

Lewis-Evans A, Jester R (2004) Nurse prescribers' experiences of prescribing. *Issues Clin Nurs* **13**: 796-805.

Leyshon J (2007) Correct technique of using aerosol inhaler devices .... art and science clinical skills: 15. *Nurs Stand* **21**(52): 38-40.

McKinley R, Middleton J (1999) What do patients want from doctors? Content analysis of written patient agendas for the consultation. *Br J Gen Pract* **49**: 796-800.

Mead N, Bower P (2000) Patient-centredness: a conceptual framework and review of the empirical literature. *Soc Sci Med* **51**: 1087-110.

National Prescribing Centre (1999) Signposts for prescribing nurses – general principles of good prescribing. *Prescrib Nurse Bull* **1**(1).

Nolan P, Haque S, Badger F, Dyke R, Khan I (2001) Mental health nurses' perceptions of nurse prescribing. *J Adv Nurs* **36**: 527-34.

Nursing and Midwifery Council (2006) *Standards of Proficiency for Nurse and Midwife Prescribers*. London: NMC.

Nursing and Midwifery Council (2009) *Standards of Educational Preparation for Prescribing from the Nurse Prescribers Formulary for Community Practitioners for Nurses without a Specialist Practitioner Qualification* – Introducing Code V150, NMC Circular 02/2009. London: NMC.

Office for National Statistics (2003) *Census 2001 Ethnicity: Population Size. National Statistics.* Available at: www.nationalstatistics.gov.uk.

Offredy M (2002) Decision-making in primary care: outcomes from a study using patient scenarios. *J Adv Nurs* **40**: 532-41.

Ogden J (1996) *Health Psychology: A textbook*. Milton Keynes: Open University Press.

Otway C, Bowskill D (2006) Prescribing for patients where English is not a first language: a pilot study. *Nurse Prescrib* **3**: 110-14.

Morran C (2007) Auditing prescribing practice in an acute setting. *J Assoc Nurse Prescrib* November: 12-13.

Rana T, Bradley E, Nolan P (2009) Survey of psychiatrists' views of nurse prescribing, *J Psychiatr Mental Health Nurs* **16**: 257-67.

Robinson F (2010) Seventh Annual Nurse Prescribing Conference: Continued challenges for prescribers. *Pract Nurse* **39**: 9.

Royal Pharmaceutical Society of Great Britain (2006) *Outline Curriculum for Training Programmes to Prepare Pharmacist Prescribers*. London: RPSGB.

Sains K (2008) Formularies: types, uses, pros and cons. *Pract Nurse* **36**: 17-20.

Sbarbaro J (2001) Can we influence prescribing patterns? *Clin Infect Dis* **33**(suppl 3): 240-4.

Schumock G, Walton S, Park H et al (2004) Factors that influence prescribing decisions. *Ann Pharmacother* **38**: 557-62.

Scott T, Stanford N, Thompson D (2004) Killing me softly: myth in pharmaceutical advertising. *BMJ* **329**: 1484-7.

Stenner K, Courtney M (2008) The role of inter-professional relationships and support for nurse prescribing in acute and chronic pain. *J Adv Nurs* **63**: 276-83.

Stenner K, Carey N, Courtney M (2010) How nurse prescribing influences the role of nursing. *Nurse Prescrib* **8**: 29-34.

Stokamer C (2003) Pharmaceutical gift giving: analysis of an ethical dilemma. *J Nurs Admin* **33**: 48-51.

Thompson D (2007) Personal reflections of pharmacist independent prescribing. *Nurse Prescrib* **5**: 311-13.

Thurtle V (2007) Challenges in health visitor prescribing in a London primary care trust. *Community Practitioner* **80**(11): 26-30.

Wells J, Bergin M, Gooney M, Jones A (2009) Views on nurse prescribing: a survey of community mental health nurses in the Republic of Ireland. *J Psychiatr Mental Health Nurs* **16**: 10-17.

While A, Biggs K (2007) Benefits and challenges of nurse prescribing. *J Adv Nurs* **45**: 559-67.

While A, Shah R, Nathan A (2005) Interdisciplinary working between community pharmacists and community nurses: the views of community pharmacists. *J Interprofess Care* **19**: 164-70.

Young D, Jenkins R, Mabbett M (2009) Nurse prescribing: an interpretive phenomenological analysis. *Primary Health Care* **19**(7): 32-6.

Chapter 4
Effective Consultation and 'the Consultation Umbrella'

Jane Rutt-Howard

Learning objectives

After reading this chapter and completing the activities within it, the reader will be able to:

1 appreciate the enormous value of therapeutic communication and the necessary investment into the non-medical prescriber and patient relationship
2 critically analyse the value of consultation models and the part that they play in helping to support safety in the process
3 demonstrate and evaluate the clinical decision-making strategies that underpin autonomous practice in assessment/examination, diagnosis and treatment

Safety is of paramount importance when considering any aspect of healthcare. It could be argued that in terms of prescribing, and particularly the novel, or novice (Benner 1984), non-medical prescriber, the tenet of safety must be paramount.

It is logical to expect that effective consultation between the patient and practitioner requires an ideal, or safe, structure, to enhance safety from the patient's, practitioner's and organisation's perspectives. From a prescribing perspective, this chapter is predominately concerned with step 1: consider the patient, although an effective consultation encompasses all the steps of the prescribing pyramid. Within the chapter, structure is facilitated via 'the consultation umbrella'.

Within this chapter, practitioner is the term used when referring to any non-medical prescriber (NMP), whether he or she be a nurse, pharmacist, physiotherapist or other health professional, and in some places the information is relevant to medical doctors. However, where necessary, distinction between practitioners is made. Use of the term 'practitioner' also includes those NMP students studying the various prescribing options: V100, V150 or V300 (independent and/or supplementary). In general, this chapter is relevant to all those studying towards the qualification or who have completed it and are prescribing.

The Textbook of Non-medical Prescribing, edited by Dilyse Nuttall and Jane Rutt-Howard.
© 2011 Blackwell Publishing Ltd

An effective consultation is something to which we should all aspire and it is something that can always be improved on (Neighbour 2005). Irrespective of our professional registration, our patients are our priority and our duty of care (Health Professions Council (HPC) 2007, General Pharmaceutical Council (GPhC) 2010, Nursing and Midwifery Council (NMC) 2008) is steeped in the ethical notion of beneficence.

It is purported that an effective consultation results in positive results (Thompson et al 2005) or clinical outcomes, or, as a minimum, acceptable outcomes for all those involved with the encounter. This chapter begins with a discussion on the discourse of the effective consultation.

For an effective consultation to happen, four key elements need to be addressed. Initially, practitioners need to understand the significance of *therapeutic communication* and how this element of caring can be honed to become more effective within a prescribing context. As we know, safety in prescribing is paramount and to this end a structure for our patient episodes will facilitate a systematic approach that enhances safety in decision-making. With regard to *decision-making*, this may be a complex multifaceted exercise or a simple task – depending on many dynamics. It was suggested (Luker et al 1998) that non-medical practitioners have greater difficulty with decision-making because of issues dealing with uncertainty. To understand these dynamics and complexities, an appreciation of the various strategies of decision-making is required. To complete this process of the patient encounter, the consultation needs to be performed in a competent and confident manner. It is not always easy, even for an expert practitioner, when embarking on, and executing, a new skill. In this instance, *consultation models* can prove very helpful.

Therefore the elements of the consultation that need to be explored within an NMP context include: the value of therapeutic communication; consultation models in context and the consultation as a skill; application/interpretation of clinical decision-making; and a shift in practice for expert practitioners taking on board a novice skill and its implications.

Within this chapter, the term 'consultation' is used to represent any patient episode. Sometimes, the medical connotations of the word 'consultation' can be misleading or off-putting for non-medical practitioners, but it could successfully be argued that any patient encounter is a consultation (to seek counsel) when taking the *Oxford English Dictionary*'s (Pearsall and Trumble (Eds) 2008) definition into consideration: 'a meeting arranged to consult, i.e. seek information or advice from'. So, patient visits, appointments, clinics, attending to a patient, all take place within the context of a consultation.

Presenting the consultation umbrella

The consultation umbrella has been constructed to help with this understanding. Take a little time to consider Figure 4.1. This umbrella provides a visual representation of a number of concepts. First, it offers protection: if its concept is integrated into routine clinical practice, it will afford a degree of safety and inclusivity. This is one of the major functions of any consultation model, as is seen below. It is also intended to demonstrate how pivotal the skills of therapeutic communication and clinical decision-making are to

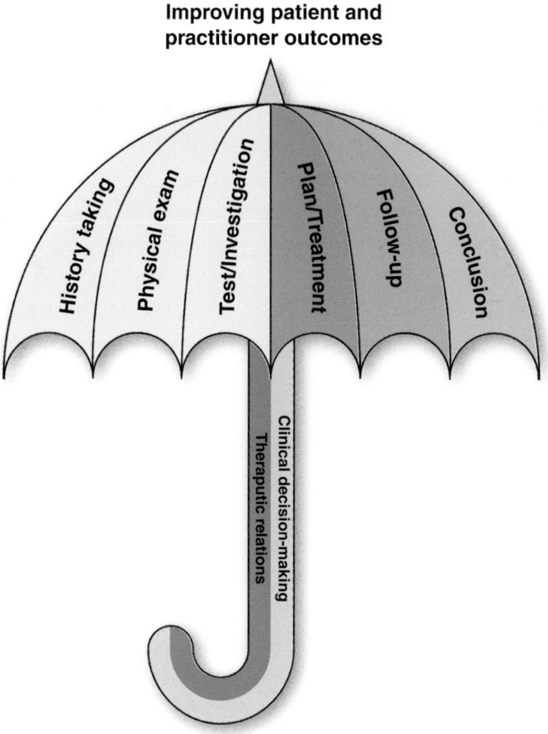

Figure 4.1 The use of colour to illustrate the similarities among three consultation models and their correlation with the consultation umbrella.

the success of the patient encounter. Finally, it is important to appreciate that a consultation model is an umbrella term for many elements of a patient encounter. Under this umbrella, for example, there are elements such as history taking and necessary investigations. To take this a step deeper, within history taking there are a number of strategies that can help with this, such as Morton's symptom analysis tool (Morton 1993).

The consultation umbrella also has a number of shades which correlate with other elements of existing consultation models, to help with consistency and analysis. This is discussed later in the chapter.

Consultation models in context

This chapter relates largely to the prescribing pyramid's first step: consider the patient (National Prescribing Centre (NPC) 1999). When this first step is executed well, the other steps can follow with increased confidence. Experience within a patient encounter, or consultation, can vary from what might be considered a straightforward process of presentation, diagnosis and prescription to a complicated process that culminates in no real end-points. The former can leave the practitioner feeling either satisfied and complete or perhaps unchallenged. The latter can equally leave the practitioner satisfied at meeting a challenge or frustrated that answers are not available. It is important to be reassured that it is the same for all practitioners and that this depends on many circumstances. The global answer is to be able to make sense of the consultation, e.g. using a consultation model, especially in a protected student environment (while training to become a registered NMP) can help to unravel the complexities and enable the practitioner to reflect, and therefore 'grow', appropriately.

Reflection on existing consultation models

To help ease the understanding of the many consultation models that have been published, it is useful to divide them into two categories. The general trend (but by no means a certainty) is that the early work around consultation models focused on understanding the communications and interactions between the players in the consultation. The latter work, while embracing the early work, tends to lean towards a task-oriented structure. More accurately, perhaps, they address the same communications and interactions but put them clearly within the structure of the consultation.

It is pertinent, at this juncture, to champion consultation models for all areas of healthcare, irrespective of the practitioner, the aim of the interaction or where the interaction takes place. It can be frustrating when some criticise the models for being too primary care focused, or just applicable to medical staff. It is argued, and defended, that, after internalisation of these models, they can easily be transferred to any setting or situation and be used by anyone interacting with patients. In fact, there is much within the body of knowledge that is easily transferred *outside* the healthcare setting.

There are many consultation models available which have been developed since the 1950s when Balint (1957 cited in Balint et al 1983) published his work *The Doctor, His Patient and The Illness*, based on observational studies of general practitioners at the notable Tavistock Clinic in London. Balint's work (1957 cited in Balint et al 1993) set the scene for doctors and all healthcare practitioners to help make sense of their interactions with their patients. He explored the way in which relationships developed between doctors and their patients, and coined such terms as: the apostolic function; the drug doctor; the sick role; and the long consultation, which are still relevant today. Interestingly, even though the shape of healthcare and the relationships between the providers and users have changed beyond recognition when compared with Balint's time, his work is still relevant. Furthermore, it almost certainly was the catalyst for our interest beyond the presenting illness or disease: it can clearly be seen that his work has a psychological underpinning.

Another notable piece of work is that of Berne (1970), who looked at more than just the patient but at the interactions between the patient and the doctor. As a result he developed three 'ego-states' that could be applied to the interactions: adult, parent and child. Later on, stroppy teenager was added. In an ideal consultation, both participants would behave in a rational and logical 'adult' state. However, the other ego states can be recognised when the consultation does not go smoothly and the practitioner begins to reflect on what went wrong: what games were being played. It is a fascinating body of work that is well worth reading – it can be used as a tool for reflection (prescribing pyramid step 7, NPC 1999) to help understand why perhaps an interaction did not go as well as it should. It can also be used, once familiar with it, to anticipate responses and ideally diffuse potential conflict, or simply to help direct a consultation in order to bring two adult states together.

Meantime, there is an analysis of three of the more contemporary models in use: Neighbour's Inner Consultation (Neighbour 2005); Pendelton et al's New Consultation (Pendleton et al 2003); and Kurtz et al's Enhanced Calgary-Cambridge Guide (Kurtz et al 2003). The backdrop of these three models will contextualise the consultation umbrella, which is intended to encompass all the models within an intuitive and diagrammatical framework.

If the constituent parts of the models are considered (Figure 4.2), it can be seen that fundamentally they are the same - or certainly they have common themes. If we consider the fact that they are all attempting to portray the practitioner-patient consultation within a framework, it could be argued that they need to be similar. All patient interactions and consultations are bound by the same aim: what is wrong and how can it be fixed (in the main).

To help contextualise Figure 4.2, it is necessary to take a brief look at Neighbour's Inner Consultation (Neighbour 2005), within which he puts the consultation into a dynamic journey. Thus, his five checkpoints are five points within a patient's journey that must be met, or reached. The content of his journey is not so obvious when reading just the checkpoint headings, but, when you appreciate the skills and activity required to move from one checkpoint to another, you understand the nuances of the model. Thus, connecting is not just about initial rapport but includes history taking, physical examination and potential investigations and/or tests. Only once this information has been gathered can the practitioner check in with summarising. Within summarising, Neighbour is diligent in mutual understanding or interpretation, in so much as the practitioner understands the patient, his or her ideas, concerns and expectations, understands the patient's interpretations of his or her symptoms, and also understands the social (including upbringing and education , as examples), economic and spiritual context of the patient. But summarising is also about ensuring that the patient understands that the practitioner understands too. Neighbour refers to the exchange of the vernacular and medical language in this shared understanding in a bid to reach mutual understanding.

Further along the journey, checkpoint 3 requires sufficient information/data to be able to do a handover - in terms of the management plan devised through the clinical decision-making process (to prescribe, or not to prescribe) and the practitioner's ability to convey this with such deftness that the patient is happy to implement the said plan. Influencing, negotiating and gift wrapping are terms that Neighbour uses to illustrate the variety of ways in which a handover can be achieved, accounting for the diverse patient base encountered in the clinical arena. Interestingly, safety netting is used to confirm what Neighbour would consider automatic, or take for granted within a consultation, yet deems it so important that it is given a checkpoint of its own. Rightly so, it is impossible to eliminate all uncertainty and therefore uncertainty needs to be accounted for and a degree of anticipatory actions are put in place, ideally before the patient's consultation is concluded.

Neighbour is onto a winner with his last checkpoint, or at least he should be! He gives credence to the fact that, as practitioners, we have a duty to look after ourselves in order to provide the best care possible. This may be the simple requirement for a break

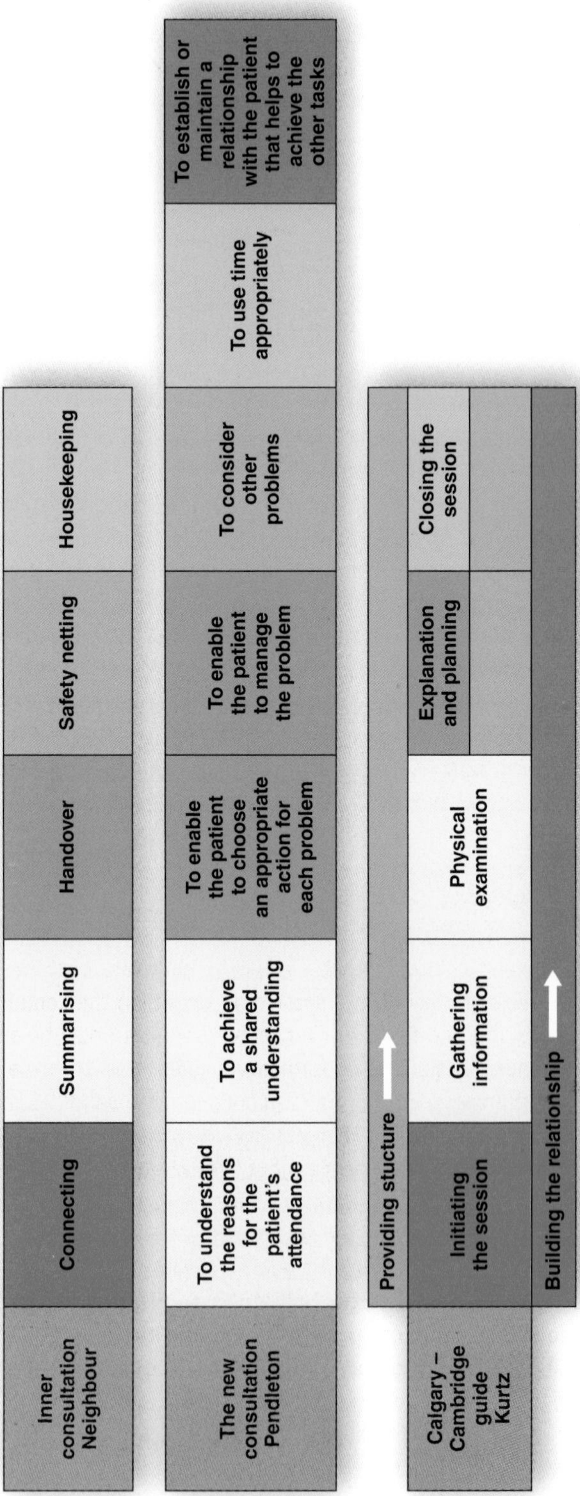

Figure 4.2 The Consultation Umbrella.

and refreshment or the time required for record keeping, documentation or reflection. We need to maintain our own 'person' in order to perform well. When we consider clinical decision-making, Croskerry (2005) recognises mismatches between the cognitive activity of the practitioner and the task in hand. When the complexity of the task is in alignment with cognitive ability, this leads to good decision-making, which in turn results in safe care. It is important to recognise when a practitioner's cognitive ability may be compromised – a busy clinical schedule, a challenging set of patients, unrealistic pressures at work, organisational frustrations or circumstances extraneous to the clinical situation, such as tiredness or hunger. As Croskerry (2005) succinctly proposes, to ensure patient safety and high-quality care, 'well-calibrated' practitioners are needed.

Often, we are asked to rationalise our actions and this is no less true in our prescribing decisions. It is purported that, by adhering to a consultation model, we invite structure and schema, thereby reducing omission and ensuring inclusivity. Also, there is a framework on which we can hang our rationale.

There would have been a time when the models of Neighbour, Pendleton et al and Kurtz et al were to be compared and contrasted but, in an attempt to do this, it was recognised that they are in fact complementary (Figure 4.2). Similar to our patients and colleagues, we are all individuals and will have a tendency to 'tune in' more so with one model than another. This tuning in could be based on the fact that it was the first model that the practitioner explored, or it may be because an existing model already closely resembles existing practice and therefore is perceived as being confirmatory. Alternatively, maybe one author's style of conveying their theory is perceived as more illuminating than another, i.e. it had a greater resonance with the individual practitioner. From experience, as you spend time researching these models in greater depth, it is advised to return to the original source where possible, before reading other opinions of them.

The value of therapeutic communication

As can be seen from the consultation umbrella (see Figure 4.1), both therapeutic relationships and clinical decision-making are the frame on which the remaining elements rely. Both need to be strong and firm in order for a consultation to be successful. The way in which practitioners and patients fulfil their roles, and the relationships that ensue, can influence a number of therapeutic outcomes (e.g. satisfaction, compliance, malpractice litigation) (McNeilis et al 1995). In other words, if you are not able to communicate effectively with your patient, you will not be able to elicit either sufficient or possibly accurate information and, without sufficient and accurate information, your clinical decisions will be fundamentally flawed and unsafe.

Neighbour (2005) highlights in his work that it is while talking with patients that a relationship evolves. As this takes place, both the patient and practitioner begin to acquire a greater sense of each other's views and positions within the presenting encounter, but a broader sense and appreciation of each other's individuality develop too. It is good to try to create a mental and emotional connection with your patient (Cohn 2007). An understanding of the patient's individuality is important, especially when it comes to interpreting the information gathered and negotiating the management plan.

Being aware of your own attributes is important (attitudes, emotions, knowledge, credibility) (Cohn 2007). To be self-aware is the first step in beginning to understand other people: it is only by being truly aware of the self that an honest connection can be established between the practitioner and the patient. This is the essence of valuing therapeutic communication within this context of non-medical prescribing because the outcomes of the decisions that need to be made with the associated degree of uncertainty rests significantly in the quality of the discourse between the stakeholders (Ellis et al 1995).

This understanding of each other within the consultation has been associated with improved health outcomes (Say and Thomson 2003) as a consequence of involving patients with the decision-making. It has been argued that relationship growth takes time and yet time is not always an available resource. Although it is recognised that evaluations of community matron roles (whose relationships with patients can develop over months and even years) demonstrate improved patient care because of the quality of the relationship and thus communication (Wright et al 2007), it is also recognised in the literature that practitioners [doctors] who see a patient for a single episode can be equally skilful at gaining a patients' trust and eliciting the necessary information (Elwyn et al 1999). This suggests that time is not a discerning factor in successful relationship evolvement and therefore must be related to other factors, e.g. the actual act of communicating. The essence of this relationship dynamism can be referred to as therapeutic communication.

Although it is appreciated that most practitioners will have a degree of underpinning knowledge regarding therapeutic communication, courtesy of pre-registration education, it needs to be reconceptualised in terms of prescribing. The apparent simple process of one person talking to another is in fact a highly complex and subtle skill (Ellis et al 1995). For many, the new skill of prescribing is the remaining frontier of the complete patient episode and this has far-reaching implications in terms of clinical outcomes and accountability. Practitioners (nurses) are happier with their clinical decision-making when the lines of accountability are clear and this is no exception with prescribing as a new skill (Luker et al 1998). Thus, therapeutic communication can enhance the consultation and result in safer outcomes that reduce uncertainty (Thompson et al 2005) and therefore help to ease the potential burden of decision-making. A revisit is worth the investment!

Therapeutic communication includes verbal communication and non-verbal communication, where verbal communication is the spoken word and non-verbal communication is concerned with body language and the impact that this has on the interaction. When discussing active listening, Cohn (2007) reiterates the concept of 'listening with all of one's sense's', not just one's ears. He is alluding to the fact that active listening also requires the use of vision: encompassing the interpretation of both verbal (hearing) and non-verbal communication (vision). Cohn claims that it is a mere 8% of communication that is conveyed within the content of a conversation and that the remaining is conveyed through the use of body language, and also the way in which the spoken word is said (use of intonation, volume, rate of speech, etc. – Williams 1997), otherwise referred to as paralinguistic features of verbal communication (Table 4.1) (Cohn 2007).

Table 4.1   Review of paralinguistic features of communication

Volume of voice	An adequate level of volume is required in order to be heard and thus understood, which is important when gathering and imparting information. This volume will need to be responsive to varying clinical situations: the volume of voice can be increased to maintain the patient's attention; it can be decreased when offering empathy or solace, as examples
Intonation	This relates to the pitch of the voice and its most significant role is in its ability to alter meaning of the spoken word
Rate of speech	When the rate of speech is just right the spoken word has clarity and accuracy. The rhythm of the sentence is optimum which enhances understanding. Too quick and clarity is clouded and there is a risk of misinterpretation. Too slow and there is the risk of the patient becoming disinterested or it may be difficult to maintain an appropriate level of concentration. Fast speech can be associated with loss of temper whereas slower speech can be associated with dominance but also when expressing sadness, as examples
Tone of voice	This is concerned with different aspects of the voice: pitch, volume, rate, quality and rhythm. In combination they convey emotion and information about attitudes. It is here that mixed messages can be illustrated when the tone of voice contradicts the words being spoken. It is suggested that the paralinguistic aspects of the conversation contain the true meaning rather than the actual words
Conversational oil	Also known as affecters, these are those phrases such as 'mm-hmm', 'that's right' and 'I see'. These are used to help the conversation progress by letting the speaker know that you are listening and also understanding (or not). Be mindful to ensure that these 'oils' are used constructively and that you are aware of how you are using them; subconsciously there is a risk that these affecters are interpreted as being negative, e.g. when using 'that's right' when it was more appropriate to disagree with the patient. This can happen when the practitioner may have been distracted or has momentarily disengaged with the conversation
Silence	The golden 2 minutes, as Moulton (2007) describes, is the first 2 minutes of the patient encounter whereby research has proved that, if the practitioner keeps silent, the patient will tell you almost everything that you need to know to draw your conclusions. This needs to be facilitated during the opening few seconds, but, if effective, can be very rewarding. Silence can be awkward and uncomfortable, yet it can also be powerful and empowering. Short silences are acceptable and can allow the patient to formulate answers or opinions, or encourage him or her to expand on certain issues, but longer silences need to be managed appropriately by the practitioner
	Silence can also be a cue to consider what is not being said, either 'conscious withholding' (e.g. not thinking that the information they have is relevant) or 'speech censoring' (e.g. when a patient holds back information unknowingly)

Adapted from Williams (1997) and Moulton (2007).

Activity box 4.1

Consider the statement:

'I'll see you in the library this afternoon.'

Ideally with a colleague, take it in turn to repeat this statement, as many times as you can, with alterations in your voice that give the statement a different meaning.

Now consider this in terms of the written word, e.g. when writing an email to a colleague.

Have you ever had an experience where the email was misinterpreted because the content was not conveyed with accompanying intonation? The reader of the email does not have the benefit of the tone of voice or body language to help with the interpretation of the meaning of the communication (Cohn 2007).

When engaging with your patients, in combination with the spoken word and its interpretation, the non-medical prescriber will need to appreciate the power of the unspoken word, i.e. non-verbal communication or body language. There is much involved with getting patients to tell you their story. There is also much to be said when conveying personal unspoken messages through the use of the practitioner's own body language – remember, communication has to involve at least two people, as a minimum (Lloyd and Bor 2004). Egan (2009) provides a useful checklist to help fine tune your body language – SOLER: sit **s**quarely in relation to the patient; **o**pen position; **l**ean slightly forward towards the patient; **e**ye contact; and **r**elax. Table 4.2 illustrates how each element interacts with our interpretations.

Developing relationships

This part of the chapter is an analysis of *developing* relationships. It is recognised that there is insufficient scope within this chapter to analyse all elements of the relationship, particularly those elements beyond the initiation of the relationship. Remember, it is the complete relationship 'package', the sum of the parts of which being equally important and worthy of investment, for the benefit of the improved clinical outcomes associated with a positive relationship.

Relationships are fundamental to understanding our interactions with patients. You may be meeting your patient for the first time where formal introductions and etiquette should be employed, especially in a non-time-critical episode. At other times, your patient may be known to you and therefore your initial 'hello' will be quite different. It is a skill in itself as to where to pitch your introductions. Too formal and you may appear intimidating, yet too informal and you may convey a feeling too blasé for the situation.

Your personality may dictate to some extent how formally or informally you portray yourself or conduct your consultations. Conversely, your patient may 'demand', by

Table 4.2 Body language

Gesture	This includes elements such as head nodding (affirmative, understanding, encouraging) or shaking (negative, insecurity, disapproval). The use of hand gestures can be powerful in helping to describe or explain particular issues. Hand gesturing can signify nervousness and anxiety. Steepling of the fingers expresses a degree of confidence, but could be interpreted as over-confident (note your patient's reaction if you do steeple your fingers and respond appropriately; alternatively, reflect on how you feel if faced with a patient using such hand gestures)
Facial expressions	Smiles (affirmative, accepting, positive), frowns (confusion, disagreement, negative), lips firmly shut (controlling; anger, sadness, humour) – notably eyes and mouth are where these data are captured
Eye contact	There is balance to be attained with eye contact: too much can be intimidating and too little may portray a notion of disinterestedness. In some cultures women believe that it is not appropriate to make eye contact, yet still need to engage in communication, which can be disarming for those of a western cultural background. In other cultures, young people are not encouraged to maintain eye contact with their elders for prolonged periods of time
Body posture	Cultural influences pervade here too: in western cultures people tend to stand just off-centre to each other, indicating friendly interactions or neutrality. This can also help to facilitate natural breaking of eye contact in a safe manner. However, some cultures have different codes of behaviour, which can lead to misunderstandings or even feelings of offence when there is a mismatch of beliefs. Generally try to sit at the same level as your patient, demonstrating equality. Also try to position your body such that arms are unfolded, legs uncrossed and back straight, ready to listen and be attentive
Body space and proximity	Don't sit or stand too near your patient which can be perceived as intimidating or threatening; don't invade his or her personal space. However, you also need to be near enough to hear, pick up on those unspoken communications and demonstrate an air of interestedness. 'Reach out and touch' is an ideal distance to place yourself (Moulton 2007)
Touch	'Touch is a potent carrier of messages' (Ellis et al 1995). Some non-medical prescribers, e.g. nurses, are more likely to be comfortable and natural about the business of touch; it could be suggested that it is an innate characteristic of being a nurse. However, it is also recognised that not all non-medical prescribers are as comfortable with this medium of conveying information. When appropriate, touch can be comforting, healing, reassuring, sympathising and emphasising. It can also be used to demonstrate power or not used to give a notion of not being connected with the patient. Of all these elements, it could be said that an unnatural use of touch could be the most transparent and that it may not be worth the sense of dishonesty if used artificially. However, trying to incorporate into usual practice can be the acquisition of a powerful tool to enhance communication, when used appropriately

Adapted from Ellis et al (1995), Shipley and Woods (1996), Lloyd and Bor (2004), Moulton (2007).

virtue of his or her dress code or accent, a more formal approach than others. Only by reading the situation, or picking up cues, will the non-medical prescriber be able to match up. This is not to say that we need to keep a wardrobe handy, but just a consideration about the way in which we respond to our patients. Just a note, a number of non-medical prescribers, by virtue of their advanced role, may not wear a uniform, so it is worth being mindful of the judgements that are made of our patients, and their attire, when choosing what to wear for work (Piasecki 2003).

Ideally, you want to try to match up the most appropriate introduction to the *individual* patient. To be able to do this, it may be that you need to rework your own usual habits. This could be considered a professional skill to be learnt, despite it not necessarily correlating with your own personal ethos. Put another way, while you may feel uncomfortable being formal in your approach because it is not your usual way, for the sake of professionalism and maximising the encounter you may need to reconsider your stance and be more adaptive. This of course works in either direction.

Activity box 4.2

Think about your own introductory style and list three reasons why it might be positive, and three reasons why it might be negative, to the success of the consultation.

Consider the ways in which you may need to modify your introductory style in order to enhance the new focus of safe prescribing.

Although the consultation is a single entity, there are many sectors within it: before you meet the patient; collecting or calling the patient; introductions and establishing the scene; 'everything in between'; and then the concluding of the consultation. The period of time before meeting the patient can be quite significant within the whole process (Moulton 2007), and yet can be dismissed as inconsequential. It is worthy of accepting this time as integral to the full episode and indeed the wider aspect of your working day. Depending on your individual place of work and the organisation of patient presentations, this period of non-patient contact will differ. Practitioners tend to use this time in different ways: revise the patient's previous records; deliberately don't revise previous notes and choose to see the patient 'blind'; pre-empt the situation and possibly begin considering some diagnostic hypothesis; or maybe spend the time engaging in some pre-encounter literature searching in anticipation of the next patient. There is no right or wrong way in which to spend this time and it will depend on your own clinical style. However, it is may be more relevant for some to appreciate that this is a defined period of time, which could be used in a more meaningful way, if the concept is new to you.

Within many clinical settings, typically either a patient is called into the consultation room/area via an intercom system connected to the waiting room or the practitioner will go and 'collect' the patient to accompany him or her back to the room/area. It is occasionally considered (Moulton 2007) an underrated segment of the consultation, yet to be able to embark upon initial patient interaction the success of this segment can determine, or certainly influence, the overall outcome.

Activity box 4.3

Take time to consider a patient episode that you have recently had where this time of 'collecting the patient', as part of the consultation, has been either maximised or, conversely, lost.

How might this affect the way in which you approach your patient interactions in the future, in terms of safe prescribing?

As eluded to earlier, the potential content of this chapter is vast. Therefore it needs to be highlighted that there are other areas of the therapeutic relationship worthy of consideration (identified in Table 4.3 and not covered specifically within this chapter).

Children and young people

Consultations with children need to be different and there needs to be an understanding of the differences in approach to the assessment of a child of a specific age, or developmental stage (Bickley and Szilagyi 2009). Table 4.4 is a useful guide relating specifically to these considerations but will be applicable only to those non-medical prescribers who actually consult with children and are competent to prescribe for them. However, it is not intended that this be a definitive guide to caring for children because this is not within the remit of this book. Legal issues, particularly in terms of consent, are covered in Chapter 2 and the physiological aspects of prescribing for children are covered in Chapter 8.

Table 4.3 Other considerations for enhancing therapeutic relationships

Patient's spiritual needs	Your own spiritual conscience
Patients from different cultural backgrounds	Your own cultural influences
Patient's first language	Is there a need for an interpreter?
Patient who may not be communicative	Chaperone requirements
Patient may be anxious or aggressive, upset or withdrawn	Is the patient capable of consent?
Patient may have hearing or speech problems	Is there a need for a person to sign?
Environmental factors	

Collated from Lloyd and Bor (2004).

Table 4.4 Consultations with children

Age	Developmental issues	Significant components of paediatric history	Approach to physical examination
Infant Up to 1 year	Stranger anxiety (7–9 months) Dislikes restraints	Birth history, prenatal history and activities of daily living (feeding, elimination, sleep) Parental coping, bonding and perception of infant's growth, development and health status	Can place on exam table before 4–6 months. After 6 months, infant mainly on parent's lap Traumatic procedures last. Parent involved if restraint necessary
Toddler 1–2 years	Egocentric Negativity Separation anxiety (peaks at 15–18 months) Development of autonomy Language skills starting Knows several body parts	Parental coping, bonding and perception of infant's growth, development and health status Issues such as tantrums, negativity and parent's response to increasing independence	Minimal physical contact initially Examine close by parent Use play to inspect body parts Parents to remove clothes Restrain only when necessary Traumatic procedures last Praise
Preschool Young child 2–5 years	Follows simple instructions Likes to help Fears bodily harm	Issues such as school readiness, discipline and sibling relationships discussed as appropriate	Keep parent close by Prefers sitting or standing. Sequencing influenced by child's behaviour Request self-undressing Use play techniques Allow equipment to be inspected Praise
School age Older child	Industrious Self-control increases Understanding of cause and effect develops	School performance Increasing participation of child in history	Privacy Head-to-toe examination. Self-undressing with gown. Explain fully Education re caring for body Praise
Teenager, adolescent	Increasing independence Future orientation	Privacy Option of parental presence Issues such as work, smoking, drugs and sexual activity	Undress in private Use gown Explain procedures and findings Emphasise normality

Adapted from Parns et al (2007)

The older person

As with children, the assessment and diagnosis for older adults require further skills and considerations, but for different reasons. Legal aspects of consent and pharmacology issues are dealt with in the respective chapters. Within this chapter, the focus is towards maximising the relationship and acknowledging the changes that occur as part of the natural ageing process. It is quite apparent that the older population are becoming more active and less disabled (Bickley and Szilagyi 2009), suggesting a need for more active healthcare than previously and for longer periods of time.

Long-term conditions are more prevalent, such as diabetes, heart disease and arthritis. This in turn means that patients are more likely to consult with their GP and/or anyone who has responsibility for their long-term care (Jerram and Newson 2007). Relationships are usually well established within the primary care setting and, at secondary care, most patients are familiar with the general routine. However, some older people may perceive healthcare intervention with scepticism (Nuttall 2008) and, at these times, therapeutic communication and negotiation will need to be employed skilfully and with care to facilitate an effective consultation.

Nuttall (2008), in her paper concerning the specific needs of the older person in prescribing and public health, recognises how the changes to the nervous, sensory and endocrine systems can affect communication, e.g. deterioration in hearing, sight and/or memory can prove challenging within the consultation process, which will require specific skills to compensate or deal with this to ensure that the overall relationship is not compromised and also that information gathered is of optimum quality.

The consultation umbrella – explained (see Figure 4.1 page 125)

History taking

As will be seen, clinical decision-making, the culmination of the consultation, is dependent on the collection of information gathered (Hardy and Smith 2008). Gathering data (Kurtz et al 2003), listening to their story (Launer 2002) or obtaining a history (Bickley and Szilagyi 2009) is the part of the consultation that is so important because many believe that it is where up to 90% (Fishman and Fishman 2005) of diagnoses are made; the remaining time within the consultation is usually spent confirming or refuting our suspicions, or hypotheses (of course not every consultation is this simple, as alluded to above). Diagnosis is fundamental to the consultation and certainly to the ultimate activity of caring for our patient with safe prescribing, or making confident decisions not to prescribe. We spend such a significant amount of our professional time listening to patients and interpreting their subjective data against our knowledge that we should do it properly (Longmore et al 2010). Launer (2002) recognises our role as *witnesses* to patient's distress and as facilitators of the quest for new meanings in their stories.

History taking is a task that we all perform; however, this does not necessarily correlate with being skilled at the task. The value of the history will depend on how effective the practitioner is at eliciting the patient's story. Furthermore, the sense made of the information elicited will grow exponentially because you are able to contextualise your understanding of the pathophysiology of the diseases that you treat, through continued exposure to patients and illnesses (Goldberg 2009). It could be suggested that no one person is fully skilled in this aspect of care, yet it is undeniable that there are practitioners who are highly skilled at it.

We obtain histories from patients whenever we have contact with them: in person, via the telephone or through correspondence. Patients' histories are their story – their perception of what has been happening to them. This is a concept with which Launer (2002) agrees within his work around narrative-based medicine. It is up to us to have sufficient knowledge within the necessary fields to either deal with it or have the where-withal to refer to someone more appropriate

History taking illustrated

From a personal perspective, the use of a template adapted from the problem-oriented medical record (POMR) (Weed 1968) as an aide memoire has proved invaluable. This can be used as a guide but over time you will find that you will establish your own style of approach or perhaps just modify your existing approach to facilitate the added skill of prescribing.

It is acknowledged that the POMR is not without its critics and its inception was not as an aide memoire. It is also recognised that many clinical areas use a 'clinical pro-forma' or 'care pathway' which has a template incorporated into it to aid the information-gathering process. Table 4.5 is just one of many options available to help ensure that, when attempting to obtain a patient's history, it is done systematically and safely – paramount in any prescribing activity.

Each of these elements requires consideration. Many practitioners will recognise from Table 4.5, or more certainly from the considerations in Table 4.6, that the information required is not new. However, what is required in this part of the chapter is to consider the shift in focus when gathering this information in order to enable safe prescribing. In other words, there is a need to consider the extra skills and decisions needed to collate the information into a meaningful document in order to be safe and credible as a prescribing practitioner. Most patients do not present with a logical and coherent set of symptoms (Moulton 2007).

Table 4.5 Aide memoire for history taking

PC	Presenting complaint
HPC	History of presenting complaint
CH	Current health
PMH	Past medical history
PSH	Past surgical history
DH	Drug history
All	Allergies
FH	Family history
SH	Social history
ROS	Review of systems
Summarise	Summary of findings, thus far
Imp	Impression

Adapted from Weed (1968).

Table 4.6 History taking

PC	Presenting complaint	Ascertain in the patient's own words, what the issue is that has prompted them to seek help or advice. However, if a patient has been asked to come and see you, then your opening question will need to be different This is the opportunity for the patient to describe their symptoms. Moulton (2007) discusses a 'golden 2–3 minutes' at the beginning of the consultation whereby, if facilitated well, you will be given almost all the necessary information required to manage the patient and the problems. It is worth letting the patient have centre stage for these few minutes The use of open-ended questions will be used here compared with further on in the consultation when the need for specific information will necessitate the use of more closed questions Your skills of active listening and interpretation of verbal and non-verbal clues are paramount at this time
HPC	History of presenting complaint	Time to explore the patient's symptoms. There are a number of symptom analysis tools available, all of which use a mnemonic system. There are three common tools, PQRST (Morton 1993), OLD CART (Goldberg 2009) and SOCRATES (Fishman and Fishman 2005). For this chapter, PQRST (Morton 1993) is used. In table 5.7 each of the letters represents two opposing, or complementing, words, which help to prompt the enquiring questions to gather the information about the symptoms as necessary **P = provocative or palliative** Provocative will prompt the practitioner to enquire about 'what makes the symptom worse'. This may include bright lights, loud noise, not taking analgesia. You may want to ask about what the patient was doing before the onset of symptoms Palliative is where the practitioner will ask about 'what makes the symptom better'. This will definitely include questions around any medication or other medicinal remedies that may already have been taken, but may also include things such as the patient's position, the use of an ice pack or abstaining from certain activities or foods – all depend on the symptom present **Q = quality and/or quantity** Quality refers to the description of the symptoms, e.g. if a patient has pain, ask him or her to describe it, using terms such as stabbing/shooting, ache, burning sensation, etc.

(Continued)

Table 4.6 (*Continued*)

Quantity is more to do with how much of the symptoms the patient is experiencing, e.g. if a patient was feeling nauseous, was it all the time, just in the mornings (possibly morning sickness), later in the day (recovering sprained ankle). This is an opportunity to establish how the patient's usual activities are being affected by the symptoms – this may well inform your management plan, including prescribing decisions

R = region/radiation/related symptoms

Region is about asking the patient where about he or she is experiencing their symptom, e.g. 'where about in your chest are you having the pain?': a generalised heaviness in the centre of the chest is indicative of myocardial infarction whereas a specific sharp pain in the right lower chest area may be more indicative of pleurisy

Radiation is most usually applied to pain too, and it is about asking if the pain radiates to other parts of the body. Or, in the case of a patient presenting with a rash, does it occur anywhere else on the body or does it spread wider than they are showing?

Related symptoms are the prompt to ask if there are any other symptoms that the patient is experiencing which may be related to the chief concern. If a patient's chief concern is a headache, it is paramount that you exclude major pathology such as a subarachnoid haemorrhage. To do this you would need to ask about any loss of consciousness or seizures accompanying the headaches, as an example

S = severity

How severe is the symptom. Is it mild, moderate or severe? This is an ideal place to attempt to measure (or objectively contextualise) how severe the symptom is. Do not underestimate the complexity of this exercise and the need to be accurate in its execution. You need to ask the patient to place the level of severity between a scale of 0 and 10, where 0 = no symptom, and 10 = the worst experience of this symptom ever. It is useful both as a baseline score and then to judge how effective a medicine (likely to be prescribed by yourself) has been in relieving the symptom. It is most commonly used to measure levels of pain but it is transferable to other symptoms too

Table 4.6 *(Continued)*

		T = timing The timing of symptoms can be very illuminating in both diagnosis and evaluation. When did the symptom(s) begin? You need to establish if the symptom is constant or intermittent? Has the patient had anything similar before? Is there a pattern to the symptom or is it indiscriminate? Is it present only during the day, or just at night? For example, when comparing asthma with chronic obstructive pulmonary disease (COPD), for diagnostic purposes, the patient's history can be crucial: a patient with asthma tends to be disturbed more in the night with episodes of breathlessness when compared with a patient with COPD who is worse first thing in the morning. In terms of prescribing, when inhalers have been prescribed, it is often the patient's symptom reduction that is used to gauge the success of the prescribing (of course, all prescribing is within evidence-based guidelines, e.g. NICE (2004)
CH	Current health	You need to ascertain the patient's usual health status before the onset of the current issues. Are they usually fit and well? Have they recently had another illness? Some illnesses have a preceding episode, e.g. a viral illness before an outbreak of chickenpox It also gives an opportunity for patients to divulge conditions such as asthma or diabetes; some patients do not always consider 'their' asthma to be 'PMH', they see it as part of their current health and not necessarily 'ill-health'. It could be argued that 'PMH' is the place to ask about these long-term conditions; however, it is also reasonable to cover these prompts here, or even at both times, depending on the situation and how proficient you are in history taking. These may be considered current 'active' medical conditions, compared with a patient's interpretation of past and/or 'inactive' conditions
PMH	Past medical history	This is about a patient's past history of medical issues. There is a mnemonic to help with this: MiTJTHREADS (Fishman and Fishman 2005). A short word about mnemonics: although they may be remembered as lists, they are made most effective when used therapeutically! Mi – myocardial infarction T – thromboembolism J – jaundice T – tuberculosis (TB) H – hypertension R – rheumatic fever E – epilepsy A – asthma D – diabetes S – stroke

Table 4.6 (Continued)

		To help ensure completeness it is worth having a few questions ready should you receive an unexpected response to a patient's past medical history, especially if that person is elderly (there is a call for judgement here). Prompts for patients may include you asking whether they see their doctor regularly, or when was the last time they saw their GP. Have they ever been in hospital before, or had a chest radiograph, or other investigations before?
		Other areas for exploration, if appropriate may include: childhood illnesses, obstetric or gynaecological history
PSH	Past surgical history	The opportunity to investigate a patient's surgical history may not seem as relevant to a prescribing decision compared with medical history, but it is. Past surgical procedures can give illuminating information regarding your differential diagnoses
		Past surgery or pending surgery is to be established, although most patients are likely to let you know if they have any surgery pending
		If there is a surgical history, in a bid to being complete, it is worth checking if there were any complications postoperatively (e.g. haemorrhage) or any problems with a general anaesthetic. If the patient has any visible scars, ask about them
DH	Drug history	This element of the history has to be comprehensive due to the implications of safety. Present medication including names of drugs, dosage is paramount. Route of administration is interesting too: oral, topical, intravenous or subcutaneous, as examples
		It is interesting from a holistic perspective to ask if patients know why they are taking the medication (this may give an overall impression of many elements of patients;"lifestyles', including their own knowledge base of the illnesses that they have and it is this that will guide you in how you respond to the patient and also give them information). You can enquire about side effects that they may be experiencing (many presentations to general practice coincide with a recent commencement of medication)
		You can also ask about previous relevant medication, e.g. recent steroid treatment or previous chemotherapy
		Immunisations are worth enquiring about too, e.g. seasonal influenza immunisation. Recent holiday immunisations. Is the patient up to date with their routine immunisations?
		There are those medications that patients don't always consider to be medication, e.g. inhalers, oral contraceptive pill, lotions or topical creams

Table 4.6 *(Continued)*

		Enquiries about alternative medication, herbal remedies or complementary therapies need to be addressed Medications bought over the counter, via the internet or borrowed from friends or a family member are another aspect to delve into Finally, there is always the sensitive approach to illegal drugs and substances – the question has to be asked and how this is done very much depends on your client base, circumstances of presentation and age of the patient. Positive therapeutic communication will help It is important to ascertain the patient's concordance status – it can be difficult for patients to take their medication as prescribed for many reasons, including complex regimens, older patients, or those who are cognitively impaired or just not too interested. This element of information can prove crucial: what may appear to be a poor response to therapy may actually be an issue of non-compliance
ALL	Allergies	It is important to ascertain any allergies that they have especially to drugs (adverse drug reaction). It is also significant to enquire about other allergies, e.g. foods (some of the drug excipients may be based on an allergic substance) or animals You need to know how the allergy manifests (simply a transient rash, or a full-blown anaphylaxis reaction). This is for two reasons: first so that you roughly gauge the severity of the allergy, but second to decide if it is a true allergy or a significant side effect – they are different but some patients perceive their sensitivity as an allergy
FH	Family history	The family history has two approaches: first you want to know if another family member has the same symptoms, e.g. gastroenteritis type symptoms or acute onset – if positive, this will increase the index of suspicion for a contagious bacterial/viral infection. You could also ask whether the patient has been in contact with other people who have had any infectious diseases, e.g. tuberculosis, meningitis or gastroenteritis The other approach is finding out about hereditary links or family trends. In particular you are looking for heritable illnesses among first- or second-degree relatives, e.g. coronary artery disease, diabetes and certain malignancies. When discussing the death of a close relative you need to ask about cause of death, age of onset of disease, age of death. All give information about risk and adds to the clinical decision-making to be made later in the consultation

(Continued)

Table 4.6 (*Continued*)

		Is there a history of consanguinity? As a result of the incidence association, it is prudent to ask black patients if there is any sickle cell disease in the family, and Mediterranean patients need to be asked about thalassaemia
SH	Social history 'Risky behaviour'	This is quite a broad topic area because it covers many possible lines of enquiry, yet not all necessarily need to be asked. This discretion will build as you increase your own proficiency. I also refer to the SAFE mnemonic as 'risky behaviour' because it can also include illicit drug use and sexual history, if relevant.

A few mnemonics to help: SAFE, HELP and HAT.

S = smoking	H = housing	H = hobbies
A = alcohol	E = employment	A = activities
F = food	L = living/dependents	T = travel
E = exercise	P = pets	

Smoking: do they smoke, what do they smoke (cigarettes, roll-up cigarettes, cigars, pipe)? How much do they smoke and for how long have they smoked? There is the 'pack-years' formula, which can be used to measure the lifetime exposure to smoking because the degree of tobacco exposure can be correlated to the risk of disease (Wood et al 2005). If they have stopped, when did they stop and why did they stop. As part of our health promotion role, if patients do smoke they should be asked about their wishes to stop smoking, but, be warned, it is one of those areas where you have to gauge the possible reaction of asking such a question against the risk that it might pose to the rapport that you have developed thus far (clinical judgement and skills of communication need to be at their finest to do this effectively). The same would be said for all the topic areas of 'SAFE'

Alcohol: how much alcohol do they consume and how often? Encourage patients to be specific. Currently we measure alcohol intake against the Government's recommended limits, i.e. men 2–3 units a day and 1–2 units a day for women. The message for us all concerns moderation; avoiding stoking up the units for 1–2 evenings a week (referred to as binge drinking). If you are concerned about the amount of alcohol patients consume, or perhaps they are being vague about the amount they drink, possibly there is a problem (or they may just not think it is your business to know!). There are a number of screening tools in clinical practice to attempt to identify 'problem drinkers'. One example is the CAGE questionnaire (Ewing 1984), consisting of four questions:

Do you ever feel you ought to **Cut** down on your drinking?

Table 4.6   *(Continued)*

Do you get **Annoyed** when other people tell you to stop drinking?

Do you ever feel **Guilty** about your drinking behaviour?

Have you ever had a drink first thing in the morning (an **Eye** opener)?

If there is one positive reply then there is an indication to enquire further. Two or more positive replies suggest that there is a drinking problem. This is relevant from two perspectives: if a patient has alcoholic liver disease the pharmacokinetics of drugs will be affected; you may need to refer the patient for specialist help with a drinking problem

Although 'covered' in the 'drug history' section, you might feel it more appropriate to ask about **illicit** drugs at this stage. However, it might also be an opportunity to revisit the subject area; illicit drug use can be strongly associated with smoking and alcohol

Again, without wanting to appear judgemental, but the evidence supports the links, you may need to enquire about **sexual history**, e.g. whether patients are sexually active, if they have a regular partner, whether they have had sexual intercourse with someone different to their regular partner recently. The gist of this information, of course, is not to be judgemental, but rather to be able to have all the necessary information to help make your prescribing practice safe and holistic. Other questions that may need to be asked include same sex relationships (particularly for men), risky practices or unprotected sex (more so for women because of the risk of pregnancy, but also men in terms of sexually transmitted infections)

Food and exercise: generally speaking this is more of a health promotion issue when considering prescribing. There are considerations of a broader context in terms of general health and risks to ill health that will impact on your considerations when making your diagnosis or reviewing a patient's ongoing situation

| SH | Social history | **Housing:** similar to the above in ascertaining a general picture of the patient and his or her circumstances: hot water, heating, electricity, telephone. What type of housing does he or she live in? |
| | | **Employment:** what is his or her job now? What does it involve? How long has he or she been off sick before seeking medical attention. All these may also be relevant in some circumstances. These answers may influence the degree of intervention that you decide on. It may be useful to find out if the patient has had other jobs and which job he or she has had for the longest (a patient presenting with respiratory symptoms, whose job is in marketing, reveals that he used to work down a mine when you asked which job he has had for the longest). |

(Continued)

Table 4.6 (Continued)

		Living: who do they live with? Have they any children (are they still at home)? Are they married or single? Is their partner well? What is their job? Is there anyone at home to help look after them (depending on severity of illness – if not there may be a need for referral to social services or even into hospital)? **Pets:** do they have any pets at home, are they new additions to family or if they have had contact with other animals? Animals can be risky from a health perspective if simple hygiene measures are not adhered to
SH	Social history	These next three also echo the above box in that you are continuing to build up a picture of the patient and his or her usual circumstances. It also helps with the continuing rapport that you have begun to develop. It is important, however, that, when asking these questions which may seem slightly irrelevant at times (to both parties), you continue to demonstrate an interest in the patient **Hobbies:** how does the patient spend leisure time, e.g. reading, watching TV? **Activities:** are there any specific activities that he or she does? This may well influence your prescribing **Travel:** ask about tropical illnesses and if the patient has been abroad in the last year – and where to. If the patient had been taking prophylaxis, e.g. against malaria, was it continued on return?
ROS	Review of systems	Of all the elements of history taking, this is possibly the most difficult to understand why the questions are asked, especially if students are new to this more broadly oriented review. The review of systems is a list of questions, organised from a body system's perspective. There is much debate around its value and also where, within the schema of the patient's story, it should be positioned. The general consensus, on the last point, is that it should be used at the end of the history taking; however, some suggest asking after PMH. It has a number of dynamic functions: as a screening tool to be asked of every patient; asked only if there was suspicion of increased risk of certain illnesses; it can be helpful in determining if there are any concurrent diseases that have been left either undiscovered or even undiagnosed thus far; it can be used as a safety net thereby reducing the chance of missing an important symptom or disease. Practice and experience will help to determine how much importance is placed on the review of systems (ROS). Practise it and 'make it yours': many practitioners prefer to use a targeted application of the ROS and believe that this strategy is more efficient and revealing, e.g. if there is a history of diabetes, you must review the patient's vascular system. As experience is gained in this element, you will be able to decide how you are going to incorporate your 'tuned' ROS into the overall strategy

Table 4.6   (Continued)

In the meantime, this is an example of a brief screening ROS, which goes from head to toe (most clinical textbooks will provide other examples):

General: usually well or unwell, fevers (night), sweats, fatigue, recent trauma, sleep

Neurological: any fits, faints or blackouts, pins and needles, headaches

ENT: any problems with hearing, nose or throat

Cardiac: any chest pain or discomfort, palpitations, dizziness, breathlessness when lying down, ankle swelling, pain in legs on walking

Respiratory: any breathlessness, cough, coughing up sputum, blood in sputum, hoarseness, wheeze

Gastrointestinal: any pains in stomach, indigestion, bowels regular, blood in stool, weight steady, appetite steady

Renal: any problems passing urine?

Female patients: (dependent on age) any irregular menstrual cycles, menopausal symptoms, vaginal discharge, do you examine your breasts monthly?

Male patients: any problems with erections, do you examine your testicles regularly?

Musculoskeletal: any problems walking, or problems with your joints?

Psychological: how is your mood, are you having feelings of sadness, do you have any memory problems?

SUM	Summary	Once all the information has been elicited, it is important to formulate a short summary of your understanding of the patient's problem or symptoms and to share it with the patient. 'Could I show this patient that I have sufficiently understood why they have come to see me?' is the culmination of Neighbour's checkpoint 2 (Neighbour 2005). This will help towards a mutual understanding of the patient's problems and helps to reduce the risk of misunderstanding. It can also be useful in a time-critical situation for other practitioners to read a summary rather than the full documentation You can end this section of the consultation by adding in extra safety netting, e.g. ask the patient is there anything else that you would like to say that has not already been covered. Do you have any questions? Is there anything that you are worried about?
IMP	Impression	This section is for you as the practitioner to make suggestions about your impression of the case thus far. You can tentatively or confidently list your differential diagnoses. It may be that there are no differential diagnoses to suggest. It may be that this section is a continuation of your summary

Table 4.7 Comparison of symptom analysis tools

PQRST	OLD CARTS	SOCRATES
P = provocative	O = onset	S = site
P = palliative	L = location/radiation	O = onset
Q = quality	D = duration	C = character
Q = quantity	C = character	R = radiation
R = region	A = aggravating factors	A = associated symptoms
R = radiation	R = relieving factors	T = time course/duration
R = related symptoms	T = timing	E = exacerbating factors
S = severity	S = severity	S = severity
T = timing		

Once our therapeutic introductions have been established, it is essential to ascertain the patient's 'presenting complaint'. Alternatively, it may be more appropriate to document this heading as 'reason for attendance' or 'reason for review' (Table 4.7). This allows consideration of the many different reasons why a person may approach a health professional/practitioner, again, discussed within the therapeutic communication section of this chapter, above.

Activity box 4.4

Make a list of five of the most common clinical presentations that you encounter and intend to prescribe for (maybe the list will be shorter – this is ok).

Using appropriate resources look up those conditions and compile a reference source for yourself, illustrating some of the key confirming symptoms and their patterns. Also ensure that you highlight key symptoms and/or patterns that may well put the diagnosis or review into question.

www.gpnotebook.co.uk and www.cks.nhs.uk are two websites that will help you begin

Physical examination

The practical aspects of this element of the consultation are covered in Chapter 7.

In terms of process and context, it is an interesting element of the consultation in that, unlike the 'history taking', there are variances in the extent to which a prescriber may need to perform a physical examination. Indeed, as Shah (2005a, 2005b) suggests, the physical examination functions to confirm or refute the patient's history. This is not to say that, in scenarios when the 'luxury' of systematic history taking followed by a physical examination is not possible, e.g. a time critical patient admitted to A&E, the history and physical examination may need to be executed in tandem. However, the ABCDE system, or primary survey, is adhered too (Greaves et al 2006) maintaining the notion of structure thus enhancing safety. Therefore, within the cognitive domain of our analysis, order does prevail and differential diagnoses are constantly being confirmed or refuted – irrespective of the circumstances of the presentation. The diagnosis is the key to accurate prescribing, taking into account the patient's individuality (Rang et al 2009), ascertained via the history.

It will depend on an individual's skill base, the role within which prescribing is to be undertaken, and of course the patient who is presenting, the extent to which a physical examination will need to be performed. What this means is that there are varying degrees of physical examination. As examples: a community nurse may need to just *inspect* a wound, in her role overseeing the care of a patient with a venous leg ulcer; a pharmacist may need to measure a patient's blood pressure, heart rate and heart rhythm as part of a GP-based hypertension clinic; and a nurse working within an advanced role on a medical assessment unit may need to perform a full physical examination in the same manner as a trained doctor would do.

Proficiency in clinical skill acquisition is paramount, if it is to be utilised. In most cases, this requires not just the psychomotor skills to perform the task, but the accompanying cognitive skills and knowledge of the relevant anatomy, physiology and pathophysiology. Without both elements being present, there is a risk of substandard execution of the skill or possibly, and more importantly, an inability to interpret or understand the implications of the information gathered through the physical examination.

Tests and investigations

Once the history and physical examination are complete, it may be that a diagnosis is still uncertain, or needs to be confirmed, and the practitioner requires further tests or investigations. It may be because there is too much uncertainty that the practitioner is unable to 'tolerate'. In non-medical prescribing, the implications of not being correct and prescribing inappropriately can be far reaching and potentially devastating. It is clinical judgement that calls the balance between the economics of investigations and the safety of certainty.

Plan/Treatment

Within the prescribing context, negotiation is important because you need to ensure that the patient agrees and cooperates with the plan, otherwise the implementation of the plan will flounder, irrespective of how 'complete and efficacious' it is (O'Connor et al 2003, Neighbour 2005). You need to convince patients that the plan is appropriate and that, when they leave your company, they intend to take responsibility for its implementation. It can be useful to engage the patient with the construction of the plan which will incorporate risk communication that leads to a better understanding and decision-making about the clinical plan (Thompson et al 2005). As Thompson et al (2005) continue, this also fulfils professional moral and ethical responsibilities when engaging patients in decisions that affect their health.

The issue of concordance versus compliance is very interesting; however, you must remember that, for patients to be compliant within the concordant relationship, they need to understand the instructions and therefore it rests with the practitioner to ensure that the plan is conveyed accurately and in a manner that patients understand. This common view about the outcome of consultation will impact on prescribing, investigation or referral decisions (Hamilton and Britten 2006).

The main decision in terms of non-medical prescribing is whether or not to write a prescription. There are many treatment options available that do not require a prescription and, as a professional, must have been considered as options (Luker et al 1998). Once again, in view of many patients' expectations for a prescription, it is a practitioner's skills in communication that can effectively convey the need, or not, for a prescription.

Another decision required is to determine whether or not the presenting condition, or patient's circumstances, are within your scope of professional practice. If not, you need to refer the patient on. To do this you need two key skills: first the knowledge of local arrangements for referral procedures and, second, to convey this message with sufficient deftness so as not to alarm the patient but also to maintain your own professional capabilities. However, as Thompson et al (2005) state, the information contained with the discussions about risk has the potential to negatively impact on a patient's motivation to change health behaviour, so it is important to support patients with their engagement with decision-making.

Follow-up

Follow-up is an element of the treatment plan in many respects. This again must be coherent and conveyed appropriately. One underpinning theory regarding the decisions that the practitioner makes when deciding on the time frame for follow-up is that the practitioner must consider the anticipated response to both the treatment (or non-treatment) and the illness/disease trajectory. This concerns the management of uncertainty by anticipating variations (Neighbour 2005). The different clinical settings may also impact on the follow-up time frames according to usual practice.

Suffice to say it is a prescriber's responsibility to ensure that prescribing decisions are monitored and that patients are exposed to the least amount of risk, taking into account every individual's situation. A patient's individual situation is incredibly broad and ascertained only through effective communication, predominately during history taking and the general discourse throughout the whole encounter. Although Barsky (2002) recognises that there will always be a degree of 'instability' in the medical history, patients' recollections of their symptoms, illnesses and episodes of care are often inconsistent, and will also be exposed to bias (Croskerry 2005). It could be suggested that the follow-up plan must attempt to reduce, or oversee, the risks associated with uncertainty. Uncertainty is inevitable; individual non-medical prescribers and patients will tolerate varying levels of uncertainty, as discussed above.

Conclusion to the consultation

The consultation needs to be concluded and again therapeutic communication is important in managing this element of the encounter. Due to time resource issues, patients must be seen but the non-medical prescriber has other demands on time: once the encounter has reached a natural, or enforced, conclusion, a patient may not be ready for it to conclude (and vice versa) and therefore will need to be sensitively addressed to avoid compromising relationships. The end of the consultation also enables a last chance to ensure concordance and understanding from both parties' perspectives (White 2002, Shah 2005b).

Table 4.8 Non-medical prescriber's and organisational responsibilities

Personal health and wellbeing	Stress management – within the consultation
Time management	Stress management – between consultations
Record keeping	Service delivery
Keeping up to date	Accountability – dealing with complaints
Personal development plan	Litigation – risk reduction
Indemnity insurance	Reflection on self and on prescribing decisions

This last segment of the consultation umbrella is also concerned with the non-medical prescriber's and organisational aspects of the consultation process. It includes issues such as those listed in Table 4.8.

 Activity box 4.5

Take time to consider Table 4.8.

Make notes on how you plan to address these issues within your prescribing practice.

Asterix those issues that you had not previously considered within your clinical practice before prescribing.

Clinical decision-making

By returning to the consultation umbrella, we also return to the handle of the 'brolly', to explore the notion of clinical decision-making (CDM).

In line with the role requirements of a prescribing practitioner, correct clinical decisions will need to be made that will ultimately consist of: identification of the problem, diagnosis and management/treatment plan; or a treatment choice made in light of an evaluation of a patient's existing problem (Offredy 1998). Even though there is an option to prescribe, not all patient encounters will require a prescription; however, there will need to be a conscious *decision* regarding this strategy.

To ensure that decisions are sound, there needs to be an understanding of what constitutes clinical decision-making and how these clinical decisions are made. They need to be considered and reflected on to appreciate how a patient's and practitioner's individuality (Thompson and Dowding 2002, Croskerry 2005, Hardy and Smith 2008) can impact on decisions and how to reduce the potential harmful and unnecessary errors that may occur (Weed and Weed 1999). Conversely, effective CDM is considered to be one of the highest attributes of (physicians) practitioners (Croskerry 2005).

Many terms are used to denote this dynamic activity (Robinson 2002) of decision-making that practitioners undertake – clinical reasoning, decision-making, diagnostic reasoning, making up one's mind, making a judgement – and they are all used interchangeably when in clinical discourse, yet fundamentally they are synonymous. In terms of decision-making in prescribing (being aware of the advanced nature of this 'task'), it is reasonable to use literature from both a medical and a non-medical perspective (Radwin 1990, Offredy 1998), to underpin the analysis. However, it could be proposed that medics and non-medical prescribers make decisions differently because of the inherent differences in respective professional training, education and their values of particular aspects within healthcare (Offredy 1998). It has been suggested that one of the main reasons for this difference is due to the threshold of uncertainty that medical training tolerates, or rather that a doctor is trained to be able to tolerate higher levels of uncertainty when compared with nurses (Fox 1979) or other health professionals. It is proposed that there is a relationship between decision-making and uncertainty, in that the more complex the decision, the greater the degree of uncertainty associated with it (Croskerry 2005).

Cognitive continuum

In a bid to make sense of CDM the literature reveals a broad cognitive approach. CDM is perceived as a continuum, with analytical strategies at one end and more qualitative or heuristic strategies at the other (Hamm 1988, cited in Luker et al 1998, p. 658). This continuum approach suggests that, while recognising that CDM is dynamic, it is also flexible and responsive. The factors on which CDM needs to be responsive are vast and can be quite complex (Croskerry 2005). This continuum has also been identified by Hammond (1990, cited in Croskerry 2005, p. R1) and Dawson (1993, cited in Croskerry 2005, p. R1) whereby they have added to the explanation such that the term 'calculation' had been added to the analytical pole, and 'informal' and 'intuition' have joined the qualitative end of the continuum.

Along this continuum, there have been specific strategies proposed to further dissect the way in which practitioners arrive at the decisions that they make. These include the hypothetical–deductive model, pattern recognition, heuristics and intuition. These are now explored together with case studies to illustrate their use.

It must be noted that there are more CDM strategies than those presented within this chapter, notably, bayesian theory, which is based on a positivist perspective, using a numerical weighting, or probability theory, to help select the 'best' decision (Hans 2007). For the more logical and quantitative non-medical prescribers, it is interesting work to read and consider, but unfortunately, there is insufficient scope to discuss this here. Clinical algorithms are another tool that can help decision-making but they are not covered within this text. Many practitioners will be familiar with their use, e.g. adult advanced life support algorithm (Resuscitation Council UK 2005), algorithm for the diagnosis of heart failure (National Institute for Health and Clinical Excellence (NICE) 2003) and a care pathway for hypertension (NICE 2006).

Hypothetical–deductive model

The hypothetical–deductive model is a method whereby hypotheses are proposed as end-points to a problem, or patient presentation, which are then confirmed or refuted through a testing process (the consultation) (Groen and Patel 1985). The hypotheses are generally identified early in the consultation so that the gathering of information can be guided (history taking predominately) accordingly. This reasoning is inductive (Buckingham and Adams 2000a, 2000b). A hypothesis list should not be too long otherwise the gathering of information can become unwieldy. As information is gathered, hypotheses will be refuted, whittling down the possible diagnosis, but it may be that other theories need to be added, or as stated: 'first principles often have to be recast as new knowledge replaces old' (illustrating an adaptive strategy). Experts in the field of psychology (Newall and Simon 1972, cited in Offredy 1998, p. 991) have suggested that, given the diversity and volume of potential information gathering from the patients, and compounded by the extensive knowledge that base practitioners have to acquire, hypothesis generation is a clinical necessity.

What this method has to offer the non-medical prescriber is that it facilitates a process beginning with an undifferentiated problem (particularly for an independent prescriber), i.e. the 'presenting complaint' and proceeds on to, as yet, an unknown endpoint. By using the skills presented earlier in this chapter, in terms of therapeutic communication, the presenting complaint can be elicited and then systematically honed down to a manageable list of possibilities, which are then tested by further data collection (deduction – Buckingham and Adams (2000a, 2000b); the consultation umbrella's history taking, physical examination and further tests). The end-result is that a single hypothesis has been confirmed, i.e. a diagnosis has been reached and an appropriate management plan can be constructed. Alternatively, there may be no firm conclusion and the list of differential diagnoses will need to remain until a point further in the future, so we sometimes use what is referred to as the 'working diagnosis'. Whatever the result, the management plan, of which there always has to be one, will need to reflect the holistic requirements or needs of the patient.

Higgs and Jones (2000) take this a step further by proposing that the process of clinical reasoning is a spiral process. Each ongoing spiral incorporates information gathering and interpretation, with further gathering and re-interpretation resulting in necessary hypothesis formation. They believe that this dynamic movement within the spiral achieves a progressively broader and deeper comprehension of the clinical presentation. The notion of a spiral can certainly help reassure the novice non-medical prescriber that clinical decision-making is a truly complex skill. This is echoed by Elstein and Schwarz (2002) who refer to a similar evolving picture.

For a new practitioner, or it could be said an experienced practitioner embarking on a significant extra element to his or her current remit, i.e. prescribing, this is a safe and systematic approach to take. It helps to keep the clinical possibilities broad. It is also useful when faced with a situation that is not as evident as initially perceived, when you are left feeling genuinely puzzled (Neighbour 2005).

Activity box 4.6

Review case study 3.

Reflect on how the hypothetical–deductive model of clinical reasoning would underpin the clinical decision making within this case.

Pattern recognition

Pattern recognition is a method using critical pieces of information (Offredy 1998). By recognising patient's key symptoms and/or signs, the practitioner will be able to match them up with previous patients who have presented with the same or similar symptoms and/or signs. Thus, it is the use of remembered patterns of diseases and illnesses that are matched against the presenting patient. This has been termed 'representativeness' by Kahneman et al (1982). However, care is needed when categorising, as Buckingham and Adams (2000b) highlight that it is more of a probabilistic relationship. It is not an exact science.

Neighbour (2005) presents pattern recognition as the 'once seen, never forgotten' principle. This would therefore suggest that this representativeness must be based on a practitioner's experience. It could be suggested that, the greater the experience of the non-medical prescriber, the more secure his or her pattern recognition will be. However, this may pose an issue for a non-medical prescriber who perhaps is not as experienced as another, and is considered one of the disadvantages of this strategy, so care must be taken – remember the concept of safety netting (Neighbour 2005).

For a non-medical prescriber working within a supplementary prescribing role, e.g. within a setting caring for patients with long-term conditions, it may be a method that resonates with some. For a practitioner who has been caring for a group of patients with, for example, heart failure, there will come a point in time when all the variations of a theme have been witnessed. Provided that they are cognitively secured and easily retrievable, a heart failure specialist practitioner will be able to recognise patterns in the disease trajectory and intervene accordingly (see case study 9).

When referring to patterns being cognitively secured, this is the realisation that these patterns will also have associated memories (Watson 1994). If the corresponding decisions that were made at the time were safe and effective, the practitioner will be more certain about the ensuing decisions. If the original situation unfolded in a negative way, the practitioner's decisions within the same set of symptoms and signs may be more cautious or the practitioner may even believe that it is 'beyond their scope of professional practice' (NMC 2008), e.g. if the above heart failure specialist treated a patient for worsening heart failure because of the development of a cough with expectoration, without even considering the possibility of a concomitant chest infection. These two scenarios occur in clinical practice and it is the duty of the practitioner to appreciate that no decision-making strategy is 100% guaranteed and that all patients are individual and liable to change and can be relatively unpredictable.

Interestingly, Offredy (1998) believes that pattern recognition can apply to either end of the cognitive continuum, perhaps supporting the notion that CDM strategy is more than either analysis or heuristics. Offredy (1998) highlights Weber et al's study (1993, cited in Offredy 1998, p. 990) which suggested that the memories of previous clinical presentations influenced the hypothesis generation of the hypothetical–deductive strategy in circumstances of similar scenarios. In fact, a number of writers insinuate at times that CDM is more to do with a person's individual behaviour (Buckingham and Adams 2000a) which is rooted in their own belief frameworks. This supports the consultation umbrella, in that all patient consultations are upheld by both therapeutic communication and clinical decision-making – they are not necessarily separate entities.

Activity box 4.7

Review case study 9.
  Reflect on how processes involved in pattern recognition would underpin the clinical decision-making within this case.

Heuristics and intuition

The remaining two CDM strategies to be presented within this chapter are possibly the least defined of them all. Heuristics has been linked to pattern recognition in the short cuts used when symptom or clinical presentation matching is used and referred to as 'rules of thumb'. It could be argued, however, that pattern recognition is a conscious process whereas heuristics and intuition are subconscious processes. It is this lack of scientific rigour that has questioned their validity. Croskerry (2005) details the rather negative aspects of heuristics: 'weak predictive power; inability to describe the process in detail; and a failure to assist physicians in improving their decision making.'

The reason heuristics and intuition have been drawn together in this chapter is that intuition suffers from similar opinions. Thompson and Dowding (2002) assert that, within the literature, there is a lack of consensus over the meaning of intuition. They provide a list of five definitions (Table 4.9). However, what is conceded is that the definitions have similarities, in so much as the authors all believe intuition to be a process that just 'happens', it is not rational and it cannot be described.

Unfortunately, when 'competing' in a medically dominated healthcare system, it could be argued that, without a rationale for a decision that has been made, there is a degree of uncertainty or unsafeness about it. Safety is paramount in caring for patients. Or more specifically, without scientific rigour there can be no scientific worth (Elstein 1976).

Table 4.9 Definitions of intuition

'Understanding without a rationale'	Benner and Tanner (1987)
'A perception of possibilities, meanings and relationships by way of insight'	Gerrity (1987)
'Knowledge of a fact or truth, as a whole; immediate possession of knowledge; and knowledge independent of the linear reasoning process'	Rew and Barron (1987)
'Immediate knowing of something without the conscious use of reason'	Schrader and Fischer (1987)
'[A] ... process whereby the nurse knows something about a patient that cannot be verbalised, that is verbalised with difficulty or for which the source of knowledge cannot be determined'	Young (1987)

Cited in Thompson and Dowding (2002).

However, Benner (1984) proposed that intuition is applicable to expert practitioners: 'intuitive judgement distinguishes the expert from the novice.' She continues to explain that the expert practitioner is able to bypass the analytical processes and rely on experiential understanding of the whole, in order to make the appropriate decisions. This was supported in her later work with Tanner (Benner and Tanner 1987) when they define intuition as 'an individual's opinion justified by their authority or experience'. This resonates with those practitioners who rely less on the hypothetical–deductive method and use pattern recognition. This also brings together those authors who claim that CDM improves with experience (Croskerry 2005), although Offredy (2005) demonstrates in her evaluation of the evidence that this is not always the case: 'greater clinical experience does not necessarily cause clinicians to converge on an optimal diagnostic strategy.' What is advantageous from an intuitive perspective is that experienced practitioners are able to make speedy decisions in light of being able to see beyond the information given or, as Meerabeau (1992) suggests, the use of 'tacit [nursing] knowledge'. Even though the history taking above is detailed, attempting to provide a vast array of potential questions that may need to be asked, as practitioners become more experienced, which in turn is related to experience within non-medical prescribing, they are able to select questions more efficiently, yet structured, to assist with their decision-making.

In terms of non-medical prescribing, although practitioners may use intuition to aid their decisions, it would be doubtful that, should a decision be brought into question, a rationale of 'I just knew' would be acceptable. Certainly at this point in time when non-medical prescribing is still in its relative infancy, any discrepancies need to be fully explained in order to maintain credibility. This is especially so while there remains scepticism of non-medical professionals taking on the skill of prescribing.

Activity box 4.8

Review case study 2.

Reflect on how the strategy of intuition underpins the clinical decision-making within this case.

Activity box 4.9

Consider a recent clinical decision that you have had to make and note the process that you think you followed in order to make that decision.

Attempt to match up the process that you followed with one or more of the CDM strategies explained above.

Discussion

The intention above was to present a selection of the current CDM strategies that are used in clinical practice, to help first to make decisions, thus enhancing the care that we provide our patients with and, second, how they could be used to reflect on the decisions that have been made.

Buckingham and Adams (2000a) argue that there are underlying similarities between all of the CDM theories and that they should be brought under a single framework. This can also be seen when reading about intuition above – when considered in their application to clinical practice, CDM strategies have many similarities. They went on to propose that this framework be constructed within a general psychological classification. Use of a psychological framework again supports the idea that CDM is dynamic and dependent on clinical relationships which, as discussed above, are also bound in both a practitioner's and a patient's own believe systems. This is supported by Simon (1986, cited in Offredy 1998, p. 992) who considers that intuitive decision-making is a component of behavioural theory.

It could be surmised that CDM can be seen as more than strategies that can be taught or learnt, in that they have a lot to do with a practitioner's behaviour and are therefore individual. CDM theory can be used only to help illustrate how practitioners make decisions rather than by learning a strategy and then applying it each time that they are in clinical practice. This dynamism is recognised by Offredy (1998) in her evaluation of the cognitive processes of nurse practitioners, which were found not to be compartmentalised but rather used a variety of approaches when arriving at a decision or diagnosis. Perhaps it is the dynamic aspects of CDM that should be facilitated, intertwined with therapeutic communication, to help non-medical prescribers to enhance their CDM skills. This would go some way to meeting and understanding the biases or influences involved when making decisions.

These influences on decision making are diverse. They range from patient perspective, personal perspectives and organisational structures within which decisions are made. There is much literature which discusses these influences (Luker et al 1998, Offredy 1998, Thompson and Dowding 2002, Higgs et al 2008) and are worthy of further consideration. As one example, in one study involving nurse practitioners, 45% of negotiations resulted in a compromise between the treatment choice and follow-up when considering the patient's social circumstances (Offredy 1998). Croskerry (2005) also acknowledges biases that influence CDM, although these seem to be portrayed from a positivist perspective whereby the rigor of CDM is questioned. From a therapeutic and qualitative perspective, it could be suggested that these 'biases' are to be embraced and considered. They perhaps should be considered value-laden decisions, recognising the patient and practitioner as individual people. This is provided that the practitioner is always acting within his or her professional framework (HPC 2007, GPhC 2010, NMC 2008).

Suffice it to say that the literature is variable in its application of the conceptual distinctions of CDM, which makes it difficult for a non-medical prescriber to make sense of the strategies as a whole (Buckingham and Adams 2000a). However, Offredy (1998) concludes from her study that the evidence is suggestive of experts using a more intuitive approach together with pattern recognition, whereas novices use more hypothetical-deductive reasoning. West and West (2002) add to this conclusion that, irrespective of how much information is gathered, there will always be a degree of uncertainty at the point when decisions need to be made. As a non-medical prescriber, the 'answer' is to ensure that as much of that uncertainty is reduced as is possible, and that the decisions can stand the medical profession's scrutiny (Hardy and Smith 2008).

Conclusion

This chapter has presented the consultation umbrella that was used to underpin the discourse of effective consultations. For an effective consultation to take place there were three key elements which were presented and analysed in the light of the current evidence base: therapeutic relationships, the consultation and clinical decision-making. Initially practitioners were helped to understand the significance of *therapeutic communication* and how this element of caring can be honed to become more effective within a prescribing context: it transcends the whole process of the consultation.

The consultation umbrella was introduced and used to facilitate the explanation of the elements of any patient encounter for any non-medical prescriber. It will also help prospective prescribers to have some insight into the necessary depth that their revised consultations will need to go. The consultation umbrella will have been a new illustration, but the elements would have been recognised by all practitioners. With regard to *decision-making*, this complex and multifaceted exercise, or simple task, was explored and a number of strategies to help arrive at safe decisions were presented.

Key themes: conclusions and considerations

Public health	The prescribing consultation provides an ideal situation for identifying and addressing public health issues, enabling the non-medical prescriber to impact on UK public health targets
	Consider the approach, model of consultation and format for recording the patient's history that you use. Does this enable or prompt you to explore public health issues?
Social and cultural issues	In adopting a holistic approach to your consultation, consideration of social and cultural issues is essential because, for some patients, the success of any prescription may be influenced by its appropriateness from a social and/or cultural perspective
	Consider how you incorporate the following factors into your consultations: • Patient's ability to take medication • Cultural acceptability of assessment and treatment
Prescribing principles	Prescribing principle 1: 'examine the holistic needs of the patient' (NPC 1999) is fundamental in safe and effective prescribing. The ability to progress through the remaining principles appropriately depends on the effectiveness of the consultation
	Consider how effective your therapeutic communication is within your next consultation by reflecting on it both during and after the consultation

References

Balint E, Courtenay M, Elder A, Hull S, Julian P (1983) *The Doctor, the Patient and the Group: Balint revisited*. London: Routledge.

Barns K, Sharu D, Rimmer M (2007) Care of the child. In: *Cross S*, Rimmer M (eds), *Nurse Practitioner Manual of Clinical Skills*. Edinburgh: Baillière Tindall.

Barsky AJ (2002) Forgetting, fabricating, and telescoping: the instability of the medical history. *Arch Intern Med* **162**: 981-4.

Benner P (1984) *From Novice to Expert: Excellence and Power in Clinical Nursing Practice*. CA: Addison Wesley.

Benner P, Tanner CA (1987) Clinical judgement: how expert nurses use intuition. In: Thompson C, Dowding D (eds), *Clinical Decision Making and Judgement in Nursing*. Edinburgh: Churchill Livingstone.

Berne E (1970) *The Games People Play: The psychology of human relationships*. London: Penguin Books.

Bickley LS, Szilagyi PG (2009) *Bates' Guide to Physical Examination and History Taking*, 10th edn. Philadelphia: Lippincott Williams & Wilkins.

Buckingham CD, Adams A (2000a) Classifying clinical decision making: a unifying approach. *J Adv Nurs* **32**: 981-9.

Buckingham CD, Adams, A (2000b) Classifying clinical decision making: interpreting nurse intuition, heuristics and medical diagnosis. *J Adv Nurs* **32**: 990-8.

Cohn KH (2007) developing effective communication skills. *J Oncol Pract* **3**: 314-17.

Croskerry P (2005) The theory and practice of clinical decision making. *Can J Anaesth* **52**: R1-8.

Egan G (2009) *The Skilled Helper*, 9th edn. Belmont: Cengage Learning Inc.

Ellis RB, Gates RJ, Kenworthy N, eds (1995) *Interpersonal Communication in Nursing: Theory and practice*. Edinburgh: Churchill Livingstone.

Elstein AS (1976) Clinical judgement: psychological research and medical practice. *Science* **194**: 696-700.

Elstein AS, Schwarz A (2002) Clinical problem solving and diagnostic decision making: selective review of the cognitive literature. *BMJ* **324**: 729-32.

Elwyn G, Edwards A, Kinnersley P (1999) Shared Decision Making: the neglected second half of the consultation. *Br J Gen Pract* **49**: 477-82.

Ewing JA (1984) Detecting alcoholism: the CAGE questionnaire. *JAMA* **252**: 1905-7.

Fishman J, Fishman L (2005) *History Taking in Medicine and Surgery*. Knutsford: PasTest.

Fox R (1979) *Essays in Medical Sociology*. New York: John Wiley & Sons.

General Pharmaceutical Council (GPhC) (2010) *Standards of Conduct, Ethics and Performance*. London. GPhC.

Gerrity P (1987) Perception in nursing: the value of intuition. In: Thompson C, Dowding D (eds), *Clinical Decision Making and Judgement in Nursing*. Edinburgh: Churchill Livingstone.

Goldberg C (2009) A practical guide to clinical medicine: history of presenting illness (online). Available at: http://meded.ucsd.edu/clinicalmed/history.htm (accessed April 2010).

Greaves I, Porter K, Hodgetts T, Woollard M, eds (2006) *Emergency Care: A textbook for paramedics*, 2nd edn. London: Saunders Elsevier.

Groen GJ, Patel VL (1985) Medical problem solving: some questionable assumptions. Cited in Higgs et al (2008).

Hamilton W, Britten N (2006) Patient agendas in primary care. *BMJ* **332**: 1225-6.

Hans C (2007) *What is Bayesian Analysis?* (online). Available at www.bayesian.org (accessed April 2010).

Hardy D, Smith B (2008) Decision making in practice. *Br J Anaesth Recovery Nurs* **9**: 19-21.

Health Professions Council (2007) *Standards of Proficiency* (online). Available at www.hpc-uk.org/publications/standards (accessed April 2010).

Higgs J, Jones M (2000) *Clinical Reasoning in the Health Professions*, 2nd edn. Oxford: Butterworth Heinemann.

Higgs J, Jones M, Loftus S, Christensen N, eds (2008) *Clinical Reasoning in the Health Professions*, 3rd edn. London: Butterworth Heinemann.

Jerram S, Newson S (2007) Care of the older adult. In: Cross S, Rimmer M (eds), *Nurse Practitioner Manual of Clinical Skills*. Edinburgh: Baillière Tindall.

Kahneman D, Slovic P, Tversky A (1982) *Judgement Under Uncertainty: Heuristics and biases*. Cambridge: Cambridge University Press.

Kurtz S, Silverman J, Benson J, Draper J (2003) Marrying content and process in clinical method teaching: enhancing the Calgary–Cambridge guides. *Acad Med* **78**: 802-9.

Launer J (2002) *Narrative Based Primary Care: A practical guide*. Oxford: Radcliffe Medical Press.

Lloyd M, Bor R (2004) *Communication Skills for Medicine*, 2nd edn. Edinburgh: Churchill Livingstone.

Longmore M, Wilkinson I, Davidson E, Foulkes A, Mafi A (2010) *Oxford Handbook of Clinical Medicine*, 8th edn. Oxford: Oxford University Press.

Luker, A, Hogg, C, Austin, L, Ferguson, B, Smith, K (1998) Decision making: the context of nurse prescribing. *J Adv Nurs* **27**: 657-65.

McNeilis KS, Thompson TL, O'Hair D (1995) Implications of relational communication for therapeutic discourse. In: Morris GH, Chenail RJ (eds), *The Talk of the Clinic: Explorations in the analysis of medical and therapeutic discourse*. Hove: Lawrence Erlbaum Associates.

Meerabeau L (1992) Tacit nursing knowledge: an untapped resource or a methodological headache? *J Adv Nurs* **17**: 108-12.

Morton PG (1993) *Health Assessment in Nursing*, 2nd edn. Philadelphia: FA Davis.

Moulton L (2007) *The Naked Consultation: a Practical Guide to Primary Care Consultation Skills*. Oxford: Radcliffe Publishing.

National Institute for Health Clinical Excellence (2003) *Chronic Heart Failure: Management of chronic heart failure in adults in primary and secondary care*. London: NICE.

National Institute for Health Clinical Excellence (2004) *Chronic Obstructive Pulmonary Disease: Management of chronic obstructive pulmonary disease in adults in primary and secondary care*. London: NICE.

National Institute for Health Clinical Excellence (2006) *Hypertension: Management of hypertension in adults in primary care*. London: NICE.

National Prescribing Centre (1999) Signposts for prescribing nurses - general principles of good prescribing. *Prescrib Nurse Bull* **1**(1).

Neighbour R (2005) *The Inner Consultation: How to develop an effective and intuitive consulting style*, 2nd edn. Oxford: Radcliffe Publishing.

Nursing and Midwifery Council (2008) *The Code: Standards of Conduct. Performance and ethics for nurses and midwives*. London: NMC.

Nuttall D (2008) Older people, prescribing and public health. *Nurse Prescrib* **6**: 357-61.

O'Connor A, Legare F, Stacey D (2003) Risk communication in practice: the contribution of decision aids. *BMJ* **327**: 736-40.

Offredy M (1998) The application of decision making concepts by nurse practitioners in general practice. *J Adv Nurs* **28**: 988-1000.

Pearsall J, Trumble B (Eds) (2008) *Oxford English Reference Dictionary* (2nd Ed Rev). Oxford: Oxford University Press.

Pendleton D, Schofield T, Tate P, Havelock P (2003) *The New Consultation: Developing doctor-patient communication*. Oxford: Oxford University Press.

Piasecki M (2003) *Clinical Communication Handbook*. Oxford: Blackwell Science.

Radwin L (1990) Research on diagnostic reasoning in nursing. *Nurs Diag* **1**: 70-7.

Rang HP, Dale MM, Ritter JM, Flower R (2009) *Rang & Dale's Pharmacology*, 6th edn. London: Churchill Livingstone.

Resuscitation Council UK (2005) *Adult Advanced Life Support Algorithm* (online). Available at www.resus.org.uk/pages/alsalgo.pdf (accessed April 2010).

Rew L, Barron E (1987) Intuition: a neglected hallmark of nursing knowledge. In: Thompson C, Dowding D (eds). *Clinical Decision Making and Judgement in Nursing*. Edinburgh: Churchill Livingstone.

Robinson DL (2002) *Clinical Decision Making: A case study approach*, 2nd edn. Philadelphia: Lippincott.

Royal Pharmaceutical Society of Great Britain (2007) *Code of Ethics for Pharmacists and Pharmacist Technicians*. London: RPSGB.

Say RE, Thomson R (2003) The importance of patient preferences in treatment decisions: challenges for doctors. *BMJ* **327**: 542-5.

Schrader B, Fischer D (1987) Using intuitive knowledge in the neonatal intensive care nursery. In: Thompson C, Dowding D (eds), *Clinical Decision Making and Judgement in Nursing*. Edinburgh: Churchill Livingstone.

Shah N (2005a) Taking a history: introduction and presenting complaint. *Student BMJ* **13**: 314-15.

Shah N (2005b) Taking a history: conclusion and closure. *Student BMJ* **13**: 358-9.

Shipley KG, Woods JM (1996) *The Elements of Interviewing*. San Diego, CA: Singular Publishing Group Inc.

Thompson C, Dowding D (2002) *Clinical Decision Making and Judgement in Nursing*. Edinburgh: Churchill Livingstone.

Thompson R, Edwards A, Grey J (2005) Risk communication in the clinical consultation. *Clin Med* **5**: 465-9.

Watson S (1994) An exploratory study into a methodology for examination of decision making by nurses in the clinical area. *J Adv Nurs* **20**: 351-60.

Weed L (1968) Medical records that guide and teach. *N Engl J Med* **278**: 593-9, 652-7.

Weed L, Weed L (1999) Opening the black box of clinical judgement: an overview. *BMJ* **319**: 1-4.

West AF, West RR (2002) Clinical decision making: coping with uncertainty. *Postgrad Med J* **78**: 319-21.

White A (2002) Practical skills: prescribing consultation in practice. *Br J Commun Nurs* **7**: 469-73.

Williams D (1997) *Communication Skills in Practice: A practical guide for health professionals*. London: Jessica Kingsley Publishers.

Wood DM, Mould MG, Ong SB. Y, Baker EH (2005) 'Pack year' smoking histories: what about patients who use loose tobacco? *Tobacco Control* **14**: 141-2.

Wright K, Ryder S, Gousy M (2007) Community matrons improve health: patient's perspective, *Br J Commun Nurs* **12**: 453-9.

Young C (1987) Intuition and the nursing process. In: Thompson C, Dowding D (eds), *Clinical Decision Making and Judgement in Nursing*. Edinburgh: Churchill Livingstone.

Chapter 5
Essential Pharmacology, Therapeutics and Medicines Management for Non-medical Prescribers

Anne Fittock, Jane Alder, Alison Astles, David Kelly, Joseph Quinn and Samir Vohra

Learning objectives

After reading this chapter and completing the activities within it, the reader will be able to:

1 define key concepts of pharmacology
2 develop their own personal formulary
3 be aware of the complexities of pharmacology with specific reference to co-morbidity, medicine interactions, adverse medicine reactions and drugs with a narrow therapeutic index
4 appreciate concordant relationships compared with compliance with medication
5 understand the constituents of medicines management

Clinicians cannot know everything about all medicines but an essential element of safe prescribing practice is learning how to find out what you need to know, in order to prescribe safely the medicines that fall within your clinical practice. This chapter directs you to resources that you will use to develop and maintain knowledge about the medicines that you intend to prescribe. We guide you through processes, developed and evaluated as successful at the University of Central Lancashire, by which you will build your knowledge of pharmacology, therapeutics and medicines management to populate your own personal formulary.

The Textbook of Non-medical Prescribing, edited by Dilyse Nuttall and Jane Rutt-Howard.
© 2011 Blackwell Publishing Ltd

Non-medical prescribing enables suitably trained and qualified practitioners to prescribe within their own competence and scope of practice (Health Professions Council 2007, Royal Pharmaceutical Society of Great Britain (RPSGB) 2007, Nursing and Midwifery Council (NMC) 2008). It is an essential component of the competence of prescribers (National Prescribing Centre (NPC) 2009) to have knowledge of both how the medicines that they prescribe work at their site of action and how the medicines are handled by the body.

Patients present with individual circumstances and the simplest scenario is that you will prescribe a medicine to an otherwise healthy person who is taking no other treatments. However, practitioners may find that this is the exception rather than the rule. This chapter directs you to resources, taking you through processes by which you can evaluate the significance of intention to prescribe, of co-morbidity and medicine interactions. Use of key resources will support you to work within your competence and determine the most appropriate course of action to: advise, prescribe, seek advice or refer.

Adverse drug reactions (ADRs), if undetected, account for significant levels of morbidity (even mortality) in patients, who can be subject to avoidable discomfort, distress or worse. In addition ADRs contribute to preventable medicine-related hospital admissions, which in 2004 were estimated to cost the NHS in excess of £500m annually (Pirmohamed et al 2004). This chapter directs you to resources and guides you through processes by which risks to patients from ADRs may be minimised.

Between a third and a half of medicines that are prescribed for long-term conditions are not used as recommended (National Institute for Health Clinical Excellence (NICE) 2009). Patients can pay a high price in unresolved illness and their own lost earnings, while the NHS wastes valuable resources. This chapter discusses issues of concordance and adherence, and guides you through processes by which negotiated consultations that result in mutual understanding are encouraged.

Maximising efficacy, minimising risks, reducing costs and respecting patients' choices are the main features of good prescribing of medicines (Barber 1995). 'Good prescribing' is supported by effective medicines management systems, where medicines management is defined as a system of processes and behaviours that determine how medicines are used by the NHS and patients (NPC 2002). This chapter discusses issues of medicines management, including how prescribing links to public health. You will be directed to resources and guided through processes to build your own medicines management support to aid safe prescribing arising from multidisciplinary teamwork.

Pharmacology as part of prescribing practice

As prescribers, you are required to 'understand the mode of action and pharmacokinetics of medicines, how these mechanisms may be altered (e.g. by age, renal impairment) and how this affects dosage' (NPC 2009). Non-medical prescribers are not expected to be pharmacologists and know everything about every medicine; however, they are required to understand the pharmacology of the medicines that they prescribe and the limits of their pharmacological competence, and apply this knowledge within their practice (NMC 2006).

Example of potential pharmacokinetic impact on patient care

Theory

Absorption is the process of medicine movement from the administration site to the systemic circulation. The amount and rate of absorption are determined by such factors as the physical nature of the dosage form, presence or absence of food in the stomach, rate of gastric emptying and concurrent administration with other medicines (Downie et al 2007).

Practice

The non-medical prescriber recognises the implications of diarrhoea and vomiting in the young woman taking oral contraceptives, because the rate of gastric emptying could affect absorption and hence whether therapeutic medicine levels necessary for contraception are maintained. Appropriate prescription and counselling advice is necessary to avoid an unplanned pregnancy.

Example of potential pharmacodynamic impact on patient care

Theory

Receptors are a target molecule that a medicine molecule has to combine with to produce a specific effect. β Blockers target β receptors and, in the cardiovascular system, relax blood vessels, slow down the heart rate and lead to an overall decrease in blood pressure (BP), which is beneficial. However, β receptors are also located in the lungs and bronchi where they help keep air passages relaxed and loose, an effect that could be antagonised by β blockers, leading to adverse effects on breathing. The Commission on Human Medicines has advised that β blockers, including those considered cardioselective, should not be given to patients with a history of asthma or bronchospasm (British Medical Association (BMA) and Royal Pharmaceutical Society of Great Britain (RPSGB) 2010).

Practice

The non-medical prescriber recognises that the patient presenting for review of BP management has been started on a salbutamol inhaler following atenolol dose increase. Blockade of β receptors in the lungs causes airway structures to become more tense and constricted, adversely affecting breathing in susceptible patients. Alternative BP management is necessary to relieve patients' breathlessness, without recourse to salbutamol.

These examples are cited to illustrate the importance, for patients, of prescribers applying an understanding of pharmacokinetics and pharmacodynamics to their clinical practice. The area that prescribers work within will determine the level of understanding of the medicines, within their personal formulary and scope of practice.

Brief introduction to pharmacological terms

To make sense of pharmacology it is necessary to refresh your understanding of physiology, because knowledge of the function of the organs and circulatory systems and the human cell is essential when making sense of how body systems handle medicines (pharmacokinetics) and where at a cellular level medicines may act (pharmacodynamics).

Activity box 5.1

Refresh your physiology knowledge and understanding of key physiological concepts including: the human cell, mechanisms of the gastrointestinal and circulatory systems, and the functions of the kidneys and liver.

This chapter does not seek to replicate what is defined in detail in the many pharmacology books available, so it gives only brief summaries of pharmacological terms. It is, however, essential that you recognise the significance of understanding pharmacological concepts in the context of the prescribing care for your patients.

Pharmacokinetics

Pharmacokinetics is what the body does to the medicines. For almost all medicines the magnitude of the pharmacological effect depends on its concentration at its site of action. This phrase is simple enough! What it means is that for a medicine to have its effect it needs to be absorbed, e.g. through skin, bronchi or gastrointestinal tract, and then distributed in sufficient quantity to its site of action, usually via blood circulation. The active medicine will not remain in the body indefinitely but will be broken down or metabolised in order to be excreted or removed. Any of the above pharmacological processes may be affected by individual patient characteristics, e.g. liver or kidney function.

Texts and reference material that discuss pharmacokinetic concepts use such terms as: absorption, bioavailability, first-pass metabolism, distribution, protein binding, metabolism, cytochrome P450, excretion, half-life.

Put simply, **absorption** is the process of drug movement from the administration site to the systemic circulation (Figure 5.1).

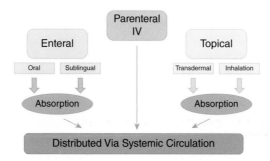

Figure 5.1 Routes of absorption.

The amount and rate of oral absorption are determined by several factors:

- Physical nature of the dosage form
- Presence or absence of food in the stomach
- Composition of the gastrointestinal (GI) contents
- Gastric or intestinal pH
- Mesenteric blood flow
- Concurrent administration with other drugs.

Most medicines are administered orally. Drug absorption is mainly in the upper small intestine, which is facilitated by the large surface area of microvilli and the rich blood supply. For drugs to pass across the lipid cell membrane they must be lipophilic, i.e. 'fat loving'. The level of mesenteric blood flow (arteries that supply blood to large and small intestines) directly affects the rate of removal of the drug from the site of absorption.

Gastric motility, constipation or diarrhoea affects the mixing in the GI tract which can alter the efficacy with which the medicines make contact with microvilli surfaces available to engage absorption. Alteration in the rate of gastric emptying will result in corresponding alterations in the rate of absorption, as in the case of diarrhoea or vomiting, which may affect whether therapeutic levels are achieved.

Activity box 5.2

Consider the effect on absorption of an analgesic or antiemetic if a patient had gastric stasis due to shock or migraine.

Consider what this may mean for the choice of route of administration and dosage form (see below) that a prescriber would select to ensure that adequate therapeutic levels could be achieved.

Dosage form refers to whether a medicine is in tablet, capsule or liquid form. The significance of the dosage form in prescribing practice is that it determines the rate and extent of absorption. Drugs in liquid dose form require no disintegration and often dissolution is already accomplished so absorption occurs more rapidly producing faster effects. For medicines administered as tablets or capsules, disintegration and dissolution of the released drug into the correct part of the GI tract are required for the drug to be adequately absorbed. Any alteration of the dosage form, e.g. crushing tablets or emptying capsules, affects the absorption process to one that has not been studied by the drug manufacturer. This should only be undertaken with expert advice where an alternative, licensed medication would not meet the patient needs (NMC 2006). Alteration of the dosage form or mixing of medicines before administration alters the pharmacokinetics of the product(s) and creates an unlicensed product (Medicines and Healthcare products Regulatory Agency (MHRA) 2009).

In 2009 the MHRA put in place changes to enable mixing of medicines before administration in clinical practice. These changes enable nurse and pharmacist independent prescribers to prescribe unlicensed medicines for their patients, on the same basis as doctors and dentists and supplementary prescribers, if part of a 'clinical management plan' (Department of Health (DH) 2009).

Bioavailability is the proportion of the administered dose that reaches the systemic circulation (Dale and Haylet 2008). It refers to the amount and rate of appearance of the drug in the blood, after administration in its initial dose form. Orally administered drug bioavailability is directly related to the individual solubility in body fluids:

Poor solubility = low bioavailability.

To produce a therapeutic effect, a drug must reach an adequate concentration in the blood. Drugs administered by the intravenous route are 100% bioavailable because they are administered directly into the blood; however, drugs administered by any other route will be less than 100% bioavailable, depending on the pharmacokinetic processes that affect them, such as first-pass metabolism.

First-pass metabolism is a defence mechanism whereby the liver protects the body from drugs (or toxins) absorbed via the GI tract by filtering them through a range of metabolic mechanisms, mediated by enzymes in the liver. All drugs taken orally, once they are absorbed, pass through the hepatic portal vein and can be subject to a degree of first-pass metabolism. As a result only part of the administered oral drug reaches the systemic circulation. This is called the 'first-pass effect'. Although there is patient variability, manufacturers take first-pass effects into account when developing appropriate dosage forms and recommending appropriate doses.

Activity box 5.3

Where in the *British National Formulary* (BNF) would you find clinicians guidance on prescribing for patients where liver disease compromises the first-pass effect?
    Propranolol and verapamil are drugs that are subject to extensive first-pass metabolism.

- What does the BNF recommend about the prescribing of verapamil in liver disease?
- What does the BNF recommend about the prescribing of propranolol in liver disease?

Distribution

The systemic circulation distributes medicines across the body and can be affected by cardiac output and regional blood flow (Downie et al 2007), e.g. a warm patient would experience better blood flow and therefore improved drug distribution compared with a hypothermic patient. Inflamed tissue has increased vascularity and permeability and therefore increased passage of drugs.

Body water is distributed into four main compartments: extracellular fluids including blood plasma, interstitial fluids, intracellular fluids, fluids within cells and transcellular fluids, such as cerebrospinal or synovial fluids (Dale and Haylet 2008). Drugs are usually distributed within each of these compartments in both free or bound form and move between compartments according to concentration. Only free drugs can be pharmacologically active, i.e. only free drugs can interact with their site of action to have an effect.

Protein binding

Drugs are bound by plasma proteins to a greater or lesser extent. The degree to which a drug binds to plasma proteins is determined by the drugs chemistry. The proportion of the drug that is bound to protein is pharmacologically inactive because the drug-protein complex is unable to cross cell membranes; however, this drug protein complex can quickly dissociate and release unbound drug into the system. The degree of protein binding will affect the intensity and duration of a drug's action.

A patient's condition and state of health may be an important consideration when thinking about protein binding because plasma proteins can be deficient in some diseases, e.g. in malnutrition, blood loss or liver disease (BMA and RPSGB 2010). Such patients could be subject to more of the drug being free to enter the tissue, and hence subject to toxicity despite a 'normal dose'.

Protein-bound drugs also provide a reservoir that may be displaced by adding another highly protein-bound drug, resulting, in a release of 'free' drug. This is a potential source of drug interactions. In practice this may be an important factor only in drugs that have high protein binding and a narrow therapeutic range, e.g. the 'fraction bound' of the anticoagulant warfarin is 97%; this means that, of the amount of warfarin in the blood, 97% is bound to plasma proteins (and is pharmacologically inactive) while the remaining 3% is the fraction that is active.

Activity box 5.4

Which BNF appendix offers the clinician guidance on drug interactions?

- Look in the relevant BNF appendix to identify which drugs interact with alcohol (ethanol).

Removal of a drug from the body occurs by two processes: metabolism and excretion.

Metabolism

Drugs are metabolised in the liver, lungs, kidneys, blood and intestines. The primary metabolic site is the liver. Metabolism is conversion of the chemistry of the drug, which requires enzymes, e.g. cytochrome P450 enzymes, to oxidise the drug (phase 1) or conjugate the drug (phase 2) in order to prepare it for excretion. The speed with which a drug is metabolised will determine the duration of the action of the drug. This, in turn, will determine how often the drug is administered. If enzyme function is inadequate, metabolism can be compromised and cause toxicity, e.g. in liver disease, or very young or very old people. Metabolic enzymes can also be induced or inhibited by drugs that could affect the metabolism and therefore the duration of the drug.

Enzyme induction is a process by which a drug initiates or enhances the activity of an enzyme.

Enzyme inhibition is a process of interference or reduction in enzyme activity. Cytochrome P450 consists of the primary metabolic enzymes in the liver which can be subject to induction or inhibition from other drugs that the patient may take. See Table 5.1 for more information about the impact of enzyme inducers and enzyme inhibitors on cytochrome P450 enzymes.

Activity box 5.5

Where in the BNF can clinicians find guidance on prescribing for patients with compromised ability to metabolise drugs?

Look at the relevant BNF drug monographs to identify what steps are advised when prescribing paracetamol or statins to a patient with liver impairment.

Excretion

How the drugs are excreted can influence prescribing decisions. Most drugs are excreted in either the bile or the urine via the kidneys. Hence, renal function is important in determining excretion and patients with compromised renal function eliminate most drugs less effectively and are therefore at risk from toxicity. For drugs to be excreted in urine they need to become more hydrophilic (water loving or soluble) than lipophilic (fat loving or soluble). When lipid-soluble drugs pass through the kidneys they are reabsorbed in the distal tubule and return to the plasma. Some reabsorption of lipid soluble drugs occurs in Bowman's capsule; these are known as metabolites, and are often less

Table 5.1 Drugs affecting the action of cytochrome P450 enzymes (Thomson 2004)

CYP450 enzyme	Inducer (2-3 weeks)	Inhibitor (2-3 days)	Substrate
1A2	Cigarette smoke, omeprazole	Amiodarone, cimetidine, ofloxacin	Clozapine, haloperidol, naproxen, theophylline
3A4, 5, 7	Phenobarbital, St John's wort	Amiodarone, cimetidine, fluconazole, verapamil	Amlodipine, atorvastatin, erythromycin, methadone
2E1	Ethanol, isoniazid	Disulfiram	Ethanol, paracetamol, theophylline

active than their parent compounds, but in some drugs contribute to the overall effect of the drug, e.g. imipramine, propranolol and diazepam.

Excretion of drugs can be affected by the urinary pH, although this is of minor clinical significance because most weak acids and bases are inactivated by hepatic metabolism rather than renal excretion. Drugs that change renal blood flow can alter the excretion of other drugs. Renal blood flow is partially controlled by prostaglandins, so drugs that inhibit the manufacture of prostaglandins, such as non-steroidal anti-inflammatory drugs (NSAIDs) may inhibit the excretion of other drugs, e.g. lithium, leading to toxicity.

Activity box 5.6

Where in the BNF can you find guidance on prescribing for patients with compromised ability to excrete drugs?

Look at the relevant BNF drug monographs to identify what steps are advised when prescribing ibuprofen or tiotropium to a patient with renal impairment.

Half-life

Drug excretion is commonly expressed in terms of the half-life ($t_{1/2}$), which is the time required for the concentration of the drug in the plasma to decrease by half of its initial value. Concentration falls as a result of metabolism and excretion. Drug half-life is variable and can be long or short. Subsequent doses are given to raise the concentration levels to a peak and maintain therapeutic effect. The optimal dosage interval between drug administrations will be determined by the half-life of the drug. If dose interval is too long, the desired effect will not be achieved; too short an interval may lead to toxicity (Table 5.2).

Table 5.2 Example of effect of half-life ($t_{1/2}$), using drug with strength of 100 mg and a 6-hour half-life

Time (h)	Dose	Accumulated dose (mg)
0	1st dose 100 mg	
6	2nd dose 100 mg + 50 mg still present from 1st dose	150
12	3rd dose 100 mg + 75 mg still present from 1st + 2nd doses	175
18	4th dose 100 mg + 88 mg still present from 1st, 2nd + 3rd doses	188
24	5th dose 100 mg + 94 mg still present from 1st, 2nd, 3rd + 4th doses	194
30	6th dose 100 mg + 97 mg still present from 1st, 2nd, 3rd, 4th + 5th doses	197

As can be seen, accumulation becomes less at each dose as 'steady state' is achieved after three to five half-lives, whereby the amount of drug absorbed with each dose is balanced by the amount of drug metabolised and excreted.

Pharmacodynamics

Pharmacodynamics is the study of what the medicine does to the body when it arrives at its site of action and how drugs exert their effect at a cellular level. How can one drug affect breathing and another alter heart rate? The answer is in the **specificity** and **affinity** of an interaction between a drug and the biological target within the body.

The four main types of biological targets within the body are commonly categorised as follows.

Receptors, ion channels, carrier molecules and enzymes (Figure 5.2)

Receptors are proteins localised on the cell membrane or inside the cell. Any molecule that binds to a receptor to produce a specific effect is known as a *ligand*. Receptors and ligands must be compatible, like two pieces of a jigsaw, for binding and for a *specific* effect to occur. The strength of a molecule binding to the receptor site is known as *affinity*. A receptor has a high affinity for a molecule if it has a strong interaction, which enables binding and subsequent biological response to occur at very low concentrations. The receptors normally bind the body's own endogenous (originating from within the body) hormones and neurotransmitters, which in turn activates the receptor and leads

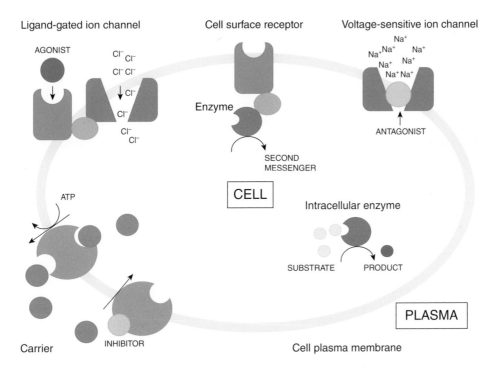

Figure 5.2 Types of targets for drug action.

to a physiological response, e.g. contraction, relaxation, secretion or enzyme activation.

If the drug's chemical structure or design is based on the structure of a specific receptor, it can selectively bind to the target receptor and produce a biological effect. The greater the specificity of the drug-receptor binding, the fewer the side effects likely to be encountered. The main types of action at receptor can be classified as receptor agonists and receptor antagonists.

An *agonist* is a drug that binds to a receptor and activates it, producing its normal biological response (Figure 5.3). An example of a receptor agonist is nicotine which is the primary alkaloid in tobacco products. It stimulates nicotinic acetylcholine receptors, naturally occurring in the body with receptors in the brain. The pharmacology of nicotine is complex, however, because it also acts as a receptor agonist in the peripheral and central nervous systems. Another effect of prolonged exposure to nicotine from tobacco smoking is a proliferation of receptors, leading to dependence and tolerance. Nicotine replacement products act as receptor agonists, which support smoking cessation by reducing cravings.

An *antagonist* is a drug that binds to a receptor without causing activation. The antagonist simply blocks the agonist from binding to the receptor and so inhibits the receptor's normal biological response (Figure 5.3). Examples of receptor antagonists include antihistamines such as loratadine and β blockers such as bisprolol.

The way that a medicine works is indicated in the nomenclature of the drug group to which it belongs, e.g. H_2-receptor antagonists block histamine H_2-receptors and antimuscarinic drugs block muscarinic acetylcholine receptors. Simply stating the facts does not, however, illustrate understanding of the pharmacology of these drugs, because it does not present the 'so what' of pharmacodynamics. If by this we mean if 'H_2-receptor

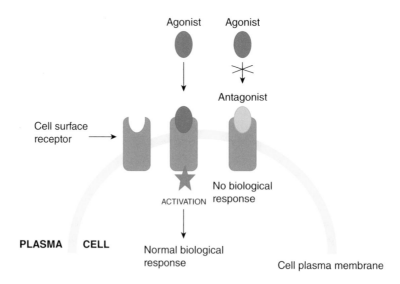

Figure 5.3 Action of the agonist and antagonist at cell surface receptors.

antagonists block histamine H_2-receptors' what does that mean for the patient? It means that the histamine H_2-receptors in the stomach which are stimulating gastric acid production are blocked, reducing the acid secretion, thus promoting healing of a gastric ulcer. As previously stated, you need to understand the pathophysiology in order to interpret the 'so what' of the pharmacology.

Activity box 5.7

If 'antimuscarinic drugs block muscarinic acetylcholine receptors' in the lung what does this mean for the patient's breathing?

Understanding the pharmacodynamics of drugs will enable you to understand and predict drug actions, interactions and toxicities.

Ion channels are gaps located in the cell plasma membrane that control the movement of electrolytes (specifically the free ions: sodium (Na^+), calcium (Ca^{2+}), potassium (K^+) and chloride (Cl^-)) in and out of the cell. There are several different types of ion channels: two of the most common ion channels targeted for drug action are the ligand-gated ion channels which are linked to a receptor and voltage-sensitive ion channels. The ligand-gated ion channels open only when the receptor is occupied by an agonist, whereas voltage-sensitive ion channels are gated by a different mechanism where the opening and closing of the ion channel are linked to voltage changes across the membrane.

When a drug behaving as a receptor agonist interacts with the receptor site at the *ligand-gated ion channels*, a conformational (or shape) change occurs and the channel opens. Large numbers of ions rapidly (milliseconds) enter the cell by moving down the electrochemical gradient; they flow from high ion concentration to low ion concentration, and initiate a biological response within the cell. A typical example of the normal biological function of this type of interaction is the action of the endogenous inhibitory neurotransmitter γ-aminobutyric acid (GABA) at the $GABA_A$ receptor on chloride channels. Drugs that act as agonists at GABA receptors or increase the amount of GABA produced commonly behave as anticonvulsants or anxiolytics, e.g. benzodiazepine tranquillisers facilitate chloride channel opening by acting at a specific benzodiazepine receptor coupled to the $GABA_A$ receptor. When the receptor is activated GABA neurotransmission is increased and chloride influx (or entry) increases, resulting in tranquillity.

Drugs can also bind directly to other parts of the ion channel, so when a stimulus arises the shape-changes that lead to the opening of the ion channel are blocked from occurring and the increase in permeability of the cell to ion influx is inhibited (or diminished). A typical example of this mechanism of drug action is the prevention of Na^+ influx by local anaesthetics, e.g. lidocaine binding to *voltage-gated channels*. The normal biological function of the voltage-sensitive ion channel is propagation (or multiplication) of nerve impulses across an excitable cell membrane (e.g. nerve cell membrane) generated by temporary changes in voltage across the cell membrane via the opening and closing of the voltage-gated Na^+, K^+ and Cl^- ion channels. Blockade of Na^+ influx by local anaesthetics prevents propagation of the membrane action potential, blocks nerve impulses and hence prevents subsequent perception of painful stimuli.

Activity box 5.8

Drugs such as verapamil block the entry of Ca^{2+} at the L-type calcium ion channels in the heart, interfering with the cardiac nerve impulses and thereby reducing contractility.

Why is co-administration of verapamil with β blockers (antagonist at β adrenoceptors such as propranolol and atenolol) listed in BNF as a potential drug interaction?

Hint: think about the combined actions of these two drugs

Carrier molecules are proteins involved in the transport of endogenous molecules across cell membranes. These carrier proteins transport molecules that would otherwise be unable to cross the cell membrane, e.g. polar (or charged) hydrophilic molecules and ions that cannot permeate the lipid cell membrane. Carrier molecules are also involved in pumping ions out of the cell against a concentration gradient, a process that requires energy. There are many examples of the normal biological function of this type of carrier in the human body including:

- transport of glucose and amino acids into the cell
- transport of Na^+ and Ca^{2+} out of the cell
- transport of neurotransmitters into nerve cells
- active reuptake of ions and molecules from the kidney nephron back into the bloodstream.

The carrier proteins contain recognition sites which ensure that only specific molecules are transported. These recognition sites can be exploited as a drug target by designing drugs with structural similarity to the endogenously transported molecule, but instead the drugs modify or block the carrier, inhibiting transport. A typical example of a drug class that inhibits using this mechanism is inhibition of the noradrenaline transporter by tricyclic antidepressants (e.g. imipramine and lofepramine). The normal biological function of the noradrenaline transporter is inactivation of the neurotransmitter noradrenaline by reuptake of noradrenaline into the nerve terminal. Inhibition of this transporter therefore leads to an accumulation of the neurotransmitter noradrenaline in the nerve cleft, which can in turn activate adrenoceptors thought to be beneficial for the treatment of depression.

Activity box 5.9

Which pump does the drug omeprazole inhibit and how does this mechanism link to the action of omeprazole?
Hint: hydrogen ions are a necessary precursor required to form gastric acid.

Enzymes are proteins that catalyse (or accelerate) most of the normal functions of the cell and are therefore obvious drug targets for therapeutic intervention. Drugs could be targeted to inhibit enzyme function, which would lead to a decrease in the amount of a product formed. An example of this type of drug enzyme inhibition is the inhibition of angiotensin-converting enzyme (ACE) by captopril. Captopril prevents the conversion of angiotensin I into angiotensin II. Angiotensin II causes arteriolar constriction and an increase in diastolic and systolic blood pressure. Inhibiting the formation of angiotensin II in hypertensive patients will therefore result in a decrease in blood pressure.

If an enzyme is inhibited (or blocked) by a drug, the pharmacological effect could be due to accumulation (build-up) of the amount of enzyme substrate, if it cannot be converted into a product (a substrate is the substance on which the enzyme acts). An example of this mechanism of action is the inhibition of the enzyme acetylcholinesterase by neostigmine which leads to an accumulation of the substrate acetylcholine. More acetylcholine is therefore present and prolonging the action of acetylcholine enhances neuromuscular transmission in patients with myasthenia gravis (severe muscle weakness).

Activity box 5.10

Using the BNF identify which enzyme NSAIDs (e.g. aspirin, ibuprofen) inhibit.
Are the effects of NSAIDs due to enzyme substrate accumulation or a decrease the enzyme product formed?

A summary of some typical examples of drug action for each of the targets mentioned is given in Table 5.3.

Guide through processes to build and develop one's own formulary, with examples

Non-medical prescribers work in a diverse range of care pathways and the study of the pharmacology of the wide range of medicines that they may prescribe must logistically

Table 5.3 Examples of targets for drug action

Drug target		Effectors	
Receptors	**Type (subtype)**	**Agonists**	**Antagonists**
	Acetylcholine (nicotinic)	Acetycholine, nicotine	
	Acetylcholine (muscarinic)	Acetycholine, pilocarpine	Atropine, hyoscine
	Adrenoceptors (α/β)	Noradrenaline, adrenaline	Labetalol
	α_1-Adrenoceptor	Phenylephrine	Prazosin
	α_2-Adrenoceptor	Clonidine	
	β_1-Adrenoceptor	Dopamine, dobutamine	Atenolol
	β_2-Adrenoceptor	Salbutamol	
	Histamine (H_1)	Histamine	Promethazine
	Histamine (H_2)	Histamine	Cimetidine, ranitidine
	Dopamine (D_1 to D_5)	Dopamine, bromocriptine (D_2)	Phenothiazine derivatives, domperidone, metoclopramide (D_2), clozapine (D_4)
	Opiate (μ)	Morphine, diamorphine	Naloxone
	Oestrogen	Ethinylestradiol	Tamoxifen
	Epidermal growth factor receptor		Trastuzumab
	$GABA_A$	GABA, benzodiazepines, barbiturates	
	$GABA_B$	GABA, baclofen, tizanidine	
	Serotonin ($5HT_1$ to $5HT_5$)	Serotonin, sumatriptan, metoclopramide	Ergotamine, methysergide, ondansetron
Ion channels	**Type**	**Blockers**	**Modulators**
	Voltage-gated sodium channels	Local anaesthetics	
	Renal tubule Na^+ channels	Amiloride	Aldosterone
	Voltage-gated Ca^{2+} channels	Divalent cations	Dihydropyridines, opioids
	ATP-sensitive K^+ channels	ATP	Sulphonylureas
	GABA-gated Cl^- channels		Benzodiazepines

Table 5.3 *(Continued)*

Carriers	Type	Inhibitors	–
	Noradrenaline transporter	Tricyclic antidepressants, cocaine	–
	Weak acid carrier (renal tubule)	Probenecid	–
	Na$^+$/ K$^+$/2Cl$^-$ co-transporter (loop of Henle)	Loop diuretics	–
	Proton pump (gastric mucosa)	Omeprazole	–
Enzymes	**Type**	**Inhibitors**	**–**
	Acetylcholinesterase	Neostigmine	–
	Cyclooxygenase	Aspirin	–
	Angiotensin-converting enzyme	Captopril	–
	HMG-CoA reductase	Simvastatin	–
	Phosphodiesterase type V	Sildenafil	–
	Dihydrofolate reductase	Trimethoprim, methotrexate	–
	Thymidine kinase	Aciclovir	–
	HIV protease	Saquinavir	–

5HT, 5-hydroxytryptamine; GABA, γ-aminobutyric acid; HMG-CoA, hydroxymethylglutaryl coenzyme A.
Adapted from Rang et al (2009) and Hopkins (1999).

be by self-directed study. Pharmacology textbooks are cited at the end of this chapter as suggested resources; the best pharmacology references for explaining these concepts and how your personal formulary drugs work are the books that make sense to you! Beyond the BNF and textbooks, there are a number of resources to help prescribers deepen their pharmacological understanding and update their knowledge, including higher education modules and courses, journal articles, e-learning resources and professional expertise such as pharmacist advice.

Summaries of product characteristics (SPC), which often include a description of the pharmacokinetic and pharmacodynamic properties of individual drugs, can be found on the Electronic Medicines Compendium which is available on the internet at the following link: www.medicines.org.uk/EMC/default.aspx

Community practitioner nurse prescribers work to a restricted formulary of preparations, which limits the choice of which medicines to study in order to develop understanding of pharmacology. However, the principle remains the same, which is to become familiar with the pharmacology of the products that you intend to prescribe.

Activity box 5.11

How should you select the appropriate medicines to study and populate your formulary?
Non-medical prescribers should reflect on:

- own area of practice
- the supporting guidelines
- any relevant local trust policies and formularies.

When you begin this process you may encounter the expression in textbooks: 'the pharmacology of this medicine is not well understood'; this is the case for a variety of medicines used empirically (historically). This is a signal to find a different example that will advance your understanding, because the pharmacology of many medicines is well understood. To start with, identify medicines from your clinical practice and, using suitable reference sources, develop an overview that represents *your* understanding of the pharmacokinetic and pharmacodynamic properties of the medicines.

Example 1

A non-medical prescriber working in a hypertension clinic in primary care would need to initially become familiar with the pharmacology of the medicines recommended for first-line use by the NICE hypertension clinical guideline (NICE 2006). Within this wide therapeutic area, the logical starting point would be with the formulary choices of their employing organisation, e.g. *bendroflumethiazide*, amlodipine, ramipril, candersartan, doxazosin.

Pharmacokinetic properties
Bendroflumethiazide is taken orally and completely absorbed from the GI tract. It is extensively metabolised with approximately 30% excreted unchanged in the urine. After an oral dose the onset of diuretic action is within 2 hours with the peak effect between 3 and 6 hours after administration. The duration of the diuretic action of bendroflumethiazide is between 18 and 24 hours. The onset of the hypotensive action is within 3 or 4 days.

Pharmacodynamic properties
Bendroflumethiazide is a thiazide diuretic that reduces the absorption of electrolytes from the renal tubules in the kidneys, thereby increasing the excretion of sodium and chloride ions, and consequently of water. Thiazides have a hypotensive effect, due to a reduction in peripheral resistance, and they enhance the effects of other antihypertensive agents.

Having gained an understanding of how one medicine works, repeat the process for the other medicines that you will commonly encounter or prescribe.

Talk to colleagues about what you have learned! Many of our students found the experience of going through this 'research' and personal formulary building process, and then explaining the pharmacology to their peers, extremely useful in consolidating and expanding their knowledge and application of pharmacology.

Understanding the pharmacokinetics and dynamics of medicines that you may prescribe is the first step, but there is greater knowledge needed of the medicines that you intend to prescribe than just the pharmacokinetics and pharmacodynamics. For each medicine, you should also use suitable reference sources to develop your knowledge of:

- indications for which the medicine may be used
- any pre-existing medical conditions that may influence the choice of medicine
- any adverse medicine reactions associated with the medicines
- any concomitant medicines that may have serious interactions
- education points for patient or family on use of medicines.

Example 2

A non-medical prescriber working in the care of painful diabetic neuropathy would need to become familiar with the pharmacology of the medicines outlined in the NICE Clinical Guideline 96: *Neuropathic Pain - Pharmacological management* (NICE 2010). The prescriber would study *duloxetine*, amitriptyline, pregabalin, tramadol, topical lidocaine.

Pharmacokinetic properties
Duloxetine is taken orally and is well absorbed from the GI tract with peak blood concentration occurring 6 hours after the dose. Food can delay the rate of and also has a slight effect on the extent of absorption but the manufacturers report that these effects have no clinical significance. Duloxetine is highly bound to plasma proteins. Plasma protein binding is not affected by renal or hepatic insufficiency. Duloxetine undergoes extensive biotransformation, metabolites being excreted mainly in the urine. Cytochromes involved in metabolism are CYP450-2D6 and -1A2. The elimination half-life of duloxetine ranges from 8 h to 17 h.

Pharmacodynamic properties
Duloxetine inhibits the uptake of both serotonin (5-hydroxytryptamine or 5HT) and noradrenaline (NA). The pain inhibitory action of duloxetine is believed to be a result of potentiation of descending inhibitory pain pathways within the central nervous system (CNS). In pre-marketing clinical trials, 50% of people experienced a 50% reduction in pain using pain assessment tools over a 12-week period. Patients not experiencing pain reduction of 30% within 60 days were unlikely to reach that level during further treatment.

Side effects
Due to the pharmacodynamic actions of duloxetine within the CNS it has a wide range of side effects that the non-medical prescriber should be aware of and should consider in relation to the individual patient each time that it is prescribed. Duloxetine should be used with caution in patients with a history of mania, a diagnosis of bipolar disorder or

a history of seizures. Duloxetine has also been associated with increased BP which can develop into clinically significant hypertension, so appropriate monitoring must be in place and due consideration taken of the potential effects of duloxetine should any changes in BP arise through treatment; for the supplementary prescriber monitoring of BP should form part of the review process for duloxetine detailed in the clinical management plan.

Drug interactions

Duloxetine potentially interacts with several medications. Due to its potential for causing dyspepsia possibly even gastric bleeding, other drugs that have a similar pharmacodynamic effect, such as NSAIDs, should be used with caution or it may be appropriate to advise on other analgesia such as paracetamol. Pharmacokinetic interactions of duloxetine include the inhibition of its metabolism by ciprofloxacin.

Education points for patient and family

The prescriber should be in a position to counsel the patient on the key issues surrounding the use of duloxetine and all the other drugs prescribed from his or her formulary. Counselling would start at the correct doses and administration times and move on to cover the main side effects to look out for; duloxetine may cause nausea and so the patient could be advised to take with food to combat this – it has been shown above that, although food delays absorption of the drug, it is not clinically significant and so this would be appropriate advice to give. Patients should be advised of potentially serious side effects that would warrant medical attention, such as the development of gastric discomfort or dyspepsia. Clinically significant drug interactions should also be covered such as that between duloxetine and ciprofloxacin; this may be an issue if the patient receives acute medical attention from a practitioner who is not normally familiar with the patient.

The process of developing knowledge of the drugs within your personal formulary will enable you to prescribe those drugs in a safe and appropriate manner and also to be able to discuss key points surrounding their use with other healthcare professionals and patients.

You will need to research, understand, update and apply the knowledge of the medicines in your personal formulary to ensure safe prescribing practice (NPC 2001, 2003, 2004a, 2004b, 2006).

BNF: practise using this essential resource

An essential resource when prescribing is familiarity with using the BNF including the appendices, which provide invaluable information on medicine interactions, co-morbidities that affect medicine handling, such as liver and renal disease, and information on cautions when prescribing to women who are pregnant or breastfeeding.

Competent use of the BNF is an essential resource for prescribers, particularly invaluable when prescribing for patients taking other medications and with co-morbidities that affect their ability to handle medicines. You cannot underestimate the importance of using the BNF efficiently and effectively. You cannot memorise the contents of the BNF but you should be familiar with its layout so that you can use it for reference, as necessary, to extract the information that you need in a timely manner.

There is a quiz on the book's website to help you become more familiar with the BNF (BMA and RPSGB 2010). Remember, it isn't about knowing all the answers but going through the process of using the BNF to find the answers.

Prescribing in co-morbidity

Co-morbidity matters to prescribers for a number of reasons and the first is that co-morbidity can affect how a patient's body handles medicines. Co-morbidity that affects absorption such as constipation or gastric surgery may affect the rate or amount of medicine entering the body, whereas co-morbidity that affects distribution, e.g. blood loss, poor circulation or shock, may affect active medicine reaching its site of action if blood flow is restricted.

Impairment of the liver or kidneys will impede a patient's ability to metabolise or excrete medicines. It is worth noting that some medicines are administered as pro-medicines and need to undergo metabolism to become active, e.g. ramipril. In this case, patients with impaired liver function may not achieve therapeutic levels if their liver is not able to convert the pro-medicine into active medicine.

More usually metabolism is the mechanism for breaking medicines down by enzymatic action in order to make them easier for the body to eliminate. Hence, patients with severely impaired liver function will be at risk from raised levels of circulating medicines, leading to possible toxicity.

Excretion via the kidneys is the main route of elimination for many medicines and co-morbidity that adversely affects patients' renal capacity will expose them to risk of increased circulating medicines, also leading to possible toxicity. Renal function declines with age and patients' ability to excrete medicines is a significant consideration when prescribing for elderly people.

The above briefly summarises why co-morbidity that impacts on pharmacokinetics, and the patient's handling of medicines, are key considerations when prescribing for patients.

Prescribers must consider the holistic needs of the patient before them and where patients have co-morbidity, reflect on their competence to evaluate where it may be appropriate to prescribe, seek advice or refer. Community nurse practitioner prescribers can take some comfort that the restricted formulary to which they work, with few exceptions, includes medicines considered safe for the indications where they are prescribed at usual doses. However, the scope and range of non-medical prescribing are vast, with non-medical clinicians prescribing within clinical competence in situations where, as examples:

- usually healthy patients, young and old, require treatment for minor conditions such as candidiasis and dry skin
- frail elderly housebound patients with multiple co-morbidities and complex polypharmacy medication regimens
- non-medical prescribers adjust doses of medicines with narrow therapeutic indices on neonatal or special care units.

Individual prescribers will need to reflect on their patient group, their personal formulary and their competence to recognise and adjust to presenting co-morbidities.

Co-morbidity and polypharmacy

Another reason to discuss co-morbidity is that patients present not only with the condition to be treated by the non-medical prescriber but also with other conditions requiring medication, which may be outside the competence of the non-medical prescriber.

When discussing co-morbidity it is useful to reflect on the scale of morbidity and the demographic changes that alter the nature of patients most frequently presenting in a modern NHS. Three out of five people aged over 60 have a long-term condition, which is over 15 million people in England (DH 2001). One in six adults in the UK has a mental illness at any one time (DH 1999). Cardiovascular disease kills more than 110 000 people in England every year (DH 2000) and 1.8 million people in the UK are diagnosed with diabetes (DH 2007).

The older population (those aged 65 and over) account for 18% of the population in the UK but for 45% of consumption of all drug prescriptions. The proportion of people aged 65 and over is projected to increase to 22% by 2031 (Office for National Statistics 2007). Given such trends, it is vital that prescribers take every opportunity to reflect on the appropriateness or otherwise of drug prescriptions particularly for elderly people.

Drug treatments need to be tailored to the individuals needs and this is especially so in the elderly population. Renal function declines with age and this can have a significant effect on the pharmacokinetics and pharmacodynamics of the drugs being used (as highlighted above). The distribution of body fat and water is altered in older people, resulting in increased risk of drug toxicity and accumulation of lipid-soluble drugs. Many acute hospital admissions of older people are due to medication side effects and drug interactions. Such side effects and interactions may lead to adverse events such as falls, postural hypotension, dehydration, confusion, gastrointestinal bleeds, or renal or heart failure.

The increased frequency of coexisting illnesses in elderly people places them at particular risk of drug–illness interactions, e.g. many elderly people have both renal impairment and osteoarthritis. NSAIDs used for pain relief can adversely affect renal function, potentially leading to renal failure. Indications for drug use may range from treatment of a condition to providing symptomatic relief or improving the quality of life. Prescribers need to maintain a careful balance, avoiding both excessive medication and under-medication.

Example 3

A non-medical prescriber working in a hypertension clinic, following NICE (2006) clinical guidance, would know that bendroflumethiazide is a first-line agent in the treatment of hypertension in patients aged over 55 years. Bendroflumethiazide 2.5 mg produces a near-maximal BP-lowering effect at this 2.5 mg dose. Increasing the dose confers no extra benefit in terms of BP reduction (a dose–response 'ceiling' effect) but increases the likelihood of adverse side effects on electrolytes, blood lipid and glucose levels. Bendroflumethiazide also affects uric acid levels and hyperuricaemia is a known side effect, which can lead to gout in susceptible patients. The prescriber would therefore take caution in selecting an antihypertensive drug for a patient who had previously had gout and would avoid bendroflumethiazide in this case.

Management and avoidance of drug interactions

Where patients are taking more than one medicine there is a potential for medicine interactions. These may be chemical, pharmacodynamic or pharmacokinetic in origin. Chemical medicine interactions occur where two medicines are chemically incompatible and can be particularly relevant when prescribing or administering medicines intravenously. BNF, Appendix 6 offers useful guidance for managing and avoiding chemical medicine interactions.

Pharmacodynamic medicine interactions occur where medicines that are pharmacologically similar or act at the same sites of action are given together. So, for example, medicines that act at the same receptors or target the same enzyme pathway may be subject to pharmacodynamic interactions. This can result in additive effects, e.g. alcohol and benzodiazepines given together may cause enhanced sedation. Alternative antagonism may occur when medicines have opposing dynamic actions or are competing at the same site of action, e.g. buprenorphine would compete with morphine at opiate receptors – leading to a pharmacodynamic interaction.

Pharmacokinetic interactions occur where the body processes of absorption, distribution, metabolism and excretion are affected.

Example 4

The non-medical prescriber is managing a patient with hypertension also treated with lithium for bipolar disorder. Lithium is a drug with a narrow therapeutic index used to treat bipolar disorder. The pharmacodynamic action of bendroflumethiazide on ion excretion causes the excretion of lithium to be reduced, so raising lithium blood levels, which if co-prescribed would put the patient at risk of lithium toxicity. The prescriber would therefore take caution in selecting an antihypertensive drug for a patient who was taking lithium and would avoid bendroflumethiazide in this case.

There is a quiz on the book's website to complement this section of the chapter.

 Activity box 5.12

Consider how many medicines a person with advanced type 2 diabetes may be taking, *before* you assess him or her within your competence and consider prescribing for any other condition with which he or she presents to you.

Tight BP control is essential to reduce morbidity associated with diabetes, so your patient may be taking one, two or three antihypertensive treatments plus a statin to reduce the cardiovascular risk and metformin or similar to manage the hyperglycaemia.

Extended example

Here are some patient scenarios to practise your BNF skills. All scenarios are separate but relate to the same patient. Imagine that Angela is consulting with you, within your competency, with the expectation of a prescription. Select a medicine (any medicine) from your personal formulary and use the BNF to check whether it would be safe to prescribe in the three scenarios.

The information you have gathered during consultation is as follows:

Patient name: Angela Patient
Date of birth: 23.03.1974
Address: 17 Any Drive, Anytown, Anywhere
Occupation: shop assistant
Married with one child
Current prescription: phenytoin
Past medical history: one full-term birth, 5 months ago
Past surgical history: none
Allergies: penicillin

Activity box 5.13

Scenario 1: Does the fact that she is taking phenytoin affect the choice of medicine that you were intending to prescribe?

You would need to check in the BNF, Appendix 1 whether there is a significant interaction between the medicine that you were intending to prescribe and phenytoin.

Activity box 5.14

Scenario 2: When you ask her if she is taking any over the counter/herbal medications, she tells you that she takes St John's wort.

Does this affect the medicine that you were intending to prescribe?

You would need to check in the BNF, Appendix 1 whether there is a significant interaction between the medicine that you were intending to prescribe and St John's wort.

Are there any other medicine-related issues that may concern you?

You need to consider carefully how you may advise Angela, within your competence, whether you would need to refer her to a colleague.

Activity box 5.15

Scenario 3: When you ask her if she may be pregnant, she tells you no because her last menstrual cycle was 1 week ago and was normal; she is, however, breastfeeding.

Does this affect the medicine that you were intending to prescribe?

You would need to check in the BNF, whether the medicine that you were intending to prescribe is safe to use in breastfeeding mothers.

Are there any other medicine-related issues that may concern you?

You need to consider carefully how you may advise Angela, within your competence, whether you would need to refer her to a colleague.

Management and avoidance of adverse medicine reactions

No medicine is risk free. All have one or more 'unwanted effects' in addition to the effect that is desired, e.g. would you want to take a medicine that had the following unwanted effects: rashes and blood disorders, which include thrombocytopenia (reduced number of platelets), leucopenia (low white blood cell count) and neutropenia (low level of neutrophils, a type of white blood cell)? You have probably taken this medicine many times in the past without giving any thought to what the unwanted effects might be. The medicine is paracetamol!

The usual term by which these unwanted effects is known is 'adverse drug reactions' or ADRs and is defined as 'A response to a drug which is noxious and unintended, which occurs at doses normally used in man for the prophylaxis, diagnosis, or therapy of disease, or for the modification of physiological function' by the World Health Organization (WHO 2002).

Confusion arises due to another common term that is often used interchangeably with ADRs and this is the term 'side effect'. This term is used in the BNF. The WHO (2002) has defined side effects as 'Any unintended effect of a pharmaceutical product occurring at doses normally used in man which is related to the pharmacological properties of the drug'.

The main difference between the two terms is that ADRs are always adverse or harmful to the patient taking the medicine, requiring discontinuation of the drug, whereas not all side effects are harmful, e.g. doxazosin may be prescribed in benign prostatic hyperplasia to relieve urinary retention but as a side effect may help a hypertensive patient by also reducing their BP.

Activity box 5.16

Look in the BNF at the Commission on Human Medicines' warnings for the following drugs: carbimazole, methotrexate, NSAIDs, the antibiotics - quinolones, trimethoprim, sulphonamides and flucloxacillin - varenicline and statins.

What action does the BNF say to take if a patient experiences the following ADRs associated with the given medicines?

- Severe muscular symptoms with statins
- Jaundice with ACE inhibitors
- Severe nausea due to nitrofurantoin
- Severe erythema and itching due to antifungals
- Liver cirrhosis with methotrexate
- Hepatotoxicity with amiodarone.

Sometimes precautions can be taken to prevent an ADR from occurring, e.g. use of sunscreen to prevent phototoxicity due to amiodarone or provision of a spacer device to prevent oral thrush due to inhaled steroid use in people with asthma.

Side effects are usually milder than ADRs and may be managed without having to discontinue the medicine, e.g. constipation as a result of opioid use can be managed with a laxative; dry mouth associated with some drugs, e.g. tricyclic antidepressants, can be managed with saliva replacements; and antimuscarinic drugs such as orphenadrine and procyclidine can be used to treat the symptoms of drug-induced parkinsonism due to antipsychotics.

Sometimes some side effects can also prove clinically useful, e.g. the constipating effect of codeine can be used to manage diarrhoea; in palliative care, hyoscine is used to treat drooling due to its antimuscarinic action, which causes dry mouth; and erythromycin, which can cause diarrhoea due to stimulation of motilin receptors, can be used to stimulate gut motility in critically ill patients.

The consequences of ADRs

As previously stated ADRs are harmful. They are responsible for a significant number of hospital admissions, inpatient morbidity, mortality and associated economic costs to the NHS (Pirmohamed et al 2004).

What do prescribers need to know?

- Factors that can influence the chance of a patient experiencing an ADR
- Steps to determine whether a drug is responsible for an ADR
- Pharmacovigilance and the reporting of ADRs.

Influencing factors

Impaired renal function

Reduced renal function can lead to the increased experience of ADRs in patients. Reduced renal excretion of the drug will give rise to accumulation of the drug in the body, leading to toxicity. This is especially serious when prescribing drugs with a narrow margin between the therapeutic and toxic dose (see below for more detail) and where renal function is the most important determinant of dosage, e.g. digoxin, which will require a reduced dose. Sensitivity to drugs may increase, so extra caution is required when prescribing nephrotoxic drugs such as NSAIDs, ACE inhibitors and methotrexate. Also, many side effects are poorly tolerated by patients with renal impairment.

Liver impairment

Changes in liver metabolism can also affect the chances of experiencing ADRs; however, liver impairment has to be severe before important changes in drug metabolism occur. Hepatotoxicity is either dose related or unpredictable (idiosyncratic). Drugs that cause dose-related toxicity may do so at lower doses in the presence of hepatic impairment than in individuals with normal liver function. Some drugs that produce reactions of the idiosyncratic kind do so more frequently in patients with liver disease. Tolcapone, used for parkinsonism and rosiglitazone, used in type 2 diabetes, should be avoided in patients with liver disease.

As elderly people have reduced renal and liver function, they are more prone to ADRs and therefore care is required when prescribing for this age group.

Multiple drug therapy

People with multiple disease states will often be on many drugs that increase their chances of experiencing ADRs. There may be various contributory factors to this such as additive effects, e.g. use of the combination treatment of isoniazid, rifampicin and pyrazinamide, all of which are associated with liver toxicity when used in tuberculosis treatment; excessive drowsiness where more than one drug has sedative effects and prescribing warfarin with NSAIDs which can increase risk of GI bleeding.

There can also be increased potential for drug–drug interactions when taking multiple drug therapy which can lead to an increased incidence of ADRs, e.g. concomitant use of simvastatin with erythromycin increases the risk of the patient having myopathy (muscle pain and weakness); clarithromycin markedly increases digoxin levels and numerous cases of digoxin toxicity have been reported.

Multiple disease states, e.g. liver and renal impairment, make the patient more susceptible to ADRs (see above).

Special attention needs to be given to elderly people who are often on multiple drug therapy. Their treatment regimens need to be simplified and non-medical prescribers need to ensure that they are only taking medicines that they actually need.

Gender

In general women appear to be at greater risk of ADRs than men (Wiffen et al 2002). The reasons for this are not clear but contributing factors include gender-related differences such as hormonal and immunological factors as well as the pattern of medicine use. In relation to the common analgesic codeine, the BNF (BMA and RPSGB 2010) advises: 'The capacity to metabolise codeine can vary considerably and lead to either reduced therapeutic effect or marked increase in side-effects.' This may be particularly important in breastfeeding mothers because there can be a risk of morphine (product of codeine metabolism) overdose in breastfed infants.

Disease states

We have already looked at renal and hepatic impairment. Examples of other disease states that can predispose to an increased experience of ADRs are: HIV-positive patients who have an increased rate of skin reactions with co-trimoxazole and antiretroviral drugs, and infectious mononucleosis (due to the Epstein–Barr virus) which greatly increases the risk of rash in patients given amoxicillin.

Ethnicity

Different racial groups have genetic differences that can affect how they metabolise drugs, e.g. glucose-6-phosphate dehydrogenase (G6PDH) deficiency is highly prevalent in individuals originating from most parts of Africa and Asia, and from Oceania and southern Europe (BMA and RPSGB 2010). Susceptible individuals could develop acute haemolytic anaemia on taking a number of common drugs, e.g. nitrofurantoin, quinolone antibiotics (refer to BNF, section 9.1.5 – BMA and RPSGB 2010).

Activity box 5.17

Find the following two drug entries in the BNF and match the entry under 'Cautions' to the correct drug: carbamazepine and isoniazid:

- Risk of Stevens–Johnson syndrome in presence of HLA-B*1502 allele in individuals of Han Chinese or Thai origin
- Increased risk of side-effects in people with a slow acetylator status

Steps to determine whether a drug is responsible for an ADR

Following three easy steps will help in determining whether or not a drug is the causative agent.

What is the timing between the start of the drug therapy and the reaction?

Some reactions can occur soon after starting drug therapy, e.g. allergic reaction to penicillin. However, some ADRs can occur after the course of the drug therapy has finished, e.g. in the case of flucloxacillin where cholestatic jaundice and hepatitis can occur up to several weeks after treatment has finished.

Does the reaction improve when the drug is withdrawn or the dose is reduced?

Most ADRs go away or improve if the causative drug is stopped, e.g. dry mouth and blurred vision due to tricyclic antidepressants and GI bleeding with NSAIDs. However, not all have this effect because damage such as renal or liver failure may continue long after the drug has been discontinued.

Is the ADR a known one?
Check the BNF or manufacturer's literature (e.g. the patient information leaflet inside the box of tablets) to see if there is any information about the ADR that the patient is experiencing.

Pharmacovigilance and the reporting of ADRs
Pharmacovigilance is the science of collecting, monitoring, assessing and evaluating reports from healthcare professionals and patients on ADRs with a view to identifying new information about the potential risks associated with medicines and preventing harm. Although all drugs undergo pre-marketing testing (clinical trials) this activity does not usually involve vast numbers of people – usually just a couple of thousand – yet millions of people may end up taking the new medicine. Therefore, not all ADRs of a new medicine may be detected during clinical trials. It is therefore important that a robust mechanism is in place post-marketing to ensure that information on the type and incidence of all ADRs is collected. In the UK this can be done using the Yellow Card scheme.

This scheme involves the completion by healthcare professionals and patients of a freepost Yellow Card (available at the back of the BNF or online at the MHRA website) which allows details of the suspected ADR to be recorded and the information sent to the MHRA which collates and processes all the information and disseminates it. Close attention needs to be paid to new drugs which are designated by an inverted black triangle symbol in the BNF (▼) and any ADR irrespective of severity needs to be reported to ensure that data are gathered and made available to other healthcare professionals.

Activity box 5.18

Have a look at the Yellow Cards at the back of the BNF and practise completing one using the following case scenario:

Mrs Edna Smith, DOB 8 August 8 1950. Commenced the drug VoArth tablets (once a day) for her arthritis. She experienced severe rash and itching, yellow discoloration of the skin 2 weeks later and was hospitalised. She was diagnosed as having suffered hepatoxicity due to VoArth. She had been prescribed para-cetamol and codeine only for pain relief for her arthritis before.

Key points for prescribers

- Consider whether drug therapy is necessary – weigh up the risks and benefits.
- Always consider whether any new symptom that the patient is experiencing is an ADR of a drug that he or she is already taking.

- Pay special attention to 'at risk' groups, e.g. elderly people, or people with renal or liver impairment.
- When possible prescribe a drug with which you are familiar. If you are not familiar with the drug consult the product literature for more information.
- Check the patient's history to determine if he or she has any documented ADRs to drugs – avoid these. Ask the patient for information on this if no documentation is found.
- Ask the patient if he or she is taking any other medicines, including herbal, complementary and bought over the counter at the pharmacy or other retail outlet.
- Give patients clear information about their medicines, e.g. how to take them, what they may experience when taking them and what to do if they suffer any harmful experience.
- Check whether there are any specific monitoring requirements before prescribing, e.g. liver function, blood counts, etc.
- If you come across a suspected ADR or side effect ensure that you complete a Yellow Card and post it to the MHRA.

Drugs with a narrow therapeutic index or range

Drugs of narrow therapeutic index are drugs, e.g. lithium, theophylline, ciclosporin or digoxin, for which there is a small range between an effective dose and a toxic dose. This means that toxic effects may happen with small increases in plasma concentration of the drug. Metabolic factors that affect plasma concentration, such as changes in renal function or hepatic enzymes, could therefore lead to toxic levels. Prescribers should be aware of these possible effects and ensure that action is taken to prevent doses reaching damaging levels.

Therapeutic drug monitoring

Therapeutic drug monitoring (TDM) is the process by which plasma levels of drugs of narrow therapeutic index are measured. This should be done only when there is a clear benefit which contributes positively to patient care, as is the case in lithium monitoring (BMA and RPSGB 2010). Situations when TDM may also be appropriate include when the patient's condition may be hard to distinguish from toxic effects of the drug, such as with digoxin therapy, or in patients with co-morbidities that are likely to affect metabolism, such as hepatic impairment.

Proprietary name prescribing

Prescribing medicines by generic name is usually considered best practice, for reasons of cost-effectiveness and ease of supply. However, there are a few medicines where bioequivalence between manufacturers cannot be guaranteed; it is recommended that these are prescribed by proprietary name, to ensure that the patient receives the same dose each time. Brand prescribing is particularly recommended for drugs with a narrow therapeutic index. The BNF (BMA and RPSGB 2010) gives advice for the specific drugs affected, but common drugs with a narrow therapeutic index that should be prescribed by brand include theophylline, ciclosporin and lithium.

Example of problems associated with drugs of narrow therapeutic index:

Drug interactions

Theophylline is metabolised by the liver, by hepatic cytochrome P450 enzymes. Drugs that induce liver enzymes will increase the clearance of theophylline and lead to lower plasma levels. Patients who smoke metabolise theophylline more quickly than non-smokers, because chemicals in smoke induce cytochrome P450 enzymes. This means that smokers may require higher doses of theophylline to achieve a therapeutic effect; conversely dose reductions may be appropriate if the patient stops smoking, so as to avoid theophylline toxicity developing. Patients should be made aware of symptoms of toxicity, such as palpitations, headache, nausea and vomiting, and the BNF (BMA and RPSGB 2010) recommends prescribing theophylline by brand name, to ensure bioequivalence.

Co-morbidity

Digoxin is excreted via the kidneys; dosage adjustments should be considered in patients with impaired renal function which should be checked before initiation. Elderly patients are particularly at risk from digoxin toxicity because their renal function declines with age. Common symptoms of toxicity include nausea and vomiting, and patients should be warned to report if such symptoms develop.

Lithium

Lithium is excreted via the kidneys; lithium levels can be influenced by a range of factors. Reduced sodium levels can increase the toxicity of lithium, so use of diuretics should be avoided. Similarly, patients should ensure adequate fluid intake and avoid any significant dietary changes that may affect sodium levels. Toxic effects of lithium can be serious – neurological effects or even death. Other signs of toxicity include GI effects such as anorexia, nausea, vomiting and diarrhoea. Proprietary name prescribing and TDM of lithium levels should be available if lithium is prescribed.

Building concordance

A key element of the medicines management process, the achievement of patient safety, is ensuring that patients receive the appropriate medicine for their condition and that they take/use the medicine correctly, with the aim of curing or stabilising their condition. Until recently, this fundamentally meant that the patient had to be compliant with the treatment regimen prescribed. However, it is acknowledged that, despite the expectation that patients will comply with the prescribed treatment regimen, non-compliance is a significant problem within all therapeutic areas and across all patient groups (Carter et al 2005). As such, it is now argued that the more collaborative approach of concordance is adopted (Bond 2004).

It is useful at this juncture to differentiate between the terms often used to debate the issues relating to concordance. There are three commonly used terms: compliance, adherence and concordance. The National Co-ordinating Centre for NHS Service Delivery and Organisation (NCCSDO 2005) defined these three terms in a manner that demonstrates their distinctions while highlighting their linkage (NCCSDO 2005, p. 12):

Compliance: 'The extent to which the patient's behaviour matches the prescriber's recommendations'

Adherence: 'The extent to which the patient's behaviour matches agreed recommendations from the prescriber'

Concordance: '... focused on the consultation process, in which doctor and patient agree therapeutic decisions that incorporate their respective views ... stretches from prescribing communication to patient support in medicine taking'

It is clear from these definitions that there is a move from a behavioural focus to a process focus; this is reiterated in the work of Bond (2004) who emphasises the need to explore the processes used to reach therapeutic decisions rather than the decision itself. In its most basic form, concordance in relation to prescribing can be defined as 'reaching a decision regarding treatment together'. Of course, the decision may be that no treatment is required or appropriate, and may instead indicate a need for health education and/or referral.

To provide a more detailed explanation, Britten and Weiss (2004) identified the key components of concordance. The first key component identified is the need for the practitioner to enable the patient to express his or her views and for the practitioner to understand them. Britten and Weiss (2004) emphasise that the patient and practitioners are equal partners whose opinions and views should form the basis of an agreed management plan. This of course relies on the practitioner articulating their view in a manner that is conducive to this process. Ultimately, it remains the patient's decision whether or not to take the medicine(s) (Britten and Weiss 2004).

The patient's health beliefs and their relation to medicines are recognised as a key factor in making the decision not to take medicines (National Prescribing Centre Plus (NPC Plus) and Medicines Partnership Programme (MPP) 2007). However, it is also acknowledged that of those patients who fail to take their medicines as prescribed, a significant proportion do so unintentionally (NICE 2009). Adopting a concordant approach to prescribing will support the practitioner not only in reaching an agreement that the patient can use, but also in enabling patient understanding.

In considering the role of non-medical prescriber, it is clear that concordance is fundamental to the prescribing consultation. Therefore, it is essential that the practitioner is aware of the concordance process and the key factors that impact on the achievement (or not) of concordance. NICE (2009) provides guidance incorporating many of these factors, yet interestingly uses 'adherence' as the chosen term for its focus. In addition, NPC Plus and MPP (2007) provide a competency framework to assist practi-

Table 5.4   Concordance: skills and actions

Focus: explain to patient that the approach used focuses on *concordance*
Approach: adopt a *non-judgemental* approach
Concerns: elicit the *patient's* concerns about medicines
Establish: the level to which the patient wants to be *involved* in decision-making
Consultation and communication: adopt a style that enables *individual* patients to express their view comfortably
Active listening: *understand* the patient's view
Remember: the patient has a *choice* not to take medicines
Education and information: ensure that the format used (verbal, pictures, leaflets, etc.) is appropriate for the individual patient (consider language barriers) so that they are able to make an *informed* decision
Strategy: *agree* the most appropriate strategy, including review schedules; employ *flexibility*   (Mnemonic devised by Dilyse Nuttall 2010)

tioners in developing the appropriate skills necessary to achieve concordance. Table 5.4 summarises, using the mnemonic 'FACECARES', the actions and skills that support and promote concordance, as identified by NICE (2009).

Activity box 5.19

Access the National Prescribing Centre Plus and Medicines Partnership Programme (2007) *A Competency Framework for Shared Decision-Making with Patients: Achieving Concordance for Taking Medicines* available at: www.npc.co.uk/ prescribers/resources/competency_framework_2007.pdf.

Identify any areas or competencies that you feel you need to develop, and develop an action plan to enable you to address any issues identified.

Using the FACECARE mnemonic, reflect on and critically analyse a recent consultation where a prescribing decision was made.

Medicines management

Medicines management has many definitions and has been described as 'a system of processes and behaviours that determines how medicines are used by the NHS and patients' (NPC 2002). This is a broad subject but the essence of medicines management is a system that promotes maximum benefit and minimal risk, from medicines, for patients. When medicines management systems are well established and implemented, more patients receive better, evidence-based and safer care (NPC 2002).

Why is it a priority?

Being prescribed a medicine is the most frequent clinical service provided by the NHS (MeReC 2002). Medicines are important to public health, with millions treated with statins and antihypertensives to prevent morbidity and mortality. Medicines account for more than 15% of the NHS revenue and there is a requirement of all prescribers to maximise value for money, within a cash-limited system (MeReC 2002). Effective medicines management frees up resources, which means that NHS money can be used for the benefit of patients. Just as prescribers cannot be expected to understand the pharmacology of all drugs, prescribers cannot be expected to be experts in pharmacoeconomics or risk-benefit ratio analysis. One contribution that the prescriber makes to effective medicines management is familiarity with and application of relevant frameworks, formularies and guidelines.

Medication problems are implicated in 5-17% of hospital admissions, with medication errors accounting for 25% of all reported harm-related incidents (Pirmohamed et al 2004). It has been estimated that medicines-related hospital admissions cost the NHS £500 million a year in additional days spent in hospital. More important than the costs to manage these adverse drug-related events are the human costs of avoidable illness or mortality. Good medicines management, timely monitoring and review have been shown to prevent hospital admissions and improve patient safety.

There is also significant waste when medicines are not managed appropriately; currently half of all patients with chronic conditions do not use their medicines as intended. Obtaining accurate and timely information about patients' medicines, concordant consultations and regular medication review are all elements that constitute processes of medicines management. Patient decision aids are recently introduced tools, increasingly used within consultations, to enable patients to better understand the pros and cons of medicine taking.

Prescribers are encouraged to reflect on what constitutes 'good prescribing.' Whilst guidance may imply that a right answer always exists, prescribers should recognise the complex trade offs that have to be made between conflicting aims. Barber (1995) proposed 'four aims that a prescriber should try to achieve, both on first prescribing a drug and on subsequently monitoring and reviewing it. They are: 'to maximise effectiveness, minimise risks, minimise costs, and respect the patient's choices' (Barber 1995). New prescribers are encouraged to read this paper, because these aims, as well as the aims of medicines management, are as relevant today as they were back then.

Other resources to support your learning

Key textbooks

Dale MM, Haylett DG (2008) *Pharmacology Condensed*, 2nd edn. London: Churchill Livingstone.
Downie G, MacKenzie J, Williams A, Hind C (2007) *Pharmacology and Medicine Management for Nurses*, 4th edn. Edinburgh: Churchill Livingstone.
Rang HP, Dale MM, Ritter JM, Flower R (2007) *Rang & Dale's Pharmacology*, 6th edn. London: Churchill Livingstone.
Sodha M, Dhillon S (2009) *Non-medical Prescribing*. London: Pharmaceutical Press.

Websites (last accessed May 2010)

Bandolier. *Adverse Drug Reactions in Hospital Patients*. June 2002. Available at: www.medicine.ox.ac.uk/bandolier/Extraforbando/ADRPM.pdf (accessed May 2010).

http://bnf.org/bnf/index.htm – *British National Formulary* (BMA and RPSGB)

www.medicines.org.uk/EMC/default.aspx – electronic Medicines Compendium, containing summaries of product characteristics (SPCs)

www.mhra.gov.uk/Aboutus/index.htm – MHRA

Key themes: conclusions and considerations

Public health	Antibiotics are a common drug prescribed by non-medical prescribers. There is proven research whereby it is evident that patients do not always complete their full prescription of antibiotics and that this is contributing to the issue of antimicrobial resistance
	Consider how, in relation to the concepts of compliance versus concordance, you can help facilitate your patient to complete their full prescription of antibiotics
Social and cultural issues	Cultural and ethnical differences have been shown to impact on the body's ability to 'handle' certain drugs
	Consider your learning needs in relation to cultural and ethical issues, and your clinical practice population and personal formulary
Prescribing principles	The prescribing principles are embedded within this chapter and especially in terms of 'considering the strategy'. Pharmacology knowledge of your personal formulary is paramount
	Consider how the risks of the chosen strategy can be alleviated, through a comprehensive knowledge base and the promotion of a concordant relationship with the patient

---

References

Barber N (1995) What constitutes good prescribing? *BMJ* **310**: 923–5.

Bond C, ed. (2004) *Concordance*. London: Pharmaceutical Press.

British Medical Association and Royal Pharmaceutical Society of Great Britain (2010) *British National Formulary 58*. London: BMA & RPSGB.

Britten N, Weiss MC (2004) What is concordance? In: Bond C (ed.), *Concordance*. London: Pharmaceutical Press, 9–28.

Carter S, Taylor D, Levenson R (2005) *A Question of Choice: Compliance in medicine taking* (online). Available at: www.npci.org.uk/adherence_to_medicines/atm/intro/resources/library_qoc_compliance.pdf (accessed 1 May 2010).

Dale MM, Haylett DG (2008) *Pharmacology Condensed*, 2nd edn. London: Churchill Livingstone.

Department of Health (1999) *National Service Framework (NSF) for Mental Health: Modern standards and service models*. London: DH.

Department of Health (2000) *NSF for Coronary Heart Disease*. London: DH.

Department of Health (2001) *NSF for Older People*. London: DH.

Department of Health (2007) *NSF for Diabetes*. London: DH.

Department of Health (2009) *Non-Medical Prescribing Programme: Changes to medicines legislation to enable mixing of medicines prior to administration in clinical practice* (on-line). Available at: www.dh.gov.uk/en/Healthcare/Medicinespharmacyandindustry/Prescriptions/TheNon-MedicalPrescribingProgramme/DH_110765 (accessed May 2010).

Downie G, MacKenzie J, Williams A, Hind C (2007) *Pharmacology and Medicine Management for Nurses*, 4th edn. Edinburgh: Churchill Livingstone.

Health Professions Council (2007) *Standards of Proficiency* (online). Available at: www.hpc-uk.org/publications/standards (accessed May 2010).

Hopkins SJ (1999) *Drugs and Pharmacology for Nurses*. Edinburgh: Churchill Livingstone.

Medicines and Healthcare products Regulatory Agency (2009) *Statement on Non-Medical Prescribing and Mixing Medicines in Palliative Care* (online). Available at: www.mhra.gov.uk/Howweregulate/Medicines/Medicinesregulatorynews/CON025660 (accessed May 2010).

MeReC (2002) Medicines Management Services – Why are they so important? *MeReC Bull* **12**(6) (online). Available at: www.npc.co.uk/ebt/merec/other_non_clinical/resources/merec_bulletin_vol12_no6.pdf (accessed May 2010).

National Institute for Health and Clinical Excellence (2006) *Hypertension: Management of hypertension in adults in primary care* (online). Available at: http://guidance.nice.org.uk/CG34 (accessed May 2010).

National Institute for Health and Clinical Excellence (2009) *Medicines Adherence: Involving patients in decisions about prescribed medicines and supporting adherence* (online). Available at: http://guidance.nice.org.uk/CG76 (accessed May 2010).

National Institute for Health and Clinical Excellence (2010) *Neuropathic Pain – The pharmacological management of neuropathic pain in adults in non-specialist settings* (online). Available at: http://guidance.nice.org.uk/CG96 (accessed May 2010).

National Co-ordinating Centre for NHS Service Delivery and Organisation (2005) *Concordance, Adherence and Compliance in Medicine Taking: Report for the National Co-ordinating Centre for NHS Service Delivery and Organisation R&D (NCCSDO)* (online). Available at: www.medslearning.leeds.ac.uk/pages/documents/useful_docs/76-final-report%5B1%5D.pdf (accessed May 2010).

National Prescribing Centre (2001) *Maintaining Competency in Prescribing: An outline framework to help nurse prescribers*. Liverpool: NPC.

National Prescribing Centre (2002) *Modernising Medicines Management: A guide to achieving benefits for patients, professionals and the National Health Service* (online). Available at: www.npci.org.uk/medicines_management/medicines/medicinesintro/library/library_good_practice_guide1.php (accessed May 2010).

National Prescribing Centre (2003) *Maintaining Competency in Prescribing: An outline framework to help nurse supplementary prescribers*. Liverpool: NPC.

National Prescribing Centre (2004a) *Maintaining Competency in Prescribing: An outline framework to help allied health professional supplementary prescribers*. Liverpool: NPC.

National Prescribing Centre (2004b) *Competency Framework for Prescribing Optometrists*. Liverpool: NPC.

National Prescribing Centre (2006) *Maintaining Competency in Prescribing: An outline framework to help pharmacist prescribers*. 2nd edn. Liverpool: NPC.

National Prescribing Centre (2009) *Competency Frameworks* (online). Available at: www.npc.co.uk/prescribers/competency_frameworks.htm (accessed May 2010).

National Prescribing Centre Plus and Medicines Partnership Programme (2007) *A Competency Framework for Shared Decision-making with Patients: Achieving concordance for taking medicines*, Liverpool: NPC Plus,

Nursing and Midwifery Council (2006) *Standards of Proficiency for Nurse and Midwife Prescribers* (online). Available at: www.nmc-uk.org/aDisplayDocument.aspx?documentID =6942 (accessed May 2010).

Nursing and Midwifery Council (2008) *The Code: Standards of conduct, performance and ethics for nurses and midwives*. London: NMC.

Office for National Statistics (2007) *Health Life Expectancy* (online). Available at: www.statistics.gov.uk/default.asp (accessed May 2010).

Pirmohamed M, James S, Meakin S et al (2004) Adverse drug reactions as cause of admission to hospital: prospective analysis of 18 820 patients. *BMJ* **329**: 15-19.

Rang HP, Dale MM, Ritter JM, Flower R (2009) *Rang & Dale's Pharmacology*. Edinburgh: Churchill Livingstone.

Royal Pharmaceutical Society of Great Britain (2007) *Code of Ethics for Pharmacists and Pharmacist Technicians*. London: RPSGB.

Thomson A (2004) Variability in drug dosage requirements. *Pharm J* **272**: 806-8.

Wiffen P, Gill M, Edwards J, Moore A (2002) Adverse drug reactions in hospital patients: a systematic review of the prospective and retrospective studies. *Bandolier Extra June*.

World Health Organization (2002) *Safety of Medicines: A guide to detecting and reporting adverse drug reactions – why health professionals need to take action* (online). Available at: http://apps.who.int/medicinedocs/en/d/Jh2992e/2.html (accessed May 2010).

Chapter 6
The Multidisciplinary Prescribing Team

Dawn Eccleston

Learning objectives

After reading this chapter and completing the activities within it, the reader will be able to:

1 discuss the meaning of the 'multidisciplinary prescribing team'
2 identify the roles of non-medical prescribers
3 critically analyse the importance of working as part of a multi-disciplinary team
4 discuss the benefits of the 'multidisciplinary prescribing team' for patients and clients
5 apply knowledge about multidisciplinary prescribing to non-medical prescribing practice

---

Defining 'the multidisciplinary prescribing team'

Non-medical prescribing is a rapidly expanding field of healthcare practice. From its constrained beginnings, when nurses were allowed to prescribe from a very limited list, the field of prescribing has now increased to include different professions and expanded to include complete use of the *British National Formulary* (BNF). To facilitate these changes and developments, there has been a distinct need for the teams in which non-medical prescribing has been undertaken to evolve. This chapter examines the meaning of 'multidisciplinary team working in prescribing' and looks at the various roles of the prescribing team members. It also considers the support processes that are provided to individual non-medical prescribers by different members of the team, in a variety of situations and circumstances.

Clark (2008, cited in Goodman and Clemow 2008, p. 140) defines a team as:

The Textbook of Non-medical Prescribing, edited by Dilyse Nuttall and Jane Rutt-Howard.
© 2011 Blackwell Publishing Ltd

… a group of people with a high degree of **interdependence** geared towards the achievement of a **common goal** or completion of a **task** … it is not just a group for administrative convenience. A group, by definition, is a number of individuals having some unifying relationship. Team members are deeply **committed** to each other's **personal growth** and **success**. That commitment usually transcends the team. A team outperforms a group and outperforms all reasonable expectations given to its individual members. That is, a team has a **synergetic** effect … one plus one equals a lot more than two. Team members not only **cooperate** in all aspects of their tasks and goals, they share in what are traditionally thought of as **management functions,** such as planning, organizing, setting performance goals, assessing the team's performance, developing their own strategies to manage change, and securing their own resources.

Activity box 6.1

Consider the words in bold print in Clark's definition and answer the following questions:

Do these words represent the ideals of a good multidisciplinary team?
What is actually meant by the term 'multidisciplinary'?

Confusion in terminology

Various terms have been used to define professionals 'working together'. Many healthcare professionals will be familiar with terms such as 'multiprofessional', 'multiagency', 'multidisciplinary', 'interagency', 'interprofessional', 'collaborative' and 'partnership working'. Although the words have different meanings ('inter' meaning 'between or among', 'multi' meaning 'many'), they are often used and interpreted differently by individual professionals and different disciplines.

In the true sense of the term, interprofessional or interdisciplinary work means that there is collaborative working and/or working together, whereas multiprofessional or multidisciplinary work means that there is more than one profession working in the same area, or with the same patient or client, but not necessarily in a collaborative fashion (Leathard 1994). The terms are, however, often used interchangeably. Leathard (1994) suggests that the term 'interprofessional' suggests only that two groups are working together, whereas 'multiprofessional' or 'multidisciplinary' implies a wider group involvement. For the purposes of this chapter the terms are interchangeable. Therefore, as long as all members of the team know precisely what is meant, then team morale and patient/client care should not be compromised. In fact, effective multidisciplinary team working can, I suggest, enhance both patient and staff satisfaction!

The drivers in multidisciplinary team working

There are various drivers to multidisciplinary working practice. McCray (2009) suggests that professionals need to work together in order to maintain Government funding. She states that 'this [government funding] is a significant factor in the shift towards multi-professional working'. Other factors, however, also contribute to the increase in multidisciplinary working practices. Increased recognition of the notion of 'vulnerability' in our society has meant that Government documents have increasingly prescribed multiprofessional working practice as essential in order to protect vulnerable people, e.g. Choosing Health, Making Healthy Choices Easier (Department of Health (DH) 2004) and *Working Together to Safeguard Children* (DH 2010b). The moves towards community-based services, nurse-led clinics and assessment services has meant that professionals increasingly have to work collaboratively in order to provide optimum care for clients/patients. Commissioners of health services are constantly looking for effective multiagency working practice, where cost can be shared between agencies.

The benefits to prescribing

In view of these issues, it is essential to consider why multidisciplinary working is essential for good prescribing practice. Hemingway (2008) states that: 'prescribing has a lot of power elements to it.' He points out, for example, that there is a real danger that prescribers may be influenced and ethically compromised by drug companies offering incentives to prescribe their products. Prescribing as part of a multidisciplinary team may go some way to minimising this risk through 'peer' regulation and monitoring. In addition, the team approach can support prescribers in making effective use of resources, particularly as it is recognised that pharmaceutical companies may be a valued resource for the prescribing team (Talley and Richens 2001).

Prescribing a model for the multidisciplinary approach

There are various models of multidisciplinary or interprofessional working practice. Ovretveit (1997) points out that the multidisciplinary team should be about planning and designing the best team for a population and/or service. Five ways of organising a multidisciplinary team are identified (Table 6.1).

In considering Ovretveit's (1997) model, it would be appropriate to suggest that the multidisciplinary prescribing team would, in most cases, be consistent with category 5. There may be various professionals, and non-professionals, working with the patient/client who need to make sure that they are approaching the patient's care from the same direction. They remain under their own managerial systems but come together to optimise the patient or client experience - producing a streamlined, coordinated service. This would seem to be the ethos of a truly multidisciplinary team and, when considering the multiprofessional team in non-medical prescribing, it clearly highlights the team as professionals coming from different disciplines but with the same goal - to optimise patient/client care and effective prescribing.

Table 6.1   Five ways of organising a multidisciplinary team

1 The *fully managed* team – a team manager is accountable for all the management work and the performance of all team members
2 The *coordinated* team – one person takes on most of the management and coordination work but is not accountable for the clinical work of the individual team members
3 The *core and extended* team – members of the team are fully managed by the team leader with extended team members (usually part time) remaining managed by professional managers in their agency of origin
4 The *joint accountability* team – most team tasks, including leadership, are undertaken by the team corporately, usually by delegating to individual members. Team members remain accountable to managers in their agencies of origin but in practice may not have strong management links with them
5 The *network association* – not a 'formal' team as such but different professionals working with the same client group who meet together on a need to share common work/clinical interest. Each practitioner remains under the management of his or her own professional manager but decisions about client care are often formulated collectively at network meetings

Ovretveit (1997) in McKimm & Phillips, 2009.

It is essential that all members of the team are aware of their own role within that team and are comfortable and confident within that role. Team members, although from varying professions, often work in the same clinical setting. Each professional has his or her own clearly defined role within the clinical/prescribing setting, although, with the advent of non-medical prescribing, these roles now, often, overlap. Where once a nurse or pharmacist may have seen a patient and referred him or her to the GP for a prescription, the nurse or pharmacist may now examine the patient, obtain a history and prescribe without referral to the GP. Historically multidisciplinary working has had some problems, not least because of the need for confidentiality and the fact that prfessionals are unaware of each other's roles. Therefore, it is beneficial, when working in a multidisciplinary team, that team members have some knowledge of and respect for each other's roles. Not only does this make for more streamlined working,but it also gives professionals access to a depth of expertise that they would otherwise be unaware of.

The barriers
Recognition of the continued drive towards multidisciplinary working must also lead one to question just how easy it is for professionals to 'work together' effectively. There are many potential barriers to multidisciplinary working, some of which are exacerbated by the addition of non-medical prescribing!

Information sharing
As has already been said, historically health professionals have been very aware of the need for patient and client confidentiality. The overwhelming notion of litigation and disciplinary action, in cases where there has been a breach of confidentiality, has made 'collaborative working' a very frightening prospect in many circumstances. Questions

have always been asked about just what and how much information can be shared. Professionals have been unsure about the extent of information sharing 'allowed'. This has been highlighted again and again in reports into child safeguarding cases, which are constantly being portrayed in the media. For most professionals this is a huge issue and an added stress. Obviously, sharing of information is not limited to safeguarding work but is relevant to all aspects of patient and client care, including safe prescribing practice. Hawley (2007) points out that clients and patients will often give information to health professionals and ask them to keep it secret. She highlights that professionals must never promise to keep relevant information secret. There must be trust, however, between all the professionals, and the patient or client, in the multidisciplinary prescribing team, that shared information is relevant to the case and confidentiality will be assured.

To prescribe safely and effectively, the prescribing professional must make it very clear to the patient or client that relevant information may be shared with the other professionals who are caring for him or her. The patient should always be at the centre of the prescribing process and, as such, should give permission for the multidisciplinary team to be involved and, therefore, for information to be shared.

Continuing professional development

Continuing professional development (CPD) is an essential part of the modern NHS career. The Department of Health's document *Modernising Nursing Careers* (DH 2006) emphasises that prescribing education should be linked to CPD. In turn CPD should be linked to career progression. Unfortunately, in the economic crisis that the NHS finds itself in, professional development and training may become victims of cost cutting. On a positive note, the Government is keen to promote nurse and midwife prescribing and research continues to demonstrate the success of this initiative. The future of nurse and midwife non-medical prescribing, therefore, looks positive and looks likely to expand.

Health service structures

Another barrier to effective multidisciplinary team working has been the 'hierarchical' approach to working within the NHS. Traditionally medical doctors have been at the top of 'the chain' and at the forefront in control of policies and procedures that impact on patient and client care. Nurses, particularly, used to be described as 'doctors' handmaidens'. This is no longer the case and most staff who care for patients and clients are expected to be responsible for their own practice. Medical practitioners are now recognising and valuing the expertise of other NHS staff. In some cases, doctors have welcomed this; in others there has been a constant 'power' struggle. However, a clearer understanding of the scope of individual practitioners' prescribing practice would go some way to overcoming these issues. This is supported by the findings of a study into perceptions of doctors and non-prescribing nurses which found that 'nurse prescribing can be acceptable to doctors and nurses so long as it operates within recommended parameters' (Stenner et al 2009).

However, as with any change in the NHS, the non-medical prescribing multidisciplinary team needs to justify its existence and demonstrate its benefits to patients and client. So far, it seems to be working well, although it is still early days. The benefits to the patient or client are addressed later in the chapter.

Activity box 6.2

Look at the following scenario and think 'outside the prescribing box'. Make a list of the people who may be involved in the general multidisciplinary team (NOT prescribing team) for this patient. Also, think about the services to whom you may refer to and with whom you would liaise:

Mrs Elliott is a 76-year-old woman who lives on her own. She is usually fit and healthy but her daughter has contacted her GP to inform him that her mother has fallen a few times and doesn't think she's been eating properly. She also seems quite confused at times. She has been going to the 'leg ulcer' café once a week for dressings to a small ulcer on her right leg. She has now presented at the surgery with an injury to her left ankle. She says she fell in the kitchen and her ankle is now swollen and painful, although she can weight bear.

Putting the 'p' in MDT

Previous discussion in this chapter has demonstrated that the ethos of 'multidisciplinary team working' is as relevant to non-medical prescribing as it is to other aspects of healthcare services. As such, there is reason to question the need for any specific consideration for prescribing in this context. However, the process of safe and effective prescribing requires a clear understanding by the non-medical prescriber of the roles of 'others' who will impact on or be influenced by the prescribing decision. The prescribing team may indeed vary from consultation to consultation, with not all members being prescribers. Only certain health professionals can undertake education programmes to enable them to prescribe, yet their prescribing role will require working with other team members in order to meet the individual needs of the patient. Regardless of the composition of each patient-specific prescribing team, the specialist process of prescribing will remain central to the team. Therefore, there is justification for utilising the term 'multidisciplinary prescribing team (MDPT)'. Table 6.2 lists those professionals who are currently allowed to prescribe, either independently or as supplementary prescribers.

Table 6.2 Professionals eligible to undertake non-medical prescribing education programmes

Pharmacists
Nurses
Specialist Community Public Health Nurses: Health Visitors, School Nurses, Sexual
  Health Advisors
Midwives
Physiotherapists
Radiographers
Optometrists
Podiatrists

Understanding roles

Up until the introduction of non-medical prescribing, prescribing had always been the prerogative of the medical doctor (or dentist). GPs in particular have 'often relied on prescribing to define their professional effectiveness' (Evans, cited in Chapter 6 of Bradley and Nolan 2008). Doctors are, therefore, sometimes reluctant to recognise the prescribing powers of other professionals. Other practitioners may also be reluctant to accept changing roles. This is a barrier that non-medical prescribers may need to overcome in order to encourage effective collaborative working practices. Therefore, it is a good idea to have some knowledge about the training that other professionals have received and the role that they play in prescribing.

Pharmacists

Pharmacists have undertaken a 5-year training programme which includes medicines management, pharmacology and pharmaceutics. Their training and subsequent practice was previously regulated by the Royal Pharmaceutical Society of Great Britain (RPSGB) and is now regulated by the General Pharmaceutical Council (GPhC). They are experts in identifying appropriate drugs and recognising the potential for drug interactions. They are an irrefutable resource for other professionals who may need advice on how to regulate and optimise drug treatments. They can give expert advice on how to avoid problems of drug interactions when there is more than one area of medicine involved, e.g. a pregnant woman who has epilepsy and diabetes. They aim to increase patients' knowledge of the medication that they are on and why they are on it, instead of just advising them to take it without expanding on information about the actual medication (Pharmacist Training 2010).

Historically pharmacists have manufactured, as well as dispensed, pharmaceutical products but, with the mass manufacture of drugs by pharmaceutical companies, their role has been under threat. Therefore, they are looking at diversification and undertaking further training in order to become prescribers themselves. They can then go on to work in primary or secondary care, as prescribing advisers or actual prescribers. Pharmacists may be employed by primary care trusts or hospital trusts, or may be employed by large companies. Some community pharmacists are employed by the primary care trust and some by the actual GP practice where they work. A study, undertaken by George et al (2006), found that pharmacists who were actually employed by the GP practice, in which they worked, felt that they were much more accepted as part of the team.

Pharmacists could also be viewed as the 'gatekeepers' of prescribing practice. They are the professionals who actually dispense the prescribed medication and they are, therefore, able to ensure that the prescription is accurate and appropriate before dispensing. They are also able to give advice to other non-medical prescribers about the appropriateness, dose and administration of pharmaceutical products and medication. In 2002, Dean et al carried out research into prescribing errors in hospital patients. Pharmacists recorded all prescribing errors in a given period and were able to identify dose errors and errors in prescribing decisions. Further studies have been carried out and in most of them (relating to prescribing errors) pharmacists represent the main source of information. In fact, Dean et al (2002) found that *all* the prescribing errors in their study were picked up by pharmacists.

The way in which patients and clients perceive pharmacists is also undergoing change. Advertising in health centres, hospitals, other NHS sites and the media is now encouraging people, with non-urgent medical needs, to access their pharmacist for help and advice, rather than the hospital or GP. People can now go to the pharmacist for a wide range of advice and help – including dietary advice, blood pressure checks, cholesterol checks, advice on minor illnesses and subsequent advice, etc. This is an extension of the pharmacists' role, for which they must be adequately trained. Their initial training means that their knowledge of pharmacology is extensive and their ability to now undertake training to become independent prescribers means that their role is constantly expanding. Of course, as with all the professionals, not all pharmacists will want to become independent prescribers, and there is a definite role for supplementary prescribing (particularly for patients with very complicated conditions), but, for those who do, the possibilities are exciting and the future prospects are encouraging. See case studies D, E and F for examples of how pharmacists use non-medical prescribing in practice.

Nurse and midwife prescribers

This title encompasses all the nurses in Table 6.2. Nurses and midwives have a minimum of 3 years' training. Some will go on to further training to become specialist nurses, such as district nurses, health visitors or specialist practitioners. They must have 3 years of experience before undertaking the non-medical prescribing course. Some will become independent prescribers, whereas others may prefer to be supplementary prescribers.

All nurses and midwives are governed by and answerable to their governing body – the Nursing and Midwifery Council (NMC). The NMC advise on and oversee their training, including non-medical prescribing. One of the '10 key roles' for nurses, highlighted in *The NHS Plan* (DH 2000) was that of prescribing. Prescribing was recommended as part of an extended role of the nurse, in order to improve and streamline patient care. In 2006, the NMC published *Standards for Prescribing*. This document made it very clear that any nurse or midwife who becomes a prescriber must prove her or his competence to diagnose and assess patients and clients before she or he is deemed fit to prescribe independently.

Problems have occurred in the past, and are still occurring in some areas today, due to the fact that some nurse prescribers undertake the non-medical prescribing course because they 'have to'. This is due to the fact that it is expected that they will be able to prescribe as part of their role, e.g. health visitors, and, more recently, community matrons. As a result, many have never prescribed or prescribe only rarely, potentially representing a waste of money in order to satisfy Government agendas and targets. Nurses have the ability, with suitable training, to assess and diagnose conditions, and to prescribe appropriately for their patients and clients. Although they may have the ability, they may lack the confidence to prescribe independently. Nurses and midwives need to be encouraged and supported in their extended prescribing roles in order for the MDPT to function effectively. Managers must consider this aspect before 'funding' nurses.

Nurses and midwives are key practitioners in managing and administering medication. They are uniquely placed to assess patients' abilities to take the required medication, their likelihood to comply with the medication regimen and their understanding of the need for their medication. Nurses and midwives are the most likely professionals to be working on an ongoing basis with patients and clients. Whether they are in a hospital or a community setting, patients and clients will often look to the nurse to explain their condition and their treatment in terms that they can understand. Therefore, it is vital that the nurse or midwife prescriber has an in-depth knowledge of pharmacology, pharmacokinetics and pharmacodynamics. Nurse and midwife prescribers must update their knowledge constantly, once they have completed the non-medical prescribing course. They are professionally accountable to the NMC and they are regulated closely. Each nurse or midwife is responsible for her or his own practice and must not carry out any procedure, including prescribing, for which she or he is nor competent. Competencies are very clearly stated by the NMC and a nurse or midwife who does not adhere to the competencies may be disciplined or even struck off the NMC register (NMC 2008). This means that they will be unable to practise as a nurse or midwife. See case studies A, B and C for examples of how nurses and midwives use non-medical prescribing in practice.

Allied health professionals

Allied health professionals use a broad range of medications and appliances. They may use supplementary prescribing, patient group directives and/or processes and protocols specific to their own profession. Specialist consultant practitioners may wish to train as independent prescribers. However, as with all changes in the NHS, this is opposed by some professionals, especially some medical doctors. This may be because of fears that the prescribing practices will not be safe or, as I have stated previously, because prescribing is viewed by some as a 'power tool' exclusive to certain professionals. Some studies have found that some medical professionals, although mainly supportive of non-medical prescribing, were reluctant to relinquish control of prescribing, preferring non-medical prescribing to have strict boundaries and protocols (Buckley et al 2006).

Whatever the reason behind the delay in training allied health professionals, many would welcome the chance to prescribe independently. This would enable them to tailor treatment to individual patient needs without the patient having to resort to waiting for a doctor's appointment before he or she can obtain medication to enable access to the correct treatment. A recent scoping exercise (DH 2009) has been carried out to determine the need for allied health professionals to become independent prescribers. The exercise also looked at and recommended the expansion of the number of disciplines of allied health professionals that should be able to prescribe, e.g. supplementary prescribing status for dieticians and independent prescribing status for physiotherapists. It will be worth keeping this in mind as you consider the MDPT.

Physiotherapists

Physiotherapists undergo 3 or 4 years of initial training, to degree level. They are experts in human movement and in helping people with physical problems caused by accident, illness or ageing. They are involved in health promotion activities and preventive healthcare as well as treatment and rehabilitation. They use various techniques including therapeutic exercise, hydrotherapy, injections, manual therapy and use of various therapy machines.

They may work in hospitals or primary care trusts or they may be self-employed independent practitioners. Many physiotherapists work closely with the medical profession and, as such, will administer certain injections under a doctor's instructions. They may specialise in paediatrics, orthopaedics, women's health, cancer care, etc. They may also work in industry, sport and leisure, e.g. football clubs, special schools and anywhere where people are at risk of injury from their activity or their job.

They are registered with the Health Professions Council. The Chartered Society of Physiotherapists issues guidelines and protocols for practitioners. They are currently allowed to prescribe as supplementary prescribers, or to use patient group directives, but there are moves to allow them to become independent prescribers. This would be useful because they need to be able to prescribe certain analgesics, etc. in order to carry pout their work effectively. The non-medical prescribing course certainly equips them to do this and it is hoped that, in the future, as part of the MDPT, they will be able to prescribe independently for their patients and clients. This would optimise the service that the physiotherapist can give to the patient or client and would result in much more streamlined care. See case study G for an example of how physiotherapists use non-medical prescribing in practice.

Radiographers

Radiographers undergo 3 or 4 years of training. They can train as diagnostic or therapeutic radiographers and are registered with the Health Professions Council. The Society and College of Radiographers oversees training and education and issues guidelines and protocols. The majority train as diagnostic radiographers. Both branches of radiography study technology, anatomy and physiology and pathology in order to qualify and register. They may undertake further training in order to become a sonographer – someone who is able to carry out ultrasound techniques. Most radiographers are employed by the NHS, although some are employed in private clinics, private hospitals and industry.

Diagnostic radiographers
Diagnostic radiographers do most of their work in hospitals and clinics. They are trained to carry out a wide range of different radiographic images, e.g. ultrasonography, magnetic resonance imaging, nuclear medicine and radiographs. They may become specialists in a particular area, e.g. computed tomography (CT).

Therapeutic radiographers

Therapeutic radiographers are usually known as radiotherapy radiographers. They work closely within the oncology team to treat patients with cancer. They deliver radiation to patients, particularly those with various forms of cancer. They work closely with the other members of the team to calculate the correct dose of radiotherapy for each individual patient, thus working as part of the MPDT.

Historically most radiographers have worked to patient group directives (PGDs) in order to administer certain drugs, e.g. contrast agents and radiopharmaceuticals. However, radiographers can now access the non-medical prescribing course to become supplementary prescribers. The prospect of radiographers being able to train as independent prescribers is an exciting one. It will open the way for diagnostic radiographers to prescribe appropriate therapy, such as analgesia, without resorting to PGDs or medical involvement. Hogg and Hogg (2006) point out that the expansion of the radiographer role in this area of prescribing fits in with the definition of an independent prescriber (DH 1999). See case study H for an example of how radiographers use non-medical prescribing in practice.

Optometrists

Optometrists undergo 3 or 4 years of degree training, with a further year of supervision and training before qualifying. They examine eyes, test sight, advise on visual problems, recommend treatments, and prescribe and dispense spectacles and contact lenses. They are expert at detecting diseases of the eye and may refer to another professional or supply various eye drugs themselves. They may undertake further training in order to practise in specialist areas such as paediatrics and sports vision.

They are registered with, and regulated by, the General Optical Council and also listed in the Register of Opticians. They can become fellow members of the College of Optometrists. To become fellow members they have to prove that their optometry practice is of a high standard, as approved by the College.

Historically, optometrists have used medicines for diagnostic purposes rather than actually 'treating' eye conditions. Restrictions were put on the use, by optometrists, of antibacterial and antibiotic medication, which are obviously essential for the treatment of eye infections. They were allowed to administer but not supply this sort of medication. This, clearly, had an impact on the way in which optometrists could help patients and clients therapeutically. They had to refer their patients to ophthalmologists in order for them to be prescribed appropriate treatment. Before 2005, optometrists were restricted to 'prescribing' chloramphenicol eye drops (no greater than 0.5%) and eye ointments (no greater than 1%) (Borthwick, cited in Chapter 7 in Bradley and Nolan 2008).

It must have been a great relief for supplementary prescribing rights to be granted to optometrists. Supplementary prescribing is most often used by optometrists when dealing with patients with long-term conditions such as glaucoma (Titcomb and Lawrenson 2006). They are now able to supply relevant 'pharmacy-only' items, which include lubricants, antimicrobial agents and anti-allergy preparations. Post-surgical management, such as analgesia and antimicrobial prophylaxis, has also been enhanced by the introduction of supplementary prescribing for optometrists.

Since June 2009 optometrists have been able to train as independent prescribers and have been able to prescribe any licensed medicines for ocular conditions affecting the eye and surrounding tissue. They cannot, however, prescribe any controlled drug independently (DH 2010a). See case study J for an example of how optometrists use non-medical prescribing in practice.

Podiatrists

Podiatrists undergo an intensive degree course. They are registered with the Health Professions Council (HPC) and become members of, and are regulated by, the Society of Chiropodists and Podiatrists. They are trained to provide preventive care, and diagnosis and treatment of a wide range of foot, ankle and lower limb problems. Clinical and assessment skills mean that podiatrists are able to help patients and clients with long-term problems, such as diabetes, to remain mobile. Their assessment and treatment can prevent severe complications, e.g. amputation in patients with diabetes. Ultimately podiatrists aim to keep patients and clients as mobile as possible. They may work in hospital or community NHS settings, private practice, retail sector, leisure industry, occupational health, and research and forensic podiatry. As with other professionals podiatrists can specialise in certain areas of practice – they can specialise in biomechanics, which looks at the development and function of the foot and its related structures. Podiatrists use their knowledge of biomechanics to diagnose and treat lower limb conditions and sports injuries. Most of the podiatrists who work in sport are self-employed practitioners. They work with individual athletes or sports teams, e.g. football clubs.

They often treat biomechanical problems with orthotics, which are custom-made insoles that aim to improve the function and position of the foot and thus reduce symptoms. They may make these themselves or they may use commercial or NHS orthotic laboratories. Other podiatrists may decide to specialise in paediatric work. Many children present with biomechanical problems that occur developmentally and it is essential that these specialist podiatrists have an in-depth knowledge of paediatric development. Working with children is known as 'podopaediatrics'. Some patients may have developed biomechanical problems due to disease processes, e.g. rheumatoid arthritis, that cause deformity of the joints. Podiatrists undertake biomechanical assessments of these patients in order to develop appropriate plans for treatment to reduce discomfort and increase stability.

Some podiatrists go on to practise podiatric surgery. There are two levels of surgical practice:

1 An HPC-registered practitioner can administer local anaesthetic in order to undertake minor surgical interventions such as nail removal and minor soft tissue surgery.
2 Some podiatrists undertake rigorous further training, lasting a number of years, in order to be able to operate on bone, joint and soft tissue disorders of the foot, e.g. bunion removal, joint straightening, neuroma removal.

Podiatrists are able to administer certain local anaesthetics and supply prescription-only medicines if they have undertaken the appropriate training. If they are qualified to administer these items they have the entitlement ('annotated') registered with the HPC. This online register is a checkpoint to ensure that they are professionally allowed to administer these medications. See case study I for an example of how podiatrists use non-medical prescribing in practice.

Activity box 6.3

Now look at the scenario again.

Mrs Elliott is a 76-year-old woman who lives on her own. She is usually fit and healthy but her daughter has contacted her GP to inform him that her mother has fallen a few times and doesn't think she's been eating properly. She also seems quite confused at times. She has been going to the 'leg ulcer' café once a week for dressings to a small ulcer on her right leg. She has now presented at the surgery with an injury to her left ankle. She says she fell in the kitchen and her ankle is now swollen and painful, although she can weight bear.

Think about:

- Which professionals might actually prescribe for Mrs Elliott?
- What might they prescribe?
- Would they prescribe independently or as a supplementary prescriber?
- How they may coordinate care as a MDPT?
- What other advice might they give

Non-medical prescribing lead

It is expected that each trust employs a non-medical prescribing lead, whose role it is to provide professional leadership and a coordinated approach to the development and maintenance of non-medical prescribing roles within that trust (South Tees Hospitals NHS Trust 2008). They help to develop strategies around non-medical prescribing and provide support for the non-medical prescribers within the trust. They liaise with the strategic health authority non-medical prescribing lead, thus linking into regional and national non-medical prescribing agendas. It is the responsibility of the non-medical prescribing lead to maintain a register of all non-medical prescribers in the trust and to advise on their continuing educational needs.

The non-medical prescribing lead works closely with commissioners of services to ensure that funding is available for potential non-medical prescribers to undertake the non-medical prescribing course. They also liaise with professionals, such as the chief pharmacist, in areas such as medicines management in order to ensure that medicines are prescribed appropriately and safely (Commission for Healthcare Audit and Inspection 2007).

The multidisciplinary non-medical prescribing team

All the above are, or could be, members of the MDPT. However, this team should also include other people, such as the patient and family or carer(s), as well as other health professionals who are involved in the patient's care. The roles of each team member must be considered when prescribing because each individual prescriber will have an impact on the practices of the others in the team. One person may prescribe but another may actually administer the prescription. That person, or someone else, may monitor the effectiveness of the medication and influence further prescribing decisions.

Consultants, doctors and GPs are also very much a part of the MDPT. They may be prescribing or they may be part of the team coordinating a clinical management plan. They also supervise professionals who are working towards gaining a non-medical prescribing qualification.

Each prescribing team member may be working as part of another team, e.g. a district nursing sister may be working as a team leader in a community setting and may be the only prescriber in that team. In support of her assessment of the patient, she may seek the observations of the healthcare assistants on her team. They may be able to provide her with current information about the patient's condition and any factors that might affect the ability to achieve concordance. She may then liaise with the GP and/or hospital consultant and may ask the pharmacist for advice – all as part of the MDPT – before generating a prescription.

The non-medical prescriber, as part of the non-medical prescribing team, should always look at a patient or client with a holistic approach. The emphasis should not just be on the actual prescription but on the whole treatment of the patient or client and his or her condition. Information about influences, such as family circumstances, lifestyle and previous medical history, may be enhanced by the inclusion of communication with other members of the multidisciplinary non-medical prescribing team. The inclusion of other non-prescribing professionals may also increase the effectiveness of the prescription, e.g. a non-medical prescriber may prescribe statins for an obese patient with raised cholesterol but the treatment will be enhanced if the patient is also referred to a dietician.

Figure 6.1 demonstrates how the patient, including the history, physical examination, family circumstances and whether concordance has been achieved, has an effect on the

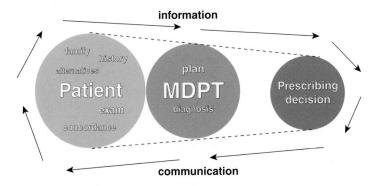

Figure 6.1 Driving the prescribing decision through multidisciplinary team working.

multidisciplinary non-medical prescribing team in order to generate a prescription. The successful prescribing decision is determined by whether the information given and communication between all parties are effective. This is a continuous process and one that should be reviewed regularly. The patient should always be the driving force and the MDPT should be informing and communicating constantly.

Benefits to patients and clients

Having considered the concept of the MDPT from the perspective of the health professional, it is important to consider the benefits for patients and clients. Case study 1 highlights some key benefits of non-medical prescribing and importantly reiterates the contribution made by adopting a multidisciplinary approach:

- In the evaluation of the service it is stated that accessibility is a significant benefit in the service that she provides.
- The other members of her team can see the benefits of Debbie being an independent prescriber and are also keen to undertake the training.
- Her patients do not have to make appointments to see multiple health professionals in order to obtain appropriate treatment.
- Debbie is able to assess patients' conditions and prescribe appropriately.
- Patients can access the appropriate healthcare, and prescription for their condition, in one place, with one professional who is able to coordinate their care.
- She can also refer to other members of the multidisciplinary team, either for advice or for further services for her patients.

The importance of patients and clients as service users is now at the forefront of many of the decisions being made in the NHS. Non-medical prescribing practice, as a relatively new concept, is in a unique position. Policies and protocols are not 'set in stone' and have not been influenced by traditional NHS drivers. The main driver for non-medical prescribing has been the need to streamline patient and client care and to ensure that there is a proper holistic view of each patient's or client's needs. Goodman and Clemow (2008) point out that the importance of communicating with service users may be easily overlooked because much of a practitioner's everyday work can often involve 'face-to-face' contact with other professionals rather than the service users themselves. Liaison with other professionals is, obviously, an essential part of multidisciplinary working but we must never forget that we should be working to improve patient and clients welfare and optimise *their* health, by *including* them!

The Royal College of Nursing (RCN 2006) state:

Service Providers and commissioners should demonstrate how they are actively and meaningfully engaging the public they serve and other stakeholders (such as staff and their representative bodies) in the design, delivery and evaluation of services regardless of the financial pressures ... (RCN 2006, p. 11)

We need to bear this in mind when looking at prescribing practice as a multidisciplinary team. Roscoe et al (2000), conducted a study into the prescribing and administration of chemotherapy, using a multidisciplinary team approach. They had highlighted inconsistencies in the way that certain drugs, such as antiemetics, were prescribed. A multidisciplinary team was formed, which resulted in the development of a manual for chemotherapy prescribing. It included guidelines and protocols, and cost-effective medication suggestions.

By working together and combining our knowledge we have provided a complete package that ensures safety in prescribing and administration of chemotherapy as well as an educational tool. Other benefits include both time and cost savings.

Roscoe et al (2000, p. 1)

Their research found the following benefits:

To the prescriber:
Clear instructions on how to prescribe each chemotherapy regimen
Guidelines on hydration requirements
Recommended antiemetics for each regimen
Likely side effects with each regimen

To nursing staff:
Easy to follow guidelines for administering chemotherapy to each protocol
Clearly written prescriptions, minimising error when interpreting the prescription
Protocol-specific patient advice which can be used as a personal education reference, or as a prompt when educating the patient

To the pharmacist:
Improved legibility of chemotherapy order, minimising error when interpreting the order
Reduced number of interventions due to the inclusion of hydration regimens, pre-medication and discharge medications on a pre-printed form
Educational reference tool for pharmacists new to the area of chemotherapy

To the patient:
Minimised the risk of error
Improved the prescribing of chemotherapy within the unit
Ensured that the chemotherapy is administered safely by providing guidelines for all personnel to follow

Roscoe et al (2000)

They found that the practice of working together to look at a multidisciplinary approach to prescribing meant that each member of the team could appreciate the expertise of the other disciplines involved in the team. They conclude that this has encouraged a team approach and an improvement in quality of care for the patient. Non-medical prescribers in a MDPT are, therefore, in the fortunate position of having access to expertise, in addition to their own, which they can use to provide optimum care and ensure appropriate prescribing for the patient or client.

Commissioning and the MDPT

Activity box 6.4

Answer the following questions in relation to non-medical prescribing:

- Who are the service providers in a non-medical prescribing multidisciplinary team?
- Who commissions the service?
- How would you evaluate the impact of the non-medical prescribing multidisciplinary team?

Having undertaken the above activity, it will be apparent that commissioners are also part of the MDPT. Their role is to commission cost-effective services that will enhance patient and client care. This may mean looking at service providers outside the NHS. It also means looking at training and staffing needs and making decisions about where money will be allocated. The prominent presence of non-medical prescribing on the Government agenda over the last decade has supported the need for training for professionals in this area. This might not always be the case, however, so it is imperative that non-medical prescribers are able to demonstrate the effectiveness and efficiency of the service. The fact that non-medical prescribing supports a multidisciplinary service further justifies its ongoing support, particularly as multidisciplinary team work, is also a Government priority.

The benefits to the patients and clients need to be constantly evaluated in order to demonstrate the effectiveness of and the need for the non-medical prescribing multidisciplinary team. Having one person coordinating the prescribing needs for a patient or client means that there is continuity and, hopefully, more clarity for the person receiving the care. Families, too, are a very important part of the MDPT. As in the case of Mrs Elliott, in the previous activities, it is very often the family who will point out changes in a patient's or client's condition. They may be responsible for administering medication or making sure that the medication is actually taken correctly by the patient or client. It is, therefore, imperative that, when considering the members of the MDPT, the family or carers are taken into account, as well as the patient. How much nicer it is for the patient or client if he or she has the benefit of expertise from different professionals but only has to deal with one 'lead' person! That lead person may be any member of the MDPT.

Activity box 6.5

Identify a patient from your caseload for whom you could prescribe.
Identify the members of the MDPT involved in his or her care.
Critically analyse their input in meeting the needs of the patient.

Problems with multidisciplinary team working!

Working as part of a multidisciplinary team can, however, result in many difficulties. What happens when professionals don't agree about a prescribing decision? What happens when they disagree about whether there should be alternative treatments or therapies? What happens if one member of the team tries to dominate the rest of the team and makes it very difficult for other opinions to be considered?

Effective communication is the key to overcoming many problems. As stated earlier, many cases, particularly in the area of safeguarding children, have highlighted gross failures in communication between services that are supposed to be caring for people. As stated earlier, studies have been carried out into prescribing errors. One such study (Nadeem et al 2001) found that prescribing errors in general practice were common, with a wide range of errors detected. Twenty-five per cent of the errors that they found consisted of 'directions not mentioned at all', highlighting that the prescribers were not communicating effectively. There can also be problems in communication between the prescriber and the patient or client. This can have serious consequences.

Activity box 6.6

Consider a prescribing error, or near miss, which you have come across.
   What part did poor communication play in this event?
   What was the effect on:

- the professional(s) involved
- the patient or client.

It is vitally important that, if a team is to be effective, the team members all have high levels of interpersonal skills, especially communication skills. Team members need to be able to communicate efficiently in order to provide the best possible outcomes for the patient or client. They also need to be experts at communicating with the people for whom they are prescribing and their families or carers.

It therefore follows that each member of the MDPT must have an exact understanding of his or her own particular role within the team. Each should be confident in that role and have points of reference about the procedures to follow in case of deviation from the 'plan' to which the team are working. The team should decide whether they are going to appoint a 'lead' professional who will coordinate the patient's or client's care (not necessarily the most senior person in the team). This is usually the professional who has most contact with the patient or client. I, therefore, prefer to call that person the 'contact' professional. The patient or client should know whom the contact professional is – they then know to whom to go if there are problems or concerns with their treatment or medication. This ensures that one professional oversees the prescribing for the patient or client, ensuring that the prescription is not changed repeatedly, etc. The contact professionals should then make sure that there is communication with other members of the MDPT – including supplementary prescribers. This is important if there is to be optimum care and benefit to the patient or client and the family. As has already been stated, the contact professional may not always be the most senior person in the team. This can cause problems with some senior personnel wanting to 'control' the prescribing situation. The fact that they may have to listen to and consider other opinions is, in some cases, a steep learning curve. It does, however, mean that the decisions about what to prescribe are often considered in more depth than they would otherwise have been. There has been much criticism in the past about drug companies giving incentives to prescribers, mainly medical practitioners, to encourage them to prescribe their product. This has long been a problem in the NHS and has contributed to the high cost of prescribing medications (National Audit Office 2007). The introduction of the MDPT should go some way to prevent this.

The cost of medicines is now taken into account by all prescribers. The individual trusts closely monitor prescribing budgets and, in today's economic climate, encourage practitioners to prescribe the most cost-effective medication possible. Therefore, the MDPT, with its ability to peer review each decision and its capacity to assess the patient or client in a truly holistic way is often seen as a means to obtaining the most lucrative process of prescribing practice. This means that, rather than the focus being on 'cheap' prescribing, evaluation of non-medical prescribing practices enables demonstration of clinical effectiveness and cost-effective prescribing.

Activity box 6.7

Look at case study 1. Think about which professionals might be involved with Harold. Imagine that you are the lead professional/patient contact in the MDPT.
  What factors would you take into account when prescribing for Harold?
  How would you communicate with the other team members?
  How would you 'manage' Harold's care, within the multidisciplinary team?
  Who do you think would prescribe?

Harold's case is ideal for inclusion in the multidisciplinary prescribing process. Many professionals and non-professionals may be involved with his care in some way. It is essential that there is excellent communication between the professionals involved, which should result in efficient and effective coordinated care for him.

Education and learning

Although there has been clear argument in support of MDPTs, it must be recognised that individual members will have different skills and different training needs. The introduction of the multidisciplinary non-medical prescribing course has resulted in a change in education practice that fits in with the 'Darzi review' (DH 2007). The emphasis in the review is on (Goodman and Clemow 2008):

the way services are delivered
how the quality of services can be improved
how access to these services can be improved
how to address inequalities in health and health care ...

These are all issues that need to be considered and addressed when thinking about the MDPT.

The Department of Health and their commissioners are now highlighting the need to plan the future workforce by looking at education and training needs that will produce clinical leaders in the future (DH 2008). As we have seen, interprofessional/ multidisciplinary working is proving to be cost-effective and beneficial to staff and patients or clients. It would, therefore, follow, that, in order for this way of working to be maximised, it would be beneficial to have 'shared' learning. Non-medical prescribing education, available to appropriate professionals, is delivered as multidisciplinary education. Various professional disciplines learn together and from each other. They share their expertise and experiences, increasing their knowledge of each other's roles and practice within the prescribing team. Goodman and Clemow (2008) propose that there are three steps to collaborative working practice, highlighting the importance of multi-disciplinary, or interprofessional, learning, leading to collaborative working.

The ultimate goal of interprofessional or multidisciplinary education in non-medical prescribing should be to prepare non-medical prescribers to work efficiently and safely in teams, to provide safe, appropriate and cost-effective prescriptions for patients and clients. Collaborative working practice, based on multidisciplinary education, will ensure that our patients and clients receive the best possible care and support with their medi-cation and treatment:

The way in which NHS staff work, and how they collaborate with each other in effec-tive teams, is key to the delivery of patient services in the NHS.

DH (2005, p. 2)

Although practitioners will remain responsible for their own professional practice, multidisciplinary education does promote 'collective' thinking and an increased under-standing of each other's roles in prescribing. This will, inevitably, increase respect for other disciplines and should result in more appropriate patient care.

Conclusion

As we have seen, the introduction of non-medical prescribing has been an innovative and challenging aspect of change in the modern NHS. The expansion of non-medical prescribing, from its origins where it was exclusively the extended role of the nurse, to include other professionals and the patient/client, their family and/or carers, is an exciting move towards total holistic care for each individual. This is an area that really can be multidisciplinary. The benefits for an overstretched NHS, with strict budgetary restraints and for the professional staff who become prescribers and, therefore have more autonomy in their work, cannot be underestimated. The benefits of a truly multiprofessional prescribing team for the patient, client, family and/or carers are huge.

As stated, the effective use of a multiprofessional prescribing team brings many benefits, albeit with a variety of challenges, which will be evaluated and tested again and as the field of non-medical prescribing expands. As different professions are 'allowed' to undertake non-medical prescribing courses and new 'team members' become qualified prescribers, the multidisciplinary team will inevitably expand. The breadth of experience available to the team will increase which, I suggest, will be of infinite benefit to non-medical prescribing professionals and patient and clients.

It will be of benefit to all professionals to be aware of the need for multiprofessional working practices. Those who do not may soon find themselves 'left behind'. All recent Department of Health's documents and guidelines call for multidisciplinary/ interprofessional working practices and see this as the way forward for the NHS.

Education practices are changing, with the changing needs of the strategic health authorities and other members of the NHS. Non-medical prescribing is expanding rapidly and there are many voices calling for an increase in the number of, and variety of, professionals eligible to become non-medical prescribers. There is, inevitably, some opposition but, as the number of non-medical prescribing teams increases and benefits are recognised, hopefully the expansion will continue.

Activity box 6.8

Take time to review the learning objectives of the chapter:

- Discuss the meaning of the 'multidisciplinary prescribing team'
- Identify the roles of non-medical prescribers
- Critically analyse the importance of working as part of a multidisciplinary team.
- Discuss the benefits of the 'multidisciplinary prescribing team' for patients and clients.
- Apply knowledge about multidisciplinary prescribing to non-medical prescribing practice
- Identify any areas in which you need to develop or increase your understanding. Devise an action plan to support this process (this may include spending some time with other members of the multidisciplinary prescribing team).

It is hoped that the roles of the various members of the MDPT have been clarified and that the importance of prescribing as a part of the team has been rationalised. This is the future of the 'caring services'!

Key themes: conclusions and considerations

Public health	Public health is a responsibility of every individual within the multidisciplinary prescribing team. However, a team approach, providing consistency in both approach and advice in relation to public health targets, will support public health initiatives. A team approach to public health facilitates effective use of skills within the team and enables the management of individual patients to better meet their needs
	Consider the targets you address as an individual practitioner. Is there opportunity to address this using a team approach?
Social and cultural issues	Individual patients may have social needs that you are unable to meet alone. Awareness of the roles of the members of the MDPT will enable you to respond to the patient's needs appropriately and effectively. This will often require interagency working as well as working with other health professionals
	Cultural issues may influence the format of an individual's prescribing team, due to acceptability of specific treatments, services and professionals. The MDPT may also include an interpreter or link worker
	Consider your patient group and the social and cultural issues that might arise. How do you address these? How does the adaptation of a holistic approach, which considers social and cultural issues, support your prescribing activity for these patients?
Prescribing principles	MDPT working can impact on each of the prescribing principles. Examples are given below: • Examine the holistic needs of the patient: sharing information, access to investigations and tests • Consider the appropriate strategy: alternative or additional treatment options available within team, support in choosing appropriate strategies • Consider the remaining principles in relation to your own practice and identify how the team supports these.

References

Bradley EJ, Nolan P (2008) *Non-Medical Prescribing*. Cambridge: Cambridge University Press.

Buckley P, Grime J, Blenkinsop A (2006) Inter and intra-professional perspectives on non-medical prescribing in an NHS trust. *Pharm J* **277**: 394-8.

Commission for Healthcare Audit and Inspection (2007) *The Best Medicine: The management of medicines in acute and specialist trusts*. London: Health Care Commission.

Crown J (1999) Review of prescribing, supply and administration of medicines. DH. Available at http://www.dh.gov.uk/en/Publicationsandstatistics/Publications/Publications PolicyAndGuidance/DH_4077151. (last accessed 3.3.10).

Dean B, Schachter M, Vincent C, Barber N (2002) Prescribing errors in hospital inpatients: their incidence and clinical significance. *Qual Safety Health Care* **11**: 340-4.

Department of Health (1999) *Final Report of the Review of Prescribing, Supply and Administration of Medicines (Crown Report)*. London: HMSO.

Department of Health (2000) *The NHS Plan: A plan for investment, a plan for reform*. London: HMSO.

Department of Health (2004) *Choosing Health, Making Healthy Choices Easier*. London: HMSO.

Department of Health (2005) *Working Time Directive Pilots Programme.Final report*. London: NM Agency.

Department of Health (2006) *Modernising Nursing Careers: Setting the direction*. London: HMSO.

Department of Health (2007) *Review of NHS Service Improvement* (known as 'the Darzi review') (online). Available at: www.dh.gov.uk (accessed 25 March 2010).

Department of Health (2008) *World Class Commissioning and the Darzi Review* (online). Available at: www.dh.gov.uk/en/Publicationsandstatistics/Publications/PublicationsPolicy AndGuidance/DH_080956 (accessed 13 April 2010).

Department of Health (2009) *Allied health professions prescribing and medicines supply mechanisms scoping project report* (online). Available at: www.dh.gov.uk/prod_consum_ dh/groups/dh_digitalassets/documents/digitalasset/dh_103949.pdf (accessed 13 April 2010).

Department of Health (2010a) *Optometrist Independent Prescribing* (online). Available at: www.dh.gov/en/Healthcare/Medicinespharmacyandindustry/Prescriptions/TheNon-MedicalPrescribingProgrammes/Optometristindependentprescribing/index.htm (accessed 25 March 2010).

Department of Health (2010b) *Working Together to Safeguard Children: A guide to inter-agency working to safeguard and promote the welfare of children* (online). Available at: www.dcsf.gov.uk/everychildmatters/safeguardingandsocialcare/safeguardingchildren/ workingtogether/workingtogethertosafeguardchildren (accessed 13 April 2010).

George J, McCaig DJ, Bond CM et al (2006) Supplementary prescribing: early experience of pharmacists in Great Britain. *Ann Pharmacother* **40**: 1843-50.

Goodman, B, Clemow R (2008) *Nursing and Working with Other People*. Exeter: Learning Matters.

Hawley G, ed. (2007) *Ethics in Clinical Practice*. Edinburgh: Pearson.

Hemingway S (2008) Prescribing within a team context: one mental health nurse's reflection on the clinical aspect of non-medical prescribing training, *Mental Health and Learning Disabil Res Pract* **5**: 119-33.

Hogg P, Hogg D (2006) Prescription, supply and administration of drugs in diagnosis and therapy. *Synergy News* March: 4-8.

Leathard A (1994) *Going Interprofessional. Working Together for Health and Welfare*. London: Routledge.

McCray J, ed. (2009) *Nursing and Multi-professional Practice*. London: Sage.

Nadeem S, Shah H, Aslam M, Avery AJ (2001) A survey of prescribing errors in general practice. *Pharmaceut J* **267**: 860-2.

National Audit Office (2007) *Prescribing Costs in Primary Care* (online). Available at: www.nao.org.uk/publications/0607/prescribing_costs_in_primary_c.aspx (accessed 13 April 2010).

Nursing and Midwifery Council (2006) Standards of Proficiency for Nurse and Midwife Prescribers. *London: NMC.*

Nursing and Midwifery Council (2008) *The Code: Standards of Conduct. Performance and ethics for nurses and midwives.* London: NMC.

Pharmacist Training (online). Available at: www.nhscareers.nhs.uk/details/Default.aspx?Id=194 (accessed 20 March 2010).

Ovretveit J (1997) How to describe interprofessional Working. In: Ovretveit, Matthias P, Thompson T (eds), *Interprofessional Working for Health and Social Care. Community Health Series.* Basingstoke: Macmillan.

Roscoe JC, Gorranson E, Slancar M, Smith J, Taylor S, Tyson S (2000) A multi-disciplinary approach to ensure safety in the prescribing and administration of chemotherapy. *J Oncol Pharm Pract* **6**(2).

Royal College of Nursing (2006) *Principles to Inform Decision Making: What do I need to know?* London: RCN.

South Tees Hospitals, NHS Trust (2008) Role of non-medical prescribing lead (online). Available at: www.southtees.nhs.uk/UserFiles/pages/3493.pdf (accessed 14 September 2010).

Stenner K, Carey N, Courtenay M (2009) Nurse prescribing in dermatology: doctors' and non-prescribing nurses views. *J Adv Nurs* **65**: 851-9.

Talley S, Richens S (2001) Prescribing practices of advanced practice psychiatric nurses. *Arch Psychiatr Nurs* **XV**: 205-13.

Titcomb LC, Lawrenson JG (2006) Recent changes in medicines legislation that affect optometrists. *Optom Pract* **7**: 23-34.

Chapter 7

Clinical Skills

Gillian Armitage and Jane Rutt-Howard

Learning objectives

After reading this chapter and completing the activities within it, the reader will be able to:

1 have the ability to assess a patient's vital signs
2 have an understanding of the principles of physical examination
3 consider differential diagnosis in physical examination
4 acquire numerical skills and confidence for safe practice

To enable the healthcare professional to effectively diagnose and subsequently monitor a patient's condition requires all the skills of the consultation, and including the skills of clinical examination in many instances. Once a medication has been prescribed (and ideally administered/taken), it is the responsibility of the non-medical prescriber to monitor the effect of their prescribing decisions, which in many cases will require a physical examination (to a greater or lesser extent) depending on individual circumstances. This chapter is a compilation of three sections: instructions on how to measure and record a patient's vital signs using a structured approach; an explanation of three complete system examinations (ear nose and throat (ENT), respiratory and gastrointestinal) underpinned by the structure and principles of physical examination (inspection, palpation, percussion and auscultation) and an introduction to examination of the cranial nerves and eliciting deep tendon reflexes; and an introduction to the importance of the skills of numeracy.

Nurse non-medical prescribers have the advantage of having been previously taught how to undertake clinical vital signs (Nursing and Midwifery Council (NMC) 2007) but, for many allied health professional and pharmacist non-medical prescribers, these skills are a new extension to their role. To become competent requires a dual approach of acquiring an understanding of the underpinning anatomy, physiology and pathophysiology of the body, together with the acquisition of new psychomotor competences.

As discussed in Chapter 4, the non-medical prescriber may be required to undertake physical examination of the patient to confirm or refute their findings as a result of the

The Textbook of Non-medical Prescribing, edited by Dilyse Nuttall and Jane Rutt-Howard.
© 2011 Blackwell Publishing Ltd

history elicited from the patient. It is beyond the realms of the chapter to address each of the physical examination systems and therefore it focuses on those as stated above. The ENT system has been chosen because many patients present with ENT problems, which non-medical prescribers are frequently exposed to, especially in primary care and accident and emergency. The respiratory and gastrointestinal systems have been chosen to illustrate the structure and techniques available. The introduction to examination of the cranial nerves and eliciting deep tendon reflexes is in response to the curriculum for training pharmacist prescribers (Royal Pharmaceutical Society of Great Britain (RPSGB) 2006).

Critics of non-medical prescribing might argue that a full physical examination of the patient should remain within the realms of the medical practitioner. However, it could also be argued that, by taking on the role of non-medical prescriber and the accountability for a patient's diagnosis (independent prescriber), to undertake the accompanying physical examination is both logical and essential. The legal position for health professionals is that, although they must practise within their level of competence and scope of professional practice (General Pharmaceutical Council (GPhC) 2010, Health Professions Council (HPC) 2008, NMC 2008), they must also gain appropriate supervision and support from a suitably qualified practitioner (NMC 2006) in the mentorship of acquiring these new skills in order to safeguard their prescribing decisions.

Further support and guidance with numerical skills has been highlighted as a development need for health professionals due to the expanding clinical roles. Mistakes made in drug calculations are a significant cause of drug errors (Warburton 2010) and subsequent patient harm (National Prescribing Safety Agency (NPSA) 2009). This book offers the reader a website to appraise and develop skills and confidence with respect to numeracy skills.

Vital signs

Vital signs are an essential element of assessing and monitoring the patient's physiological status: 'Important information gained by assessing and measuring vital signs can be indicators of health and ill health' (Royal College of Nursing 2007) and the practitioner should practise the art of monitoring and recording vital signs until they can master each skill. In addition to the skill, the practitioner needs to know the normal and abnormal parameters of each of the vital signs. Many decisions about a patient's treatment are made on baseline, and trends, of vital sign recordings – it is important that standards are maintained in the measuring and recording of these vital signs in order to maintain standards and safety in care delivery.

In terms of vital signs, this section addresses the skills required to perform and understand a patient's health status: conscious level, respiration status, temperature, pulse, blood pressure, pain, pulse oximetry, pupil dilatation and peak flow.

Conscious level

The first skill is to assess the patient's level of consciousness, or mental status, if there is any suspicion of altered consciousness. The AVPU scale is a four-part scale

(Table 7.1), which is a simplified method of assessing a critically ill patient compared with the Glasgow Coma Scale (GCS) (Mahadevan and Garmel 2005):

A   Awake and aware
V   Responds to verbal stimuli
P   Responds to noxious stimuli
U   Unresponsive

An AVPU response of P or U is an indication of significant intracranial injury or 'assault'. During this rapid AVPU assessment of the patient, the practitioner should additionally undertake examination of the pupils (see below) for size and reaction (Greaves et al 2006).

The GCS score comprises three parameters – best eye response, best verbal response and best motor response – and should be used in a full assessment (Table 7.2). It is a complex scale compounded by a slowness and complexity in its measurement compared with AVPU (Mahadevan and Garmel 2005). However, it has its function in less time-critical situations or in complex care delivery circumstances, e.g. within an intensive care setting, when a more formal assessment of conscious level is required. A GCS score ranges from 3 (completely unresponsive) to 15 (fully alert and oriented) with

Table 7.1   AVPU

A – Alert – ascertain if alert and coherent; if they are, status is 'A'. If confused, consider if this is a long-standing problem or of recent/acute onset
V – Responds to voice – if not fully awake, check the response to your voice, if they do respond they are status 'V'
P – Responds to pain – if no response to voice, administer a painful stimulus (pinching above the clavicle), if there is a response, status is 'P'
U – Unconscious – status is 'U' if no response

Adapted from Mahadevan and Garmel (2005).

Table 7.2   Glasgow Coma Scale

Eye opening response	Best verbal response	Best motor response
1 – No eye opening	1 – No verbal response	1 – No motor response
2 – Eye(s) opening to painful stimuli	2 – Incomprehensible sounds	2 – Extension to pain
3 – Eye(s) opening to verbal command	3 – Inappropriate words	3 – Flexion to pain
4 – Eye(s) open spontaneously	4 – Confused	4 – Withdrawal from pain
	5 – Oriented	5 – Localising pain
		6 – Obeys commands

Adapted from Greaves et al (2006).

intermediate scores of 13 or higher being associated with a mild brain injury, 9-12 a moderate injury and 8 or below a severe brain injury (Greaves et al 2006).

If there is an altered conscious level, it is important to establish the cause: check for medical alert bracelets or if medical notes are available review the medical history or presenting complaint. Check for signs of head injury (e.g. Battle's sign - Greaves et al 2006), hypoglycaemia (blood glucose monitoring), or alcohol or other drug-induced intoxication (use your skills of 'inspection' for clues).

Respirations

A patient's respiratory rate is the number of breaths counted in 1 minute and is usually counted by observing the patient's chest rise for each breath. It is best measured when a patient is at rest. When assessing the rate of breathing it is also necessary to note the depth, rhythm, symmetry and effort of the breathing pattern. It is known that an unobserved respiratory rate is more accurate and reflective of the patient's normal breathing pattern compared with the data collected when the patient is aware of your actions. Thus, try to record respiratory rates covertly: the respiratory rate is one of the few signs that can be altered voluntarily by the patient (Cox and Roper 2005): you cannot tell someone to 'breath normally,' normal breathing is involuntary (Bickley and Szilagyi 2010). To do this, you could measure the respiratory rate immediately before or after you have assessed the patient's pulse, without letting him or her know that you have moved on; you can keep holding the patient's wrist to give the impression of monitoring the pulse.

Aside from visual inspection, there is much information to be gained from auditory clues, i.e. listening to the patient's breathing. Pathologies such as wheezing, grunting, snoring or stridor can be noted, all of which may indicate difficulty in breathing. Beyond difficulty in breathing the patient may become significantly distressed and display signs such as nasal flaring, cyanosis, intercostal recession, use of accessory muscles and acute confusion. Depending on each individual patient, the clinical situation and your scope of professional practice, your prescribing decisions will be influenced by any of these abnormal findings. As an example, an asthma specialist nurse may be confident to prescribe a course of prednisolone for a patient with asthma presenting with a wheeze, but, for a less experienced non-medical prescriber, the identification of a wheeze may be an indicator to refer to a doctor.

Table 7.3 shows normal respiratory rates according to age - note the wide range of 'normal'. Cox and Roper (2005) comment on how difficult it is to decide on an abnormal

Table 7.3 Normal breath rates according to age

Age	Average breaths/min
Newborn	44
Infant	20-40
Pre school	20-30
Older children	16-25
Adult	12-20

respiratory rate when the margins are so wide and research is not definitive. It is as well that a respiratory assessment does not rely solely on rate and that all the factors above are collated to make the judgement in terms of decision-making.

In terms of respiratory rates and abnormal findings, bradypnoea is the medical term for a slow rate (less than 12 breaths/min for an adult). There are many pathologies associated with bradypnoea including depressed respiratory drive secondary to narcotic medication (which could be a side effect/toxicity from prescribed anaesthetics or a consequence of overdosing on illicit drugs (opioids, alcohol or sedatives), again depending upon each clinical situation), a diabetic coma, severe hypothermia or neurological dysfunction (affecting the respiratory centres in the brain stem).

Tachypnoea is fast breathing (more than 20 breaths/min) and is a normal response to activity. Additionally tachypnoea occurs with fever, illness, pain, anxiety, shock, anaemia, lung and heart disease and with other medical conditions (Talley and O'Connor 2009, Bickley and Szilagyi 2010).

In terms of respirations the final three medical terms worthy of note in this chapter is dyspnoea, orthopnoea and paroxysmal nocturnal dyspnoea (PND). The first is the term used to describe a patient being short of breath, orthopnoea is shortness of breath when lying flat and PND is when breathlessness wakes the patient from sleep. The rationale for knowing this distinction is to do with patient assessment and monitoring of a patient's status. For a non-medical prescribing example, you may decide to increase a patient's diuretic treatment if he or she starts to complain of PND, or indeed decrease his or her diuretics if the PND resolves (National Institute for Health Clinical Excellence 2003), when caring for a patient with heart failure.

Pulse oximetry

To complement a patient's respiratory effort, pulse oximetry can be used to assess the effectiveness of this effort. Pulse oximetry is a non-invasive technique used to monitor arterial oxygen saturation. It is based on the difference in light absorption between oxyhaemoglobin and deoxyhaemoglobin (Wyatt et al 2006). Ventilation or PCO_2 (CO_2 partial pressure) is not reflected in pulse oximetry. Although it has many advantages over clinical methods of assessing oxygenation, there are a number of pitfalls to appreciate (Table 7.4).

Table 7.4   Pitfalls of pulse oximetry

Poor circulation (shock)
Carbon monoxide poisoning
Skin, dirt and grease
Nail varnish (dark and metallic colours only) or synthetic fingernails
Hypothermia
Increased temperature
Excessive movement
Fluctuating light levels

Adapted from Greaves et al (2006), Wyatt et al (2006).

The pulse oximetry probe can be placed on a finger, toe, ear or nose. Acceptable normal ranges are from 95% to 99% and readings under 90% are classed as severe hypoxia. It is noteworthy to appreciate that tolerance of pulse oximetry differs with age (oxyhaemoglobin dissociation curve, (Kumar and Clark 2004): children are less tolerant of reduced saturations, quickly deteriorating as their percentage saturations drop, so quick and safe clinical decision-making is a priority. However, due to the pitfalls above, never assimilate the pulse oximetry in isolation; always correlate with clinical findings (Wyatt et al 2006).

Peak flow (peak expiratory flow rate)

The peak expiratory flow rate (PEFR) can be measured using a peak expiratory flow meter (Table 7.5). The PEFR is the maximal flow rate of expired air and thus begins after the patient has taken a full inspiration. The key to an accurate reading is to facilitate the patient to blow as hard and fast as possible into the meter. This facilitation is maximised by clear instructions and often a demonstration too.

In conditions such as asthma, when small airways are obstructed, the PEFR is reduced. An element of asthma diagnosis and management is based on a patient's peak flow readings (British Thoracic Society 2009).

The **best** of three readings is used and recorded on graph paper charts together with a record of symptoms - a peak flow diary.

Table 7.5   Procedure for measuring peak flow

Check that the pointer is at zero
Stand or sit in a comfortable, upright position
Hold the peak flow meter level (horizontally), keeping fingers away from the pointer
Take a deep breath and close lips firmly around the mouthpiece
Blow as hard as you can - as if you were blowing out candles on a birthday cake
  - it is the speed of your blow that is being measured
Look at the pointer and note the reading
Reset the pointer back to zero
Do this three times and record the highest reading

Temperature

The body's temperature is kept at a steady 36-38°C by homeostatic mechanisms that are controlled by the hypothalamus (Wyatt et al 2006) within an average of about 3°C (Bickley and Szilagyi 2010). The medical term for an elevated body temperature or fever is pyrexia where hyperpyrexia is an extreme elevation, >41°C and hypothermia refers to those temperatures <35°C (Kumar and Clark 2004).

As a non-medical prescriber, there will be a number of reasons for needing to know a patient's temperature. Predominantly there will be a need for a baseline temperature and then subsequent recordings to help evaluate any treatment initiated, continued or stopped, charting a patient's trends. An elevated temperature is a positive sign of infection (with or without an associated fever), inflammation or an abnormality of the central nervous system.

There are a number of factors to consider when assessing a patient's temperature including any recent exercise, hormone production (thyroxine and adrenaline increase heat production), food intake, menstrual cycle (in females) and age (very young and old people have greater difficulty in regulating their body temperature – Cohen 2009). The time of day that it is recorded can have an impact, with relatively lower recordings in the morning compared with the evening due to reduced muscle activity and food intake over night (Cohen 2009). Another consideration is the place where you obtain the recording from, e.g. axilla (cooler), rectal (warmer), mouth (unreliable) or tympanic (quick, safe and reliable) (Bickley and Szilagyi 2010).

To monitor and record an oral temperature, accurate placement of the thermometer is essential and should be placed at the sublingual pocket at the base of the tongue. The patient must then close the mouth and retain a 'seal' around the probe – the rationale being that this area is close to thermoreceptors which respond rapidly to changes in core temperature. When using electronic thermometers, this may take about 10 seconds (Bickley and Szilagyi 2010).

Rectal temperature monitoring is used only in certain specialised clinical situations and does not need to be addressed in terms of non-medical prescribing: you will either be competent already or use a less invasive procedure.

Tympanic membrane temperature is becoming increasingly popular in clinical settings, not least because it is quick and relatively safe (Wyatt et al 2006, Bickley and Szilagyi 2010). Placement is important in that the probe is securely placed in the external auditory canal and the infrared beam is aimed towards the membrane itself. It is ideal to ensure that there is no significant wax build-up (cerumen) to obscure the tympanic membrane and thus produce a lower temperature recording. It takes about 3 seconds and reliably measures core body temperature (it shares the blood supply of the hypothalamus), which is higher than the usual oral temperature by approximately 0.8°C (Bickley and Szilagyi 2010). Table 7.6 gives procedure guidance.

Temperature can be a significant finding in many clinical presentations and can also be a key decision aid, e.g. in a patient presenting with a productive cough, pyrexia may be the defining reason for prescribing antibiotics in the absence of any other significant clinical findings. The Centor criteria use 'history of a fever' as one of four criteria to guide antibiotic treatment for a patient with a sore throat (National Prescribing Centre

Table 7.6 Ear thermoscan procedure

Explain procedure to the client
Ensure that you have good access to the client's ear
Apply the disposable cover to the thermoscan
Straighten auditory canal
Press the 'on' button, note the digital display on
Place the probe in the ear
Press the sensor to take a temperature reading
Record the reading

Table 7.7 Guidelines for non-ritualistic monitoring of temperature

1	In patients with disorders which affect metabolic rate, e.g. hypothyroidism or hyperthyroidism
2	In patients who are critically ill or postoperative. Trends and baseline recordings are significant in these situations
3	In patients who are immunosuppressed and therefore at greater risk of infection, e.g. patients undergoing chemotherapy or radiotherapy.
4	In patients receiving blood transfusions
5	In patients with an infection requiring monitoring of temperature to assess development or regression or the infection

2006). Rather than ritualistically monitoring a patient's temperature, see Table 7.7 for guidelines on when to monitor temperature.

Pulse

The pulse represents an impulse transmitted by contraction of the left ventricle of the heart and felt by palpation where an artery crosses a bone, e.g. the radial artery at the wrist. The composition of arteries results in them having two key properties: elasticity and contractility. The ejection of blood into the arteries causes them to stretch to compensate for the increased pressure as the blood flows from the left ventricle. This wave of expansion is felt through the palpation of certain arteries at selected sites (see below and Activity box 7.1) and is termed 'pulse'. When you palpate the pulse you are feeling the wave of expansion in the artery, not the blood flowing through it. The palpation of a pulse involves using your fingertips to gently press an artery against a bony prominence. The most commonly palpated pulse is the radial artery because it is extremely accessible: it can easily be located in a 'gutter' between flexor carpi radialis and abductor pollicis longus (Abrahams et al 2003). For alternative pulse locations see Activity box 7.1.

 Activity box 7.1

www.gla.ac.uk/ibls/US/fab/tutorial/generic/sapulse.html
   Access this website and make notes on the anatomical locations and clinical procedures for locating the pulses in the lower limbs.

   Other locations of pulses include the temporal artery superior and anterior to the pinna of the ear and palpated against the bone of the skull. Carotid artery is located lateral to the larynx/trachea and medial to the sternocleidomastoid muscle in the neck (palpate one at a time; never try to palpate both carotid arteries simultaneously). The brachial artery is located in the antecubital fossa on the anterior surface of the elbow joint (Abrahams et al 2003). Finally there is the apex beat, or the palpation of the heart

Table 7.8   Normal pulse rate values according to age

Infant	100–160/min
Child	70–120/min
Child over 10 years and adults	60–100/min

Table 7.9   Summary of abnormal findings

Abnormal heart rates	Differential diagnosis
Tachycardia (>100 beats/min)	Haemorrhage, fever, dehydration, hyperthyroidism, supraventricular tachycardia, medication such as adrenaline
Bradycardia (<60 beats/min)	Increased intracranial pressure, sinus bradycardia, heart block, hypothyroidism, medication such as β blockers (e.g. atenolol) or digoxin
Rhythm	
Regularly irregular	Sinus arrhythmia, second-degree heart block, ventricular ectopics
Irregularly irregular	Atrial flutter with varying block, Arial fibrillation
Volume	
Weak and thread like	Haemorrhage, shock
Bounding and full	Hypertension, heart failure, aortic valve regurgitation, chronic kidney failure, anaemia

itself. This apex beat is located in the fifth intercostal space in the midclavicular line. This pulse is more like a tapping feel than the other pulses, which feel more like a waveform.

When palpating the pulse you need to consider the rate (Table 7.8), rhythm, volume, state of the vessel wall and character of the pulse. See Table 7.9 for a summary of some abnormal findings and possible differential diagnoses.

In terms of non-medical prescribing, the theme continues in that the pulse can inform your decision-making. It can be used to aid the initiation of treatment, e.g. when atrial fibrillation has been diagnosed, or it can be used to evaluate an issue of side effects, e.g. in a patient who has recently been started on β blockers and is now feeling light-headed.

The pulse can also be used to aid decisions, in combination with a patient's temperature, for example, because an increase in temperature and heart rate is a stronger indication of infection than either in isolation. Conversely, a reducing pulse and temperature is a good indicator that the infection is abating.

Blood pressure

Blood pressure is the force exerted by the circulating blood on the walls of an artery and is expressed in terms of the systolic pressure and diastolic pressure, e.g. 120/80 mmHg.

Systolic pressure is measured at the peak pressure in the arteries, at contraction, and diastolic pressure is measured at the minimum pressure in the arteries at rest. Blood pressure constantly changes in response to bodily functions, diseased states, drugs/ medication, exercise and external influences. It is also subject to circadian variations.

Before the safety issues associated with the use of mercury sphygmomanometers were identified, blood pressure was measured using such a device. More recently, however, there has been a necessary increase in the use of aneroid and electronic devices, although a millimetre of mercury (mmHg) is still the unit of measurement expressed.

The electronic devices are relatively easy to use, provided that they are employed according to the manufacturer's instructions, and are just as accurate as sphygmoma- nometers (O'Brien et al 2003). However, students are still taught how to take a blood pressure using a manual technique. See Tables 7.10 and 7.11 for guidance on measuring blood pressure using either a mercury device or a digital device.

Activity box 7.2

www.bhsoc.org/bp_monitors/ESH_BP_rec.pdf

This web link provides access to the 2003 article: 'European Society of Hypertension recommendations for conventional, ambulatory and home blood pressure measurement.'

Take time to read this and consider its implications for your own clinical prac- tice in terms of both your own training needs and the clinical needs of your patients.

Table 7.10   Measuring blood pressure using a mercury blood pressure device

The patient should be seated for at least 5 min, relaxed and not moving or speaking
The arm must be supported at the level of the heart. Ensure that no tight clothing constricts the arm
Place the cuff on neatly with the centre of the bladder over the brachial artery. The bladder should encircle at least 80% of the arm (but not more than 100%)
The column of mercury must be vertical, and at the observer's eye level
Estimate the systolic BP beforehand:
Palpate the brachial artery
Inflate cuff until pulsation disappears
Deflate cuff
Estimate systolic pressure
Then inflate to 30 mmHg above the estimated systolic level needed to occlude the pulse
Place the stethoscope diaphragm over the brachial artery and deflate at a rate of 2-3 mm/s until you hear regular tapping sounds
Measure systolic (first sound) and diastolic (disappearance) to nearest 2 mmHg

From O'Brien et al (2003).

Table 7.11 Measuring blood pressure using a digital device

The patient should be seated for at least 5 min, relaxed and not moving or speaking

The arm must be supported at the level of the heart. Ensure that no tight clothing constricts the arm

Place the cuff on neatly with the indicator mark on the cuff over the brachial artery. The bladder should encircle at least 80% of the arm (but not more than 100%)

Most monitors allow manual blood pressure setting selection where you choose the appropriate setting. Other monitors will automatically inflate and reinflate to the next setting if required

Repeat three times and record measurement as displayed

Initially test blood pressure in both arms and use arm with highest reading for subsequent measurement

From O'Brien et al (2003).

Additional vital signs

The 'fifth vital sign' is the term referred to when assessing a patient's pain.

This is an interesting and incredibly complex symptom that a patient experiences. It is also interesting because it is the *absence* of pain that is the desired outcome compared with the preceding signs that are 'vitally' important to be present. Within secondary care, pain is the main area of prescribing for non-medical prescribers (Courtenay and Gordon 2009)

Pain cannot be assessed objectively because it is a symptom, an experience (multidimensional: physical and emotional) that is unique to every individual. However, as a non-medical prescriber, it is important to be aware of the various tools available to help facilitate a patient to describe pain and allocate a degree of objectivity to it.

Qualitatively, Morton (1993) developed a mnemonic to help practitioners assess a patient's pain, namely PQRST. Many 'presenting complaints' have specific symptom patterns, e.g. appendicitis usually begins with a vague dull ache in the umbilical area (visceral pain) and, as it progresses through its trajectory, it becomes more localised to the right lower quadrant of the abdomen, and is more of a discrete experience – sharp and more intense (somatic or parietal pain). Without intervention, the appendix is liable to rupture resulting in peritonitis, which often produces pain in the tip of the shoulder blade (referred pain) (Mahadevan and Garmel 2005). As a prescriber, without knowing the pattern of pain in a patient with appendicitis, and without a thorough exploration of the patient's experience, there is potential for misdiagnosis that will automatically result in unsafe prescribing and management. Another example of careful exploration and interpretation based on sound anatomical knowledge is a patient presenting with abdominal pain that reveals it to be pain from a diagnosis of pneumonia: T9 distribution of neurons is shared by the lung *and* abdomen. There are a number of similar tools available to explore a patient's symptom(s) of pain and these are discussed in further detail in Chapter 4.

Included within the narrative of the patient's story about pain experience, there is an attempt to measure the degree of pain using, in the main, a numerical scale (British Pain Society 2008). The link directs you to downloadable pain scales for use in your clinical practice, together with multiple language versions: www.britishpainsociety.org/pub_pain_scales.htm.

Activity box 7.3

www.britishpainsociety.org
   This web link provides access to the British Pain Society's website homepage.
   Navigate the website → publications → professional → the assessment of pain in older people: National Guidelines (2007) → appendix 3
   Take time to 'digest' this algorithm and next time that you need to assess an older person's pain, try to follow the algorithm. Alternatively, use the algorithm as a tool for reflection (especially if a new algorithm and time are critical) to guide an improved assessment in the future.

When assessing children, the situation can be compounded by their ability to understand the concept of numbers to reflect their pain experience. Thus, a paediatric pain scale has been developed (Wong et al 2001). The scale is made up of six expressions on pictured faces, ranging from a happy face to a grimacing face suffering from pain that is intolerable (sixth face).

Activity box 7.4

http://pain.about.com/od/testingdiagnosis/ig/pain-scales/Wong-Baker.htm
   This web link takes you to a website with a successive list of six different pain scales that can be used with adults and children.
   Take a look at the various scales and decide which would be the most appropriate for your own clinical setting, be it primary care, accident and emergency or intensive care, as examples.

Once a patient's pain has been assessed, the non-medical prescriber will need to make sense of the pain, contextualise it within the patient's usual health status and make decisions about the most appropriate management, be it pharmacological, non-pharmacological or a combination. The World Health Organization (WHO) developed a pain relief ladder to help with this decision-making in patients with cancer pain (WHO 2010). For non-cancer pain, control of the situation could be less complex. As Wood (2008) comments: 'The diagnosis of acute pain and interventions are usually simple, but this is not usually the case with chronic pain, as the processes of investigation, diagnosis and management are often complex and lengthy.' This raises another issue for non-medical prescribers and their level of knowledge to be able to discern between chronic and acute pain.

Activity box 7.5

www.nursingtimes.net/nursing-practice-clinical-research/assessment-of-pain/1861174.article
   www.nursingtimes.net/nursing-practice-clinical-research/investigations-and-pain-management-guidelines/1861192.article
   These two web links takes you to two articles in the *Nursing Times*, written by Wood (2008).
   They can be used to supplement this section of the fifth vital sign.

The management of pain requires a sound knowledge base of pharmacological interventions: non-opioid, opioid and adjunctive analgesics. Knowledge is required of the various behavioural and physical therapies available as well. Many of the analgesic medications produce side effects, which also need to be managed accordingly, so knowledge of these pharmacological and non-pharmacological interventions will be required. Bickley and Szilagyi (2010) suggest the use of the four As to monitor patient outcomes, which might be useful to consider: **a**nalgesia, **a**ctivities of daily living, **a**dverse effects and **a**berrant drug-related behaviours.

Clinical examination

> ... unless you take the time to build a solid foundation, you will never have confidence in the accuracy and value of what you can uncover with a sharp mind, agile fingers and a few simple tools!'
>
> Goldberg (2009)

Those tools include a systematic approach to any clinical examination, however brief or comprehensive. It is the process by which the practitioner investigates the body of a patient for *signs* of disease whereas the history taking leans towards an exploration of the patient's *symptoms*. Clinical examination is structured by using the 'inspection, palpation, percussion, auscultation' approach.

   Before you embark on your clinical examination, the importance of a thorough history from your patient cannot be emphasised enough, as discussed in Chapter 4. This will guide and inform your clinical examination, enabling safer and more accurate clinical decisions about diagnosis and treatment.

Principles of clinical examination

Before the non-medical prescriber begins any degree of clinical examination, assent should be gained, hands washed, and the patient should be as comfortable as possible, privacy respected, confidentiality assured and the presence of a chaperone offered and provided as appropriate. At all times, explain to the patient what you are doing, or about to do (Gleadle 2003). If any abnormality has been reported, always examine the good side first, e.g. if a patient complains of right ear pain, examine the left ear (cautiously assuming that the left ear is 'normal') first so that you can then compare the normal with the abnormal – effectively you are using the unaffected side as a control for the affected side.

Inspection

This is a thorough and unhurried visualisation of the patient using all the senses: sight, hearing, smell and touch. You should stand back at a slight distance (e.g. the foot of the bed) and take a look at the patient, as a whole. Observe for clues, e.g.: oxygen mask, cigarette packets, vomit bowl, walking stick, obvious signs of pain or discomfort. Correctly position the patient according to the element or part of body to be examined (e.g. lying supine for an abdominal examination or sitting at a 45° angle for a respiratory or cardiovascular exam) and ensure appropriate exposure of the patient. When nearer the patient, observe for obvious abnormalities, such as lumps, unconsciousness, wounds. More careful inspection may reveal less obvious abnormalities such as fine tremor or a vague rash. You can also begin to 'test' the patient, or more accurately your suspicions, by asking the patient to undertake specific movements, e.g. if your history was leading you to suspect a hernia, you could ask the patient to cough while you observe the area of suspicion: a hernia becomes more prominent on coughing (Talley and O'Connor 2009), although it must be noted that this is not the only way to discern a hernia.

Palpation

This is essentially the practitioner touching and feeling the patient. Tactile pressure from palmar fingers or fingerpads is used and the practitioner feels the size and shape, or firmness, or location of something – organs and/or masses. Palpation can also be used to evaluate the presence and extent of any oedema, palpation of pulses and a crude assessment of temperature.

Always begin lightly and gently (this also helps the patient to trust you and to relax), then repeat using firmer pressure. Palpate painful areas last – so ask if the patient has any pain or remember from your history.

Percussion

This is used to find out about changes in the thorax or abdomen, in the main. It is done by tapping on the surface of the skin to determine the underlying structure. The middle finger of the right hand taps on the middle finger of the left hand (a more detailed description of the technique is provided below, on page 242).

Auscultation

This is the technical term for listening to the internal sounds of the body, usually using a stethoscope. Information to be gained includes: location, timing, duration, pitch and intensity of the sounds heard. Again, technique is a large part of success, together with taking the time to listen.

A further note before embarking on the three selected clinical examinations is the concept of red flags. Hopcroft and Forte (2007) explain how most presentations in primary care are self-limiting, or non-urgent. However, they also recognise that for each presentation there are red flags, or significant findings, that should 'set alarm bells ringing'. These aspects of a patient's symptoms (or signs, in clinical examination) are suggestive of significant pathology and therefore should not be missed or not acted upon.

It is a similar case throughout all areas of healthcare but, interestingly, these red flags may differ in urgency according to an area of speciality (or an individual's level of confidence/competence) or provision of immediate intervention, whereby tolerance of red flags could be increased or decreased. Alternatively, other health professions, e.g. physiotherapists, use 'yellow flags' when social aspects of a patient's illness are a cause for concern.

Finally, it is a good idea, to help with the examinations below, to have an appropriate level of anatomy and physiology textbook for reference. Many of the terms used below may be new to many new non-medical practitioners, but it is important that, as your prescribing skills develop, you appreciate that there will be adjunctive skills to be learnt in tandem, not least an increased anatomy, physiology and pathophysiology knowledge. There are also many clinical examination books available, some of which include relevant anatomy that is sometimes easier to understand in the first instance due to its conceptuality. The website http://meded.ucsd.edu/clinicalmed/index.htm is an excellent resource (and is used throughout the next section) to support a detailed explanation of all clinical examinations of all the body systems.

Examination of body systems

Ear, nose and throat examination

Due to the anatomical closeness of these organs, it is safest always to examine all elements despite a patient possibly complaining only of otalgia (earache), as an example. (Table 7.12) This is because pain may be referred or there may also be a concurrent throat infection of which the patient is unaware, yet will still need to be treated. For greater detail, the following website is worthy of a 'few clicks' http://meded.ucsd.edu/clinicalmed/head.htm#Ear.

Safe auroscope technique
The auroscope enables the examination of the external ear, external canal, tympanic membrane (ear drum) and a few inner ear structures.

To begin, have your seat at the same height as the patient (safety) and, after inspecting the external auditory meatus, select an appropriately matched, similarly sized speculum, to attach to the auroscope. Turn on the light source and examine the unaffected ear first.

The position of the auroscope is important to ensure safety for the patient. If there is sudden movement of the patient and an incorrectly held instrument the tympanic membrane could be accidentally perforated. The scope should be held so that your little finger is in constant contact with the patient's cheek, providing a buffer, or stabilisation – so that, if there is sudden movement, your finger position will enable the scope to travel with the patient, preventing further insertion of the speculum.

Once the scope is in position in your hand, gently, but with confidence, place the speculum into the opening of the external canal (do this under direct vision, not through

Table 7.12   Examination of the ear (note no percussion or auscultation)

Inspection	Both ears (pinna) Observes for Battle's sign	Assess for shape, size, symmetry, scars, colour (redness may indicate inflammation: infection or trauma; blueness may indicate cyanosis) or discharge (purulent foul-smelling discharge could indicate a suppurative otitis media or foreign body). A bloody or clear ear discharge is a red flag, suggestive of a skull fracture. Look at pinna for abnormalities such as asymptomatic cancers (basal cell, melanoma, squamous cell) Battle's sign is a red flag (indicating urgent referral) suggesting base-of-skull injury or fracture
Palpates	Both pinna Mastoid bones	For tenderness, swelling or nodules. Tenderness over the tragus may indicate otitis externa (infection of the external auditory canal) Tenderness over the mastoid area could indicate mastoiditis
Inspects	Both auditory canals Tympanic membranes	Demonstrates safe auroscope technique (see below) Inspect the canal for discharge, scaling, excessive redness, lesions, foreign bodies and cerumen (wax) – excessive or impacted cerumen can press against the tympanic membrane and/or occlude the canal causing impaired hearing, tinnitus, vertigo and otalgia The tympanic membrane should be translucent, pearly grey in colour with no perforations. You will need to be able to recognise and name the normal landmarks of the tympanic membrane (see website in text) In cases of otitis media (middle-ear infection) the eardrum becomes red and the light reflex is lost. You may also be able to see a fluid collection behind the drum which may cause it to bulge outwards

the scope). Next, hold the top of the pinna and pull up and backwards, facilitating a straightening of the canal which allows easier passage of the scope and greater visualisation of the tympanic membrane. In children, due to anatomical immaturity, the pinna is pulled down and backwards.

Revert your eyes to look through the viewing window of the scope. Slowly and gently advance the speculum (scope) moving in small stages, employing a smooth movement to reduce the risk of irritation or pain: the external canal is sensitive. Continue until the tympanic membrane is visualised (or the patient becomes intolerant of the procedure). Move to the other side of the body and examine the affected ear, noting that the hand position is reversed. Note your findings, take the necessary action and document appropriately.

Auditory acuity is another element of the examination of the ear and a detailed explanation of these associated tests: crude hearing test and the Rinne and Weber tests can be found via this web link: http://meded.ucsd.edu/clinicalmed/head.htm#Ear. In general, most non-medical prescribers would need to refer patients with any degree of hearing deficit or abnormality unless they were working within the clinical field. However, relevant to non-medical prescribing, there are a number of medications that can affect hearing, including aminoglycosides, aspirin, non-steroidal anti-inflammatory drugs, quinine, furosemide and others (Bickley and Szilagyi 2010).

Tables 7.13-7.15 show how to examine the nose and sinuses, mouth and neck, respectively.

Table 7.13 Examination of the nose and sinuses (note no percussion or auscultation)

Inspection	Both nostrils Inferior turbinates	The nose is inspected for size, shape, symmetry and patency, as well as obvious abnormalities, previous fractures, scars or lesions. In a similar way to the pinna of the ears, the nose is at risk of complications of sun exposure. Nasal flaring is an indication of respiratory distress and is considered a red flag: urgent referral. To visualise inside the nasal vestibule, a light source and speculum can be used. Membranes should be pink and moist without excessive secretions. In viral rhinitis, the mucosa is red and swollen compared with allergic rhinitis which may be pale, bluish or red. Septal deviations can be assessed, as can polyps, perforations or inflammation, if present. If there are excessive or abnormal secretions they need to be examined in terms of clear/purulent/offensive odour/blood. A malignancy must be suspected if an older person presents with a blood-stained discharge, with further suspicion if unilateral
Palpates	Frontal and maxillary sinuses	The paranasal sinuses are air-filled cavities within the skull bones and it is just the frontal and maxillary sinuses that are accessible for clinical examination. If tenderness is suspected or infection, it is best to palpate for confirmation. To do this you gently press up on the frontal sinuses from just under the orbital ridge, or under the eyebrows (ensuring that no pressure is put on the eyes). The maxillary sinuses are palpated by pressing up on the maxilla, or cheek bone. Acute sinusitis is characterised by local tenderness, together with pain, fever and nasal discharge

Table 7.14 Examination of the mouth (note inspection only)

Inspection	Mouth and pharynx	Use a pen torch and tongue depressor to inspect mouth and pharynx, commenting on tonsils, tongue, mucosa and dentition. If the patient has dentures, ask them to be removed for a thorough inspection
		Look at the *lips* for colour and moisture while observing for abnormalities such as cracking (vitamin deficiency, dehydration), lumps, ulcers or sores (herpes simplex). Swollen lips may be due to infection or possibly angiodema (a red flag). A bluish tinge to the oral mucosa can indicate a compromised respiratory and/or cardiovascular system. While inspecting the *mouth*, it is important to note colour, ulcers, white patches or nodules, which can be signs of disease in isolation, or systemic signs of other disease processes, e.g. mouth ulcers may be indicative of ulcerative colitis. Make a note of any halitosis or fetor – many odours can be specific, e.g. the fruity breath of ketoacidosis; however, halitosis may also be a consequence of diseases of the oral cavity, nasal passages, sinuses or respiratory tract, or of an oesophageal origin. The mouth contains gums, teeth, a hard palate and the tongue, which all need to be inspected and any abnormalities accounted for or investigated. Beyond the oral cavity, the soft palate, uvula, tonsils and pharynx itself can be found. You may need to use a tongue depressor to fully visualise the necessary structures. To test the integrity of the tenth cranial nerve, you need to assess the rising and falling of the soft palate – if there is an abnormality, the uvula will deviate to the opposite side of the lesion
		Please note: you should never examine the pharynx if you suspect epiglottitis because this may worsen the condition – it is a red flag situation

Examination of the respiratory system

The following web link is a good point of reference to progress to after this section. It supplements this concise explanation of the respiratory examination with detailed notes, anatomy and other resources http://meded.ucsd.edu/clinicalmed/lung.htm.

This examination follows the systematic approach of inspection, palpation, percussion and auscultation, with no exceptions (unlike ENT which has no percussion or auscultation and in an abdominal examination, auscultation is performed after inspection, and before percussion and palpation).

Ideally the patient needs to be lying at a 45° angle and have the ability to sit forward for examination of the posterior chest. However, in acute situations, patients with respiratory disease may not be able to sit back; they often adopt a 'tripod' position of sitting

Table 7.15 Examination of the neck, including lymph glands and thyroid gland

Inspection	The neck	Note symmetry, masses and scars. Parotid and submandibular glands are more easily observed if enlarged. Also within this area lie the great vessels, trachea and thyroid gland, in terms of significant structures
		The trachea can be directly visualised for assessment of possibly deviation. A central trachea (normal) would have equal space between the lateral edge of the trachea and the medial edge of the sternomastoid muscle
		A goitre is an enlarged thyroid gland and can be a consequence of either hyper- or hypothyroidism. The thyroid should rise and fall in correlation with swallowing (offer a drink of water)
Palpation	Lymph nodes	Take a look at the website link http://meded.ucsd.edu/clinicalmed/head.htm#Lymph and familiarise yourself with the anatomical location of the lymph glands (to help with correct palpation). To palpate, you need to use the pads of all four fingertips and, with gentle pressure, using a circular motion, palpate all 10 groups of lymph nodes (submental, submandibular, tonsillar, preauricular, postauricular, occipital, posterior cervical chain, anterior cervical chain, deep cervical chain, although difficult to feel due to the overlying sternomastoid muscle, and supraclavicular). Lymph nodes are not usually palpable in a healthy person. Note the size and location of palpable nodes and whether they are soft/hard, tender/non-tender, mobile/fixed. During times of infection they can enlarge and are usually tender. If lymph nodes are enlarged secondary to a malignancy, the glands tend to be painless and hard or fixed. Any unexplained enlarged or tender nodes require re-examination of drainage regions and re-examination of other lymph nodes to distinguish between regional or generalised lymphadenopathy (medical term for enlarged lymph nodes)

forward and leaning on a table for support. If mechanically ventilated, the patient is likely to be supine (lying flat with face upwards). As your skills and knowledge develop, you will become able to deal with these situations and make clinical decisions, taking the patient's position into account. The guidance in Tables 7.16-7.19 is documented in a systematic order, but, in clinical practice, you will find it easier to inspect, palpate, percuss and auscultate the anterior chest first and then repeat the sequence for the posterior chest, the reason being that it is more convenient for the patient, especially if he or she has respiratory disease which can be fatiguing, without having to be sitting forwards and backwards three or four times.

Table 7.16 Examination of the respiratory system

| Inspection | General appearance
Hands
Face
Anterior chest wall
Posterior chest wall | Start the exam with monitoring of vital signs. Look around the patient for clues: sputum pot, oxygen mask, inhalers/nebuliser, evidence of smoking. Look at the patient for signs of distress (dyspnoea, agitation) or discomfort. Comment on general appearance: pallor, flushing, cyanosis and effort of breathing, including pattern, rate and length of expiration (prolonged in obstructive disease), and audible sounds, e.g. wheeze
There are a number of signs present on the hands that can indicate respiratory abnormalities: clubbing, cyanosis (check capillary refill time), anaemia, tremor, tar-stained fingers (beware of jumping to conclusions because the degree of staining does not necessarily correlate to the number of cigarettes being smoked)
For signs of cyanosis, pursed lips characteristic of obstructive pulmonary disease. Is there any facial swelling, suggestive of superior vena cava obstruction: a lung malignancy? Inspect the neck: are the accessory muscles in use, suggesting abnormality: is the trachea central?
Note the shape of the chest, which tends to alter with age. The width of the chest wall is larger than the depth with a ratio of 2:1 in a healthy person. Look for any deformities (kyphosis, scoliosis as examples), retraction of the intercostal spaces during inspiration (a red flag). The chest wall should rise and fall equally when breathing; there should be no lag or impaired movement. Note any scars or lesions, areas of tenderness |
| Palpation | Chest expansion
Lymph nodes
Anterior and posterior chest | The aim of chest expansion is to compare the two sides, noting any reduction in expansion on one side. Place your hands on the chest wall, at the level of the lower ribs, with fingers gripping the lateral aspect and the thumbs meeting midline. Then ask the patient to take a deep breath in while you gauge the movement of your thumbs. Normally they should be displaced laterally, about 2-3 cm, equally on both sides (accounting for the differences between sizes of patients). If one thumb moves less than another, this indicates reduced expansion on that side, suggestive of active disease (e.g. pneumonia, pleural effusion, pneumothorax). Bilateral expansion can be reduced in severe airflow limitation |

(Continued)

Table 7.16   (Continued)

		During a respiratory examination it is essential to palpate associated lymph nodes, employing the same technique as described in the ENT examination. Refer to an anatomy text for the location of the nodes
		Ask if there are any painful areas on the chest, to guide your approach and firmness of palpation. Identifying any underlying abnormalities, such as bruising over a fractured rib, tenderness over inflamed pleura, subcutaneous cysts, surgical emphysema
Percussion	Anterior chest wall Posterior chest wall	This is a skill that relies on examiner technique and it is worth investing time to master it. Place your left hand on the patient's chest wall with your middle finger aligned in an intercostal space. Then hyperflex the remaining fingers and thumb to ensure that as little of your hand is actually making contact with the patient's skin (this helps to elicit an improved note by reducing impedance) except for the last joint line of your finger. When in position, use the middle finger of your right hand, the tip of (not the pad of the finger – you will need short fingernails), to strike the dorsum of the middle finger over the last interphalangeal joint. This striking motion needs to occur at right angles between the left middle finger and right striking finger. While making the striking motion, listen to the noise being made (when proficient, you will be able to feel the note too). Always percuss the chest wall using a 'ladder technique' (Bickley and Szilagyi 2010, p. 301) which enables a smooth movement down the chest wall while always comparing sides (do not do one side of the chest wall first and then cross the midline to percuss the other side) to help confirm unilateral abnormalities. Percuss from the apices down to the bases of the lung fields (appreciating that the posterior lung surface is relatively low), including the lateral/axillary aspects (note lung anatomy to rationalise this). When percussing the posterior chest ask the patient to bring the arms across the chest wall to help displace the scapula, increasing the available space for percussion. Note, percussion only penetrates about 5–7 cm into the chest, so cannot help detect deep-seated lesions. See Table 7.17 for possible percussion notes to denote whether the underlying tissues is air filled, solid or fluid filled

Table 7.16   (*Continued*)

Auscultation	Anterior chest wall Posterior chest wall	Auscultation requires the use of the stethoscope and predominately it is the diaphragm that is used to listen for breath sounds and any adventitious sounds (added sounds). The bell can be used to auscultate the apices of the lungs: because of its smaller diameter and the surface anatomy overlying the apices it is easier The systematic approach to auscultation is the same as percussion, using a ladder technique to be able to compare sides and placement of the stethoscope firmly in the intercostal space. When in position with the stethoscope, ask the patient to breathe in and out through an open mouth (reduces added sounds from turbulence of air travelling through the noisy nasal passages). Listen for at least one full cycle of inspiration and expiration in each location of the lungs. Adventitious breath sounds are superimposed on breath sounds and you need to listen to both the nature and the timing of the breath sounds. Refer to Table 7.18 and 7.19 for notes on normal breath sounds and adventitious sounds, respectively

Table 7.17   Percussion notes with related pathology

Percussion note	Relative intensity	Relative pitch	Relative duration	Example of location	Pathological examples
Flat (stony dull)	Soft	High	Short	Thigh	Large pleural effusion
Dull	Medium	Medium	Medium	Liver	Lobar pneumonia
Resonance	Loud	Low	Long	Normal lung	Simple chronic bronchitis
Hyperresonance	Very loud	Lower	Longer	None if normal	Emphysema, pneumothorax
Tympanic	Loud	High		Gastric Air Puffed out cheek	Large pneumothorax

Bickley and Szilagyi (2010, p. 300).

Table 7.18 Characteristics of breath sounds

Breath sound	Duration of sounds	Intensity of expiratory sound	Pitch of expiratory sound	Locations where heard normally
Vesicular	Inspiration (I) > expiration (E)	Soft	Relatively low	Over most of both lungs
Bronchovesicular	I = E	Intermediate	Intermediate	First and second intercostal anterior + intrascapular
Bronchial	I < E	Loud	Relatively high	Over manubrium, if at all
Tracheal	I = E	Very loud	Relatively high	Over trachea in the neck

Bickley and Szilagyi (2010, p. 303).

Table 7.19 Adventitious breath sounds

Adventitious sound	Sound	Causes
Crackles Result from a series of tiny explosions when small airways, deflated during expiration, pop open during inspiration	Intermittent non-musical sounds *Fine crackles* – soft, high pitched and brief *Coarse crackles* – louder, lower in pitch, not as brief. Occur from fluid in large bronchi *Late inspiratory crackles* – may begin in first half of inspiration but must continue into late inspiration. Usually fine crackles. Appear first at the base of the lung but as the disease worsens they spread upwards *Early inspiratory crackles* – appear soon after start of inspiration and do not continue into late inspiration. Coarse and usually few in number	Lungs (pneumonia, fibrosis, early CCF) or of airways (bronchitis, bronchiectasis) Early CCF, fibrosis, pneumonia Bronchitis, bronchiectasis
Wheezes Suggest narrowed airways	High pitched, have a hissing or shrill quality. Commonly expiratory. High pitched suggests disease of small airways	Asthma, COPD, bronchitis, CCF, partial obstruction of bronchus by tumour or foreign body
Rhonchi Suggest secretions in large airways	Low pitched and have a snoring quality	Bronchitis
Stridor	A wheeze that is predominantly inspiratory. Often louder in the neck than the chest wall	Partial obstruction of larynx or trachea
Pleural rub	Creaking sound – walking in snow. Both inspiratory and expiratory	Pleural inflammation – pneumonia, pulmonary embolism

CCF, congestive cardiac failure; COPD, chronic obstructive pulmonary disease.
Bickley and Szilagyi (2010, p. 319).

Abdominal examination (Tables 2.20 and 2.21)

The following web link is a good point of reference to progress to after this section. It supplements this concise explanation of the abdominal examination with detailed notes, anatomy and other resources: http://meded.ucsd.edu/clinicalmed/abdomen.htm.

As discussed in Chapter 4 and above, the patient's history remains essential and ideally is obtained before examination, or at least simultaneously, where possible.

This examination follows the systematic approach of inspection, auscultation, percussion and palpation to ensure that the abdominal contents remain undisturbed before palpation, helping to reduce the risk of false interpretations. However, the four principles are still maintained.

Ideally the patient needs to be lying supine (lying flat with face upwards) with the arms resting at the side. A pillow under the patient's knees can be a comfort and also helps to relax the abdominal wall, enabling an easier and more informative examination. Encourage the patient to empty the bladder before commencing. The abdomen should be exposed from midchest to the symphysis pubis, when you are performing the exam, so attention to the warmth of the room and your hands would always be appreciated. Always be looking at the patient's face for signs of undisclosed pain and, in relation to pain, begin the exam from the point furthest from the pain.

Activity box 7.6

There are many resources with information about abdominal pain, including many of those in the reference list of this chapter. Using either of the categorisations below, research the physiology of abdominal pain that best suits your own clinical practice. Having a reference for abdominal pain and its characteristics is very useful for diagnostic purposes and therefore will guide treatment too.

Mechanism of pain	Anatomical location
Visceral	Upper right quadrant
Parietal or somatic	Upper left quadrant
Referred	Epigastric area
	Umbilical area
	Lower right quadrant
	Lower left quadrant

The abdominal system has a number of specific tests that can be conducted depending on your suspicions, or differential diagnoses, and the need to confirm or refute specific pathology. Examples include: assessing for guarding, rebound tenderness, e.g. at McBurney's area, percussing and palpating for hepatomegaly and/or splenomegaly. There may be a need to ballot the kidneys or perform a direct rectal examination or bimanual vaginal examination. Any of these specific and relatively specialist examination procedures can be found on the website above and the references for further

Table 7.20 Examination of the abdominal/gastrointestinal system

Inspection (and smell)	General appearance Hands Face Abdomen (Inspect tangentially)	Start the exam with monitoring of vital signs. Take note of the patient's general condition: obese, anorexic, dehydrated. Note obvious abnormalities: jaundice (liver disease); pallor (anaemia); flushing (infection, inflammation or pain); abdominal masses (hernias, pregnancy, tumour, ascites, as examples). Environmental clues in relation to this system could be a nearby vomit bowl, medication list with aperients or other GI-related treatment Inspect for evidence of: palmer erythema, a redness to the palmar aspect of the hand that can be a normal variant; however, it is also related to high output states, e.g. pregnancy, and it can be associated with liver disease; finger clubbing (poorly understood but an abnormal sign associated with malignancy and respiratory disorders particularly) in ulcerative colitis or Crohn's disease; asterixis is the medical term for a liver flap and is a coarse tremor seen in hepatic failure Look for signs of jaundice, a yellowness to the sclera of the eyes (although, in black people, their sclera tend to have a yellow tinge as normal, so be careful in your interpretations). Inspect the conjunctiva for paleness indicative of anaemia and to do this you need to gently lower the lower eyelid and look at the conjunctiva, where if the patient is anaemic the usual red anterior third will be pale, losing a demarcation line. Some GI diseases have malodours emanating from the patient's mouth, e.g. hepatic foetor or gingivitis' a faecal smell can occur with prolonged vomiting especially when associated with intestinal obstruction. Inspect the mouth noting dentition, ulcers, tongue condition Observe the exposed abdomen for: scars, stria, hernias, asymmetry, spider naevi, linea nigra, ascites, pulsations, peristalsis

(Continued)

Table 7.20 (*Continued*)

Auscultation	Bowel sounds Bruits: aorta, iliac, renal, femoral arteries Friction rub	Place your stethoscope gently on the abdomen and listen for sounds. noting frequency and character. The bowels are generalised and easily transmit across the abdomen, so listening in one area is sufficient. Normal bowel sounds are heard between 5 and 34 a minute and sound like 'clicks and gurgles'. 'Borborygmi' is the term given to prolonged gurgles similar to the sound of a stomach growling. An ileus presents with absent bowel sounds whereas they are enhanced and tinkling in bowel obstruction (Longmore et al 2004) Auscultate for bruits that can be abnormal findings indicative of turbulent blood flow through an artery and the sound it makes is like a 'whooshing' noise. A pathological bruit can be associated with either partial arterial occlusion or arterial insufficiency Is a high-pitched sound heard over the liver or spleen and can indicate inflammation of the peritoneal surface of the organ, from tumour, infection or infarction, for example
Percussion	The four quadrants or nine areas of the abdomen (see Table 7.21)	Using the same technique as described within the respiratory examination, and for the same purpose (to help decide on air-, fluid- or solid-filled areas). Again underlying anatomical knowledge is essential to appreciate the organs and structures over which you are percussing. Tympanic notes usually predominate because of the amount of gas within the bowel. However, there should be intermittent areas of dullness over the liver, faeces within the bowel or fluid. Abnormalities or unexpected notes are heard in cases of pregnancy, tumour, distended bladder or hepatomegaly

Table 7.20   (*Continued*)

Palpation	Light palpation Deep palpation	Light palpation is to discern any abnormalities within the surface structures of the skin. To palpate the abdomen, ensure that hands are warm and gently lay your left palm of hand on the abdomen, furthest away from any pain, if reported. Then gently depress your finger into the abdomen to about a depth of 1 cm. Progress throughout the four areas of the abdomen using gentle circular movements trying to keep your hands in constant contact with the patient, to help reassure and provide comfort. Once you become confident you will be able to do this without looking at the patient's abdomen and can focus on the face for signs of pain or discomfort. The aim of palpation is to identify any areas of tenderness (varying degrees of pain from mild discomfort through to excruciating pain of peritonitis), muscle resistance and any superficial masses. If muscle resistance is present, try to distinguish between voluntary (patient anxiety or fear) and involuntary (peritoneal inflammation) guarding (can herald life-threatening complications) Repeat the process of palpation but use two hands, one on top of the other, to penetrate to the deep structures and organs of the abdominal cavity, or perhaps if the patient is obese. Also, repeat only if necessary (significant findings on light palpation do not require deep palpation for confirmation). If an abnormality is suspected, note its site, size, border, consistency, tenderness, mobility, movement with respiration, percussion note, pulsatility, overlying temperature and bruit (Cox and Roper 2005, p. 162)

Table 7.21 Anatomical mapping areas of the abdomen

Four quadrants of the abdomen	Nine areas of the abdomen
Right upper quadrant	Left and right hypochondriums
Right lower quadrant	Epigastric
Left upper quadrant	Left and right lumbar
Left lower quadrant	Umbilical
	Left and right iliac fossa
	Suprapubic/hypogastric

Provided that you are able to visualise the underlying structures and organs, it does not matter which mapping method you use (Goldberg 2009).

information. These tests would also need to be closely supervised while the non-medical prescriber is a novice because most are used when significant pathology is suspected so risks are high – the designated medical practitioner (DMP) should be the first place of contact for a student.

Neurological examination (Table 7.22)

The neurological examination is a complex examination and is multifaceted. It includes an assessment of a patient's mental status, *cranial nerves*, motor system, sensory system, coordination, gait and *reflexes* (Bickley and Szilagyi 2010, p. 672). Knowledge, especially anatomical and physiological, and experience are fundamental. For the purpose of this chapter, there is coverage of the cranial nerves and the use of the tendon hammer as stated in the *Outline Curriculum for Training Programmes to Prepare Pharmacist Prescribers* (RPSGB 2006). Once again, the following link is invaluable: http://meded.ucsd.edu/clinicalmed/neuro2.htm. In addition, you will find that your DMP is a very useful resource to help you acquire the necessary skills to perform the test or, alternatively, he or she will be able to guide you towards a colleague if he or she feels that would be more suitable.

Cranial nerves

To remember their names and some key information can be very useful when attempting to remember all that is needed and the use of Table 7.23 with the mnemonic may help.

Reflexes

The testing of deep tendon reflexes is useful to test both sensory and motor pathways and function. Their integrity can assure the examiner on many different levels (see Activity box 7.7). This is a skill that is worthy of practice (and necessary) because first it is not easy to elicit all necessary reflexes and second when you do there is a strong sense of achievement, especially if they are normal.

Table 7.22 Cranial nerve information

On	Old	Olympus'	Towering	Top	A	Finn	And	German	Viewed	Some	Hops
Olfactory	Optic	Oculomotor	Trochlear	Trigeminal	Abducens	Facial	Acoustic	Glossopharyngeal	Vagus	Accessory	Hypoglossal
I	II	III	IV	V	VI	VII	VII	IX	X	XI	XII
Some	Say	Marry	Money	But	My	Brother	Says	Bad	Business	Marrying	Money
Sensory	Sensory	Motor	Motor	Both	Motor	Both	Sensory	Both	Both	Motor	Motor

Table 7.23 Cranial nerve checklist

No.	Name	Sensory ± motor	Function and information Test
I	Olfactory	Sensory	Responsible for the sense of smell Can be lost due to trauma, infection, ageing. Smell important component of taste 1. Identify familiar odour – coffee, orange
II	Optic	Sensory	Various tests possible, usually dependent on integrity of optic nerve(s). 1. Inspection of pupils 2. Ophthalmoscopy 3. Test visual acuity 4. Visual fields by confrontation 5. Pupillary reactions reflexes
III	Oculomotor	Motor	1. Inspection 2. Extraocular muscle movement – cardinal directions of gaze
IV	Trochlear	Motor	1. Extraocular muscle movement
V	Trigeminal: optic maxillary mandibular	Both	Sensory divisions and motor to muscles of mastication 1. Touch to three divisions 2. Corneal reflex 3. Test temporal and masseter muscle
VI	Abducens	Motor	1. Extraocular muscle movement
VII	Facial	Both	Muscles of facial expression, stapedius muscle, taste to anterior two-thirds of tongue, parasympathetic nerve to lacrimal gland Lower motor neuron lesions affect all muscles on that side; unilateral upper motor neuron lesions spare the forehead. 1. Show teeth 2. Purse lips and then resist them being opened 3. Blow out cheeks and stop them being pushed in 4. Close eyes tightly and resist them being opened 5. Open eyes as wide as possible
VIII	Acoustic	Sensory	Hearing and balance 1. Screen hearing 2. Weber and Rinne test 3. Gait

Table 7.23   (Continued)

No.	Name	Sensory ± motor	Function and information Test
IX	Glossopharyngeal	Both	Sensory to posterior third of tongue, pharynx and middle ear Motor to stylopharyngeus Autonomic to parotid salivary gland 1. Gag reflex
X	Vagus	Both	Sensory to tympanic membrane, external auditory canal, external ear. Motor to muscles of palate, pharynx and larynx Autonomic to afferents from carotid baroreceptors, Parasympathetic supply to and from thorax and abdomen 1. Inspect uvula and ask patient to say 'ahh' 2. Note voice quality and note swallowing
XI	Accessory	Motor	Each cerebral hemisphere supplies ipsilateral sternomastoid muscle and contralateral trapezius – so a lesion on one side can give rise to signs on both sides 1. Sternomastoid 2. Trapezius
XII	Hypoglossal	Motor	Motor to the intrinsic muscles of the tongue 1. Open mouth 2. Pull out tongue 3. Waggle tongue 4. To test power – patient resists examiner, pushing tongue away from wall of cheek 5. Listen to articulation

Patient instructions and cooperation are paramount so be clear and confident in your articulations. Demonstration is good and also reassurance: you need the patient to relax and this may mean that you take the weight of the patient's arm or leg. Generally patients want to help the examiner and take their own weight.

All you need is a reflex hammer and sound anatomical knowledge. Once you have your patient in the correct position (Table 7.24) and they have the relevant limb relaxed, hold the hammer loosely between your thumb and index finger, allowing a free swinging motion necessary to knock the tendon. Then strike the slightly taut tendon briskly and firmly (but without causing pain). It needs to be purposeful and quick, not hesitating. Note the speed, force and amplitude of the reflex response (Bickley and Szilagyi 2010,

p. 696) and grade using Table 7.25. Compare sides to help with your judgement/ interpretation, based on the same principles as for the respiratory system.

If it appears that the patient's reflexes are diminished or absent, you can use *reinforcement*, a technique to help increase reflex activity. When testing arm reflexes, you could ask the patient to clench their teeth or if testing leg reflexes, ask the patient to lock fingers and pull against each hand. Instruct the patient to clench or pull just before you strike the tendon. This action will detract the patient from your action of striking their tendon, thus a reflex may be easier to elicit.

Activity box 7.7

Using this web link – http://meded.ucsd.edu/clinicalmed/neuro3.htm – locate information about reflexes. Use the information and links within the web pages to help you understand the physiology of a reflex. This understanding will in turn help with your interpretation and decision-making.

Numeracy skills

Numeracy skills are essential. Once a diagnosis (or review) has been made (based on your therapeutic communication, ability to elicit a patient's story and clinical examination skills) a treatment plan will need to be devised, using your clinical decision-making skills further. Decisions will remain about specific pharmacological intervention, or not, depending on your decision-making. In those situations where the decision is to prescribe, there will be a need for some degree of mathematical calculation.

Numeracy is embedded within the V100, V150 and V300 training programmes, as stipulated by the NMC (2006) and supported by the HPC and RPSGB. This is supported by a nationwide website the pages of which have links to numeracy supervision: www.nmplearningnw.org/precourses/Drug_Calculation.html.

They reassure the non-medical prescriber, or prospective non-medical prescriber, by stating that complex equations or calculus will not be expected. However, they do highlight that confidence will be required for 'SI unit conversion, basic calculation skills for drug dosage and pack size, along with consideration of cost', as detailed in the web site directly above.

To emphasise this point, in the north-west region at least, prospective students are required to undertake a pre-course numeracy exam and, within the training programme, there is also a numeracy examination. The important message to take from this is not fear or trepidation about existing skills, but an appreciation that prescribing depends on safe and correct drug calculations: there is no room for error.

Every prescription written will have a degree of mathematical calculation attached to it and in order to do this correctly a prescriber needs to have in-depth knowledge of their personal formulary (discussed in Chapter 5) in order to have a reasonable

Table 7.24 Deep tendon reflexes

Name of reflex	Nerve root	Position of patient	Muscle innervated	Effect expected
Brachioradialis/supinator	C5 and C6	Rest the hand on the patient's lap with forearm slightly pronated (like holding a drink can). Strike the radius about 4–5 cm above the wrist	Brachioradialis	Supination and flexion lower arm
Triceps	C6 and C7	Flex the arm at the elbow with palm facing towards the body and pull it across the chest. Strike the tendon just above the elbow (outer aspect)	Triceps contracts	Elbow/arm extension
Biceps	C5 and C6	Arm flexed at the elbow with palm down and place your thumb over the tendon and then strike your thumb	Biceps contract	Elbow/arm flexion
Patella/knee	L3 and L4	This is easiest if the patient is able to sit with the knee flexed, with free movement (not with feet resting floor). Briskly tap the tendon just below the patella	Quadriceps	Lower leg extends
Posterior tibialis/Achilles	L5 and S1	Probably easier if the patient is lying on the bed. Flex one leg over the other leg's shin and dorsiflex the foot at the ankle joint and strike the Achilles tendon	Hamstrings/calf muscle	Plantar flexion of the foot
Plantar reflex	L5 and S1	With the foot exposed, stroke the lateral aspect of the sole of the foot from the heel to the ball of the foot, continuing across towards the base of the great toe	Great toe extensor (extensor hallucis longus) tendon contract	In normal adult, great toe plantar flexion

From Bickley and Szilagyi (2010, p. 697).

Table 7.25 Grading of reflexes

Grade	Description
0 or −	No response or absent
1+ or ±	Present with reinforcement, somewhat diminished
2+ or +	Normal, average
3+ or ++	Brisk but normal, brisker than average
4+ or +++	Abnormally brisk (hyperreflex), with clonus (rhythmic oscillations between flexion and extension)

Cox and Roper (2005, p. 211), Bickley and Szilagyi (2010, p. 696).

Table 7.26 The basic arithmetic skills required of non-medical prescribers

Adding
Subtracting
Multiplying
Dividing
Simplifying fractions
Changing decimals to fractions and vice versa
Using proportions
Using percentages

recollection of the range of strengths, forms and routes of the most frequently pre-scribed medication. All prescribers will have an up-to-date *British National Formulary* (BNF) to back up any clinical decisions and prescriptions that need to be written. The front of the BNF also provides guidance on the written prescription, reminding the prescriber to include dose, route of administration, strength of drug, frequency of administration and total quantity required. If the dose of the drug that has been decided on depends on body weight or surface area, the patient's weight and height should also be included on the prescriptions. All these elements demand a confident numeracy aptitude to safely and accurately write the full prescription. Also, as a non-medical prescriber, the professional body to which registration is made require clear lines of accountability in the actions we make (GPhC 2010, HPC 2008, NMC 2008).

These calculations referred to require an understanding of essential arithmetic (Table 7.26) and knowledge of the metric system (Table 7.27).

The book website will be your next port of call because it offers practical examples to help confirm your current numeracy status. The example calculations can either reassure you that you are competent, provided that you answer them correctly, or offer practice examples through which you can develop your skills and become more competent.

Once it is understood that our professional responsibilities dictate the need for com-petent numeracy skills, there are two other aspects that need to be considered. Our

Table 7.27 The metric system

Weight (mass)	Volume	Length

1 kilogram = 1000 grams
1 gram = 1000 milligrams
 	
1 milligram = 1000
  micrograms
1 microgram = 1000
  nanograms
	1 litre = 1000 millilitres
	1 millilitre = 1000
	  microlitres
		1 metre = 1000 millimetres
		1 centimetre = 10
		  millimetres

patient safety is paramount and our professional credibility needs to be upheld. Warburton (2010) reminds the reader that serious incidents are invoked as a result of drug errors in terms of wrong doses. This statement is compounded by the fact that much of the research around this issue suggests that medication errors are largely preventable. Poor numeracy skills are responsible for a proportion of drug errors. This is a particular issue within paediatrics where the NPSA (2009) have audited that almost half of reported medication errors are related to the wrong strength or dose of medicine. Interestingly, in Tudor times, the Swiss physician, Paracelsus (1567) noted that:

> All substances are poisons; there is none which is not a poison. The right dose differentiates a poison from a remedy.

Clearly medication 'errors' are not a new concept, but that is not to say that our professional integrity and patient advocacy duty compel numeracy skills to be a paramount competency of a non-medical prescriber.

Conclusion

This chapter has provided insight into measuring vital signs, the theoretical and systematic approach to clinical examination, and a discussion in relation to the rationale for competency in numeracy for a non-medical prescriber.

Vital signs are elements of clinical examination that all non-medical prescribers need to be skilled at in order to assess their patients and make safe clinical decisions as a consequence. They are also fundamental to the monitoring responsibilities that prescribers have in response to the prescriptions written. Vital signs are also used to assist decisions about the cessation of treatment.

Some practitioners will require additional clinical examination skills and, although it is not the intention of this chapter to equip practitioners with all the skills necessary, it was intended for an introductory illustration of the principles of clinical examination. This was followed by a more detailed (though not definitive) explanation of certain body system examinations: ENT, respiratory, abdominal/gastrointestinal, cranial nerves and deep tendon reflexes. This section used a key website to provide further support, along with the recognition of the DMP for practical advice and support within the clinical field. It is of great value that Dr C Goldberg, the author of the website, has allowed his website to be used in this way.

The final section of the chapter discussed the essential nature of numeracy and the rationale for all healthcare practitioners, not least non-medical prescribers, to be confidently competent in order to ultimately safeguard our patients against the potential harm of medications: to prescribe in appropriate doses to ensure a therapeutic effect with the least toxic side effects. There is also the issue of professional integrity and professional accountability, both requiring protection via competence.

Key themes: conclusions and considerations

Public health	Clinical skills are fundamental to safe prescribing practice, whether they aid decisions about diagnosis or support accurate prescription writing. From a public health perspective, it is important that the non-medical prescriber is able to identify the skills and tools needed to enable him or her to address relevant public health issues
	Consider the specific public health targets that you are most likely to encounter. Identify the clinical skills and tools required to address these targets. Consider the actions necessary to address any limitations identified
Social and cultural issues	Sensitivity to social and cultural differences is essential in undertaking clinical skills
	Consider the clinical skills you use to support your prescribing practice and identify any social and cultural issues that could impact on their efficacy
Prescribing principles	Prescribing principle 1: 'examine the holistic needs of the patient' (NPC 1999) is fundamental in safe and effective prescribing, as too is prescribing principle 3: 'consider the choice of product'
	Consider how these two principles interact, e.g. how a physical disability or illness can impact on the choice of product and what strategies you have within your clinical practice to help in fulfilling these aspects of prescribing

References

Abrahams PH, Marks SC Jr, Hutchings RT (2003) *McMinn's Colour Atlas of Human Anatomy*. Edinburgh: Mosby.

Bickley L, Szilagyi PR (2010) *Bates' Guide to Physical Examination and History Taking*, 10th edn. Philadelphia: Lippincott, Williams & Wilkins.

British Pain Society (2008) Pain scales in multiple languages (online). Available at: www.britishpainsociety.org/pub_pain_scales.htm (accessed June 2010).

British Thoracic Society (BTS) (2009) *British Guideline on the Management of Asthma: A national clinical guideline*, London: BTS.

Cohen BJ (2009) *Memmler's The Human Body in Health and Disease*, 11th edn. Philadelphia: Lippincott, Williams & Wilkins.

Courtenay M, Gordon J (2009) A survey of therapy areas in which nurses prescribe and CPD needs. *Nurse Prescrib* **7**: 255–62.

Cox NLT, Roper TA (2005) *Clinical Skills*. Oxford: Oxford University Press.

General Pharmaceutical Council (GPhC) (2010) *Standards of Conduct, Ethics and Performance*. London. GPhC.

Gleadle J (2003) *History and Examination at a Glance*. Oxford: Blackwell Science.

Goldberg C (2009) *A Practical Guide to Clinical Medicine: Introduction* (online). Available at: http://meded.ucsd.edu/clinicalmed (accessed June 2010).

Greaves I, Porter K, Hodgetts T, Woollard M (2006) *Emergency Care: A textbook for paramedics*. Edinburgh: Saunders.

Health Professions Council (HPC) (2008) *Standards of Conduct, Performance and Ethics*, London: HPC.

Hopcroft K, Forte V (2007) *Symptom Sorter*, 3rd edn. Oxon: Radcliffe Medical Press Ltd.

Kumar P, Clark M, eds (2004) *Clinical Medicine*, 5th edn. London: Saunders.

Longmore M, Wilkinson IB, Rajagopalan S (2004) *Oxford Handbook of Clinical Medicine*, 6th edn. Oxford: Oxford University Press.

Mahadevan SV, Garmel GM (2005) *An Introduction to Clinical Emergency Medicine: Guide for practitioners in the emergency department*. Cambridge: Cambridge University Press.

Morton PG (1993) *Health Assessment in Nursing*, 2nd edn. Philadelphia: FA Davis.

National Institute for Health and Clinical Excellence (NICE) (2003) *Chronic Heart Failure: Management of chronic heart failure in adults in primary and secondary care*. London: NICE.

National Prescribing Centre (1999) Signposts for Prescribing Nurses – General Principles of Good Prescribing, *Prescribing Nurse Bulletin*, Vol. 1, No. 1.

National Prescribing Centre (2006) Sore throat. *MeReC Bull* **17**(3).

National Prescribing Safety Agency (NPSA) (2009) *Safety in Doses: Improving the use of medicines in the NHS*. London: NPSA.

Nursing and Midwifery Council (NMC) (2006) *Standards of Proficiency for Nurse and Midwife Prescribers*, London: NMC.

Nursing and Midwifery Council (2007) *Essential Skills Clusters (ESCs) for Pre-registration Nursing Programmes*, Annexe 2 to NMC Circular 07/2007.

Nursing and Midwifery Council (2008) *The Code: Standards of Conduct, Performance and Ethics for Nurses and Midwives*. London: NMC.

O'Brien E, Asmar R, Beilin L (2003) European Society of Hypertension recommendations for conventional, ambulatory and home blood pressure measurement. *J Hypertens* **21**: 821–48.

Royal College of Nursing (RCN) (2007) *Standards for Assessing, Measuring and Monitoring Vital Signs in Infants, Children and Young People*. London: RCN.

Royal Pharmaceutical Society of Great Britain (RPSGB) (2006) *Outline Curriculum for Training Programmes to Prepare Pharmacist Prescribers*, London: RPSGB.

Talley NJ, O'Connor S (2009) *Clinical Examination: A Systematic Guide to Physical Diagnosis* (6th edn) New South Wales: Churchill Livingstone.

Von der Besucht P (1567) All substances are poisons. In: Trautmann N (2005) *The Dose Makes the Poison – Or Does It?* (online). Available at: www.actionbioscience.org/environment/trautmann.html (accessed June 2010).

Warburton P (2010) Poor numeracy skills must be tackled to cut medication errors. *Nurs Times* 9 March.

Wong DL, Hockenberry-Eaton, M, Wilson, D, Winkelstein ML, Schwartz P (2001) *Wong's Essentials of Paediatric Nursing*, 6th edn. St Louis: Mosby Inc.

Wood S (2008) Investigations and pain management guidelines. *Nurs Times* 18 September.

World Health Organization (2010) *WHO's Pain Relief Ladder* (online). Available at: www.who.int/cancer/palliative/painladder/en (accessed June 2010).

Wyatt JP, Illingworth RN, Graham CA, Clancy MJ, Robertson CE (2006) *Oxford Handbook of Emergency Medicine*, 3rd edn. Oxford: Oxford University Press.

Chapter 8
Prescribing for Specific Groups

Janice Davies and Dilyse Nuttall

Learning objectives

After reading this chapter and completing the activities within it, the reader will be able to:

1 identify the needs of specific groups in order to support safe and effective prescribing
2 critically analyse prescribing practice in relation to meeting the needs of specific groups

It is acknowledged that different groups, such as those with hepatic and renal impairment, pregnant and breastfeeding women, older people and children, require specific attention to ensure that the physiological differences and related risks are recognised and considered when prescribing (British Medical Association (BMA) and Royal Pharmaceutical Society of Great Britain (RPSGB) 2010). In adapting a holistic approach to non-medical prescribing, it is essential to consider not only the physiological presentation of the condition but also the psychological and social impact. In addition, it must be recognised that other groups, such as young people, men, travelling families and black and minority ethnic (BME) groups, have specific needs that can impact on the ability of the non-medical prescriber to prescribe safely and effectively. This chapter explores the needs of these individual groups in relation to safe and effective prescribing practice.

Prescribing in liver disease

The importance of considering the patient's liver function must be recognised by all prescribers, regardless of their speciality or personal formulary. The assessment of the patient must incorporate consideration of the patient's liver function before any drug treatment is prescribed because adverse effects and drug interactions are more common

The Textbook of Non-medical Prescribing, edited by Dilyse Nuttall and Jane Rutt-Howard.
© 2011 Blackwell Publishing Ltd

in people with liver impairment (BMA and RPSGB 2010) (see also Chapter 5). As most drugs pass through the liver on their journey around the body, changes in both pharmacokinetics and pharmacodynamics can occur in liver disease. Therefore, so that an appropriate judgement on choice of drug and dose can be made, consideration of the patient's liver function is essential.

Unfortunately the assessment of liver impairment is not simple, because (unlike in renal disease) there is no single biochemical marker for grading liver function. The extent of a patient's liver impairment should be holistic and is usually assessed using a combination of three factors (Lewis 2008) although, taken individually, none of these is specific to liver disease:

Liver function tests

Although liver function tests (LFTs) are an important tool in the development of a picture of the patient's overall liver function, routine isolated LFTs are often a poor guide to the capacity of the liver to metabolise drugs. As such, it is not possible to predict in an individual patient the extent to which metabolism of a particular drug will be impaired (BMA and RPSGB 2010). Table 8.1 explains the individual elements of the screening undertaken in LFTs. It is worthy of note that, although not automatically reported with LFTs, the clotting screen is also a useful indicator of liver function because the international normalised ratio (INR) is often raised in liver disease (Lewis 2008).

Signs and symptoms

In approaching the assessment of liver function from a holistic perspective, it is important also to consider signs and symptoms in the three-factor approach. Table 8.2 lists the non-specific signs and symptoms that are suggestive of liver disease. However, it is again important to recognise that, in isolation, these cannot be considered as indicative of impaired liver function because each could have a variety of other causes (Lewis 2008).

Table 8.1 Liver function tests explained

> The transaminase enzymes aspartate transaminase (AST) and alanine transaminase (ALT), are both released from damaged liver cells, but are found in other organs as well
> Bilirubin is formed from the destruction of red blood cells and is conjugated (a process involved in metabolism) in the liver but several other diagnoses can lead to raised levels
> Albumin is a protein that is manufactured in the liver and is a measure of the capacity of the liver to synthesise, but low albumin levels are found in various conditions, e.g. malignancy and malnutrition

From Lewis (2008).

Table 8.2   Signs and symptoms of liver impairment

Jaundice
Pale stools and dark urine
Gynaecomastia
Spider naevi
Ascites
Oesophageal and gastric varices
Hepatic encephalopathy
Dupuytren's contracture
Finger clubbing
Pruritis

From Lewis (2008).

Diagnosis

There are hundreds of different types of liver disease and these can manifest them-selves as mild and self-limiting or severe with high mortality, or anywhere in between (Lewis 2008). Liver disease does not necessarily mean liver dysfunction, because the liver may compensate and still be functioning well, despite being diseased (Lewis 2008). Therefore, a diagnosis of a specific liver disease will provide a clearer indication of its likely impact. Every drug is handled differently by patients with different liver condi-tions, but a combination of the factors above is used to assess the extent of liver disease in order to assist in choosing the correct drug and dose. The decision to adjust doses or avoid certain drugs depends upon:

- the nature and severity of disease
- the route of elimination for the drug.

Activity box 8.1

The current edition of the BNF is an essential source for checking whether or not drugs should be avoided, or prescribed in a lower dose, depending on whether disease is mild, moderate or severe. The summaries of product characteristics (SPCs) available at www.medicines.org.uk contain further information on the use of individual medicines in liver impairment.

Identify three drugs that you prescribe or are likely to prescribe. Access the BNF and SPCs to determine the actions to be taken in the event of liver impair-ment. Use this information to support your personal formulary.

Pharmacology in liver disease

To prescribe safely in liver disease it is necessary to have an understanding of both pharmacokinetics and pharmacodynamics. The principles of both these elements of pharmacology are explained in detail in Chapter 5. However, it is pertinent to identify the specific issues relating to pharmacokinetics and pharmacodynamics in liver impairment.

Pharmacokinetics

The liver plays an essential role in pharmacokinetics because most drugs pass through it. Patients with liver disease often need lower doses of drugs primarily because of an increase in bioavailability and a decrease in systemic clearance, both of which increase the average steady-state plasma concentration (Waller et al 2005).

Absorption and bioavailability

Although the rate of absorption from the gut is not greatly affected by liver impairment, bioavailability can be increased for many drugs, especially those that normally undergo extensive hepatic first-pass metabolism (Waller et al 2005). For many drugs, after an oral dose, a proportion is removed by the liver before it enters the systemic circulation. This process is first-pass metabolism and the extent of absorption is referred to as the bioavailability. A drug that undergoes extensive first-pass metabolism will have low bioavailability. A patient with liver disease may have reduced first-pass metabolism and this will lead to increases in blood levels of these drugs, increasing bioavailability and necessitating a lower dose.

Distribution

Once a drug is in the systemic circulation, its distribution to the tissues depends on a range of factors including its lipid solubility, plasma protein binding and tissue binding. For drugs to be active they must be free; when they are bound to proteins they are not free to exert an effect. In liver disease there may be changes in plasma proteins as the liver is the main source of albumin, the predominating plasma protein. This means that less of the drug is protein bound, and more is free to exert an effect (and generate side effects), so the patient may need a lower dose. Drugs affected include warfarin, phenytoin and prednisolone. Severe liver disease often leads to the development of ascites (accumulation of fluid in the peritoneal cavity) and an increase in plasma volume, and this will increase the response (and side effects) of water-soluble drugs such as gentamicin.

Elimination

The liver has an important role in elimination of drugs from the body. This may occur through either excretion into bile or hepatic metabolism. For the latter, the determining factors involved in clearance are blood flow to the liver, access to hepatic enzymes and enzyme activity. Blood flow to the diseased liver may be reduced due to the development of 'shunts', in which blood bypasses the congested liver. With less blood entering the liver for metabolism, plasma levels of drugs will be raised and a reduction in dose may be necessary.

The liver is the main site for metabolism and excretion for many drugs. Most drugs presented to the liver undergo metabolism, and the water-soluble metabolites are then excreted in either bile or urine. The process depends on the activity of hundreds of different enzymes, the effect of which varies depending on the type of liver disease. If the activity of the enzymes is reduced or if there are too few liver cells to produce enzymes, the metabolism of drugs will be reduced, and a reduction in dose may be required. Patients with liver disease may also be more susceptible to drug interactions as a result of impaired metabolism.

Some larger drug molecules and their metabolites are excreted in bile and a reduction in bile formation can lead to a reduction in clearance of these drugs (e.g. rifampicin and fusidic acid are eliminated unchanged in bile) Reduced elimination of drug metabolites in bile can affect enterohepatic circulation; and reduced bile production could reduce the absorption of fat-soluble vitamins (Waller et al 2005).

Pharmacodynamics in liver disease

In addition to altering the pharmacokinetics of the drug, liver disease can affect the pharmacodynamics, making effects and side effects more pronounced. The complications of liver disease may also increase the risk of developing side effects.

Ascites

Some drugs can cause fluid retention and these should be used with caution because they can exacerbate ascites and oedema. These drugs include diuretics and sodium-containing medicines (including some soluble formulations).

Reduced clotting

Bleeding disorders are a common complication of liver disease. Synthesis of clotting factors takes place in the liver and, if this function is impaired, the INR will be raised and the patient will be at increased risk of bruising and bleeding. In addition, sensitivity to oral anticoagulants will be increased. Any drug that increases the risk of bleeding should be avoided or used with caution in liver disease. Table 8.3 provides examples of these drugs.

Hepatic encephalopathy

Hepatic encephalopathy is due to the accumulation of toxins in the brain. Drugs affecting the central nervous system (CNS) should be either not prescribed or used with caution in patients with this complication. Drugs such as these can cause or worsen sedation and confusion, and if their metabolism is also impaired there is an increased risk of further side effects. The following are examples:

Table 8.3 Drugs that increase bleeding risk

Non-steroidal anti-inflammatory drugs
Aspirin
Clopidogrel
Dipyridamole
Warfarin
Heparin
Selective serotonin reuptake inhibitors
Corticosteroids

- Opioids
- Tricyclic antidepressants
- Sedating antihistamines
- Hypnotics
- Antipsychotics.

In addition, drugs that lower the seizure threshold should be prescribed with caution because severe encephalopathy can lead to convulsions. The following are examples:

- Tramadol
- Pethidine
- Antidepressants
- Sedating antihistamines
- Antipsychotics.

Constipation

Constipating drugs should be avoided, or prescribed with a laxative, in patients at risk of encephalopathy, in order to ensure adequate clearance of waste products through the bowel. Constipation can lead to these toxins accumulating, crossing the blood–brain barrier, and causing or worsening encephalopathy (Lewis 2008)). Some drugs that commonly cause constipation are as follows:

- Opioids
- Tricyclic antidepressants
- Sedating antihistamines
- $5HT_3$ antagonists (triptans)
- Calcium channel blockers
- Drugs with anticholinergic properties (examples include hyoscine, some drugs used in Parkinson's disease and any drugs with anticholinergic side effects listed in their side-effect profile)
- Aluminium-containing antacids
- Loperamide.

Pharmacodynamics and prescribing

Liver disease may affect the response to drugs in several ways as indicated above. The reserve of the liver is large and. therefore, the functioning of the diseased liver may range from normal to severely compromised. As such, it is important to know the patient's liver function status in order to avoid side effects and drug interactions. In severe liver disease, this is best achieved by keeping prescribing to a minimum.

A holistic approach to prescribing for patients with liver impairment

Many patients diagnosed with liver disease or impairment will require long-term interventions, ranging from regular monitoring to organ transplantation. The physical impact of liver disease is often apparent through the manifestation of physical signs and symptoms. However, it has also been recognised that there is often a significant psychological impact (Collis and Lloyd 1992). Unsurprisingly, in considering the physical limitations that can result from increased liver impairment, the psychological, and indeed social, impact has been linked to related quality-of-life issues (Martin et al 2007). The Department of Health (DH 2010), Scottish Government (2009) and Long Term Conditions Alliance

Table 8.4 Considerations in liver disease

A full and holistic assessment to determine presence and severity of liver
  impairment (including liver function tests, symptoms and diagnosis)
Assessment to include psychological and social impact of both the condition and of
  any treatments/interventions
Ensure that drug doses are adjusted (where indicated) to ensure safety when
  prescribing for patients with liver impairment
Keep prescribing to a minimum in severe liver disease
Review and monitor patients regularly
Refer patients to other agencies where appropriate (e.g. psychological support)

Northern Ireland (2008) demonstrate a clear recognition of the importance of addressing the psychological needs of patients with long-term conditions. Indeed, this is supported by the National Institutes for Health and Clinical Excellence (NICE 2009) which
identified that depression is significantly more common in patients with a chronic physical health problems than in those in good physical health. Importantly, it is recognised
within the NICE (2009) guidance that recognition and treatment of psychological problems in these patients can increase both their quality of life and their life expectancy.

In view of the potential for patients with liver disease to develop a range of problems,
there is clearly a need for a holistic approach to assessment and treatment planning.
Non-medical prescribers are able to undertake a number of actions, summarised in
Table 8.4, to ensure that the needs of these patients are met.

Prescribing in renal disease

Assessment of renal function

Many drugs or their metabolites are excreted by the kidney. Knowledge of a patient's
renal function is essential in order to determine whether or not the drug should be given
in a lower dose or avoided altogether. The cornerstone of any alteration of drug dosage
is the estimation of the glomerular filtration rate (eGFR). This is now the routine method
of estimating renal function in adults and information on dose adjustment in the BNF
is now mostly expressed in terms of eGFR rather than the traditional creatinine clearance (CrCl).

Activity box 8.2

Annette (case study 5) has approached you requesting help to give up smoking.
She has tried to stop on numerous occasions using willpower alone, but has only
ever managed to stop for 1 week.

What action would you take? Provide an evidence-based rationale for your
decision.

GFR is estimated using the modification of diet in renal disease (MDRD) formula which uses serum creatinine concentration, age, sex and ethnic origin. However, it is normalised to a standard body surface area of $1.73\,m^2$, so for patients at the extremes of body weight eGFR should be converted to the patient's absolute GFR using the following formula (BMA and RPSGB 2010):

$$GFR\ absolute = eGFR \times Body\ surface\ area/1.73$$

NICE Clinical Guidance 73 (NICE 2008) should be consulted for the classification of stages of chronic kidney disease (CKD).

The MDRD formula is not validated for use in children, and the BNF (BMA and RPSGB 2010) advises that CrCl should be used to adjust doses of potentially toxic drugs with a narrow therapeutic index (NTI) (see Chapter 5). The dose regimens in the BNF should be regarded only as an initial guide to treatment for drugs with an NTI, with subsequent dosing adjusted according to plasma concentration levels and clinical response (BMA and RPSGB 2010). Where an accurate GFR is deemed necessary, e.g. in chemotherapy prescribing, an isotope GFR determination should be performed. Serum creatinine is sometimes used as a measure of renal function but it is only a very rough guide to dosing. The following example illustrates why this is so:

- 70-year-old woman, ideal body weight (IBW) 45 kg, serum creatinine 149 micromol/L
- 30-year-old man, IBW 75 kg, serum creatinine 149 micromol/L.

Even though serum creatinine is the same, the first patient has a degree of renal impairment, whereas the second patient has normal kidney function (Wright et al 2006). Renal function declines with age. Many elderly patients have renal impairment but because of reduced muscle mass this may not be indicated by a raised serum creatinine. It is wise to assume at least mild renal impairment when prescribing for elderly people.

The extent to which dosage of a drug needs to be altered depends on the pharmacology of the drug and degree of renal impairment. The BNF (BMA and RPSGB 2010) guides dosage alteration based on the severity of renal impairment. Specialist literature, e.g. the *Renal Drug Handbook* (Ashley and Currie 2008) provides more detailed information.

Pharmacokinetics in renal impairment

The pharmacokinetics of many drugs is altered in renal impairment, particularly in those that are excreted by the kidney. However, renal impairment can also affect other aspects of pharmacokinetics.

Absorption and bioavailability

Several factors may lead to a reduction in absorption of drugs:

- Nausea, vomiting and diarrhoea as a result of uraemia and gut oedema
- An increase in gastric ammonia with a resulting increase in pH; alterations in pH can affect the absorption of some drugs, e.g. iron, digoxin

- An oedematous gut may result in a decrease in local blood flow, reducing the rate of absorption (Barber and Willson 2007).

Additionally, the regular use of phosphate binders and calcium resonium in kidney disease may impede the absorption of some drugs and alter the absorption profile of slow-release or enteric-coated products (Barber and Willson 2007). Drug doses need not be routinely altered to allow for these factors alone, but a change in the route or dose may be considered if the desired therapeutic effect is not being achieved (UK Medicines Information (UKMi) 2010).

Distribution

The state of hydration of a patient will affect the volume of distribution of water-soluble drugs, e.g. a patient with ascites or oedema may need a lower dose of gentamicin because the volume of distribution of the drug will be increased. Another factor affecting the volume of distribution in kidney disease is reduction in protein binding caused by decreased serum albumin concentrations, reduction in albumin affinity for drugs, and competition for binding sites from accumulated metabolites and retained endogenous substances. This can be significant for highly protein-bound drugs such as phenytoin because the proportion of free, and therefore active, drug will be increased (UKMi 2010).

Metabolism

A small number of drugs are metabolised in the kidneys. This is important for the degradation of insulin and the conversion of vitamin D to its active form. In CKD stages 4 and 5 either calcitriol or alfacalcidol should be prescribed because these do not require hydroxylation by the kidneys. Renal impairment affects some metabolic processes, e.g. hydrolysis and reduction are slower. This may increase serum concentrations of the parent drug and subsequent toxicity (UKMi 2010).

Elimination

Water-soluble drugs or their water-soluble metabolites which are mainly excreted by the kidney may have a prolonged half-life in renal impairment and accumulation may occur, which can cause toxicity (UKMi 2010). It may be necessary to prescribe a lower dose if a large proportion of the drug is normally excreted by the kidney and also if the drug has a low therapeutic index.

Pharmacodynamics in renal impairment

The clinical response to some drugs can be altered in renal impairment, e.g. one of the aims of the treatment of CKD is to slow its progression and prevent symptoms such as hyperkalaemia from developing. However, some drugs can cause hyperkalaemia, particularly in the presence of renal impairment. These include potassium-sparing diuretics, angiotensin-converting enzyme (ACE) inhibitors, angiotensin receptor blockers (ARBs), digoxin overdose, NSAIDs, ciclosporin and trimethoprim.

Sensitivity may be increased even if elimination is unimpaired (BMA and RPSGB 2010), e.g. greater sensitivity to drugs acting on the central nervous system (CNS), such as benzodiazepines, antihistamines and codeine (UKMi 2010). This is thought to be due to an increase in the permeability of the blood–brain barrier (Barber and Willson 2007). There is also an increased risk of gastrointestinal bleeding or oedema with non-steroidal anti-inflammatory drugs (NSAIDs) or warfarin (Barber and Willson 2007, UKMi 2010).

Nephrotoxicity

Nephrotoxic drugs should be avoided in renal impairment because the consequences are likely to be more serious if renal reserve is already reduced (BMA and RPSGB 2010). ACE inhibitors and NSAIDs are the most frequent causes of drug-induced reduction in GFR. For patients receiving dialysis, the adverse effects of nephrotoxic drugs on the kidney is not a factor because the kidneys have already been irreparably damaged; however, care should still be taken to consider other adverse effects.

Dosing

There are two approaches to altering drug maintenance doses in renal impairment (UKMi 2010):

1 The standard dose can be given but at extended intervals (this approach should be used for drugs that must reach a specific peak serum concentration, such as gentamicin).
2 A reduced dose is given at the usual intervals (this approach should be used for drugs that require maintenance of a serum concentration over the whole dosing interval).

Loading doses should not usually be changed because a rapid therapeutic response may be needed, and a prolonged half-life means that it would otherwise take a long time to reach therapeutic levels. It is suggested that a drug with the following characteristics is chosen when prescribing for patients with renal impairment (UKMi 2010):

- Wide therapeutic index
- Does not require renal metabolism to the active form
- No or minimal nephrotoxicity
- Active drug or active metabolites not renally excreted
- Not highly protein bound
- Low side-effect profile
- Action unaffected by altered tissue sensitivity
- Unaffected by fluid balance changes
- Able to reach site of action in high enough concentrations in the presence of renal impairment.

Most drugs will not meet all the above criteria but, if a drug has an NTI with no potential for monitoring potential renal adverse effects, or serious dose-related adverse effects, an alternative should be found.

Prescribing and renal impairment: summary

In summary, the factors in Table 8.5 should be considered before prescribing a drug to a patient with renal impairment (UKMi 2010).

Table 8.5 Factors to consider before prescribing in patients with renal impairment

> Use drugs only when there is a definite indication
> Choose a drug that has no or minimal nephrotoxicity
> Use recommended dosage regimens for renal failure
> Use plasma concentration measurements to adjust dosages where possible
> Monitor the patient carefully for evidence of clinical effectiveness and toxicity.

Table 8.6 Considerations in renal disease

> A full and holistic assessment to determine presence and severity of renal
> impairment (including estimated glomerular filtration rate (eGFR) or creatinine
> clearance (CrCl) as appropriate)
> Assessment to include psychological and social impact of both the condition and
> any treatments/interventions
> Use drugs only when there is a definite indication
> Choose a drug that has no or minimal nephrotoxicity
> Use recommended dosage regimens for renal failure
> Use plasma concentration measurements to adjust dosages where possible
> Review and monitor the patient carefully for evidence of clinical effectiveness and
> toxicity
> Refer patients to other agencies where appropriate (e.g. psychological support)

A holistic approach to prescribing for patients with renal impairment

As previously discussed in relation to patients with liver impairment, there is a clear need to adopt a holistic approach to care provision for long-term conditions. Renal disease is one such long-term condition that often has a significant impact on all aspects of the patient's daily life. As was shown to be the case in liver disease, renal disease can have a significant impact not only physically but also psychologically and socially (White and Grenyer 1999, Hutchinson 2005, Davison 2007). This supports the need for a holistic approach to assessment and treatment planning for these patients. Non-medical prescribers are able to undertake a number of actions, summarised in Table 8.6, to ensure that the needs of these patients are met.

Activity box 8.3

Annette (case study 5) recently had routine blood tests that indicated a need for further investigation. She has just been informed that she has moderate renal impairment.

Consider Annette's current drug regimen and identify any changes necessary as a result of this new diagnosis.

Prescribing in pregnancy

All drugs should be avoided in pregnancy unless they are essential; however, it is estimated that 80% of women still take between three and eight medicines, either prescribed or over the counter, before they realise that they are pregnant (Lee et al 2000). In addition, prescribing in pregnancy is sometimes necessary because pregnancy can be associated with medical problems that require treatment (Waller et al 2005), and some conditions such as psychosis, diabetes, hypertension and epilepsy require treatment because the risk of not treating is hazardous to both mother and fetus.

Teratogenicity

A drug is a teratogen if it causes abnormalities in the fetus, or in the child after birth, which may not be seen until later in life (Lee et al 2000). The timing of drug exposure is important in determining whether it is likely to cause harm. The fetus is most at risk of structural malformations such as cleft palate or spina bifida during the first trimester. During the second and third trimesters drugs can affect the growth and functional development of the fetus, or they can have toxic effects on fetal tissue. Drugs taken shortly before term or during labour can have adverse effects on labour or on the neonate after delivery (BMA and RPSGB 2010). Most drug effects will be evident at, or before, birth. One infamous example is that of the drug thalidomide, which was prescribed to pregnant women in the 1950s and 1960s to alleviate morning sickness, yet caused severe limb abnormalities in the fetus. Although this incident resulted in better recognition of the need for caution in prescribing in pregnancy, it has been suggested that both pregnant women and health professionals are sometimes overcautious, failing to use drugs even though they are clearly needed (Elliott 2007). Other drugs can have delayed effects, appearing years later. Diethylstilbestrol is a synthetic oestrogen that was used in the treatment of threatened spontaneous abortion between the 1940s and early 1970s (Waller et al 2005). Female fetuses exposed to this drug have an increased risk of adenocarcinoma of the vagina or cervix in later life (Waller et al 2005).

Pharmacokinetics

The placenta does not provide a barrier to the passage of drugs, so the fetus is inevitably exposed (Lee et al 2000). Nearly all drugs, except those with a very high molecular weight such as insulin or heparin, cross the placenta to the fetus driven primarily by the concentration gradient. Lipid-soluble, unionised drugs cross more rapidly than polar drugs. In practice, nearly all drugs have the potential to affect the unborn child (Lee et al 2000). Table 8.7 summarises the physiological changes during pregnancy that cause the pharmacokinetics of some drugs to be altered, particularly during late pregnancy.

These changes mean that the maternal drug concentration is often lower than that in non-pregnant women given the same dose. Care needs to be taken in the interpretation of data from therapeutic drug monitoring using plasma samples because the total concentration may be decreased, which could be interpreted as needing a higher dose, but if this is due to decreased protein-binding the active free concentration may be

Table 8.7 Physiological changes impacting on pharmacokinetics during pregnancy

Absorption	
Gastrointestinal motility	Decreased
Lung function	Increased
Skin blood circulation	Increased
Distribution	
Plasma volume	Increased
Body water	Increased
Plasma protein	Decreased
Fat deposit	Increased
Metabolism	
Liver activity	Increased
Excretion	
Glomerular filtration	Increased

Adapted from Lee et al (2000) and Waller et al (2005).

unaltered (Waller et al 2005). In addition to the changes indicated in Table 8.7, the following factors affect exposure of drugs to the fetus:

- The degree of drug metabolism that takes place in the placenta
- The ability of the fetus to metabolise drugs
- Reabsorption and swallowing of drugs by the fetus from the amniotic fluid.

Prescribing principles in pregnancy

Lee et al (2000) suggests that the following principles be adhered to when considering prescribing in pregnancy:

- Consider non-drug treatments
- Avoid all drugs in the first trimester if possible
- Avoid drugs known to have harmful effects (if potentially harmful drugs must be used, a discussion of the potential risks must take place)
- Avoid new drugs
- Avoid polypharmacy
- Use the lowest effective dose for the shortest possible time
- Consider the dose changes and therapeutic drug monitoring for some drugs.

Finding information

Women are generally advised to avoid all drugs in pregnancy because their safety is uncertain and the study of drugs in pregnant women is usually unethical. However, it is important that this does not compromise any existing medical conditions. Vickers and Brackley (2002) stress the importance of pre-pregnancy counselling for patients who require drugs to stabilise medical conditions. In addition, they emphasise the need to ensure that, while considering the effects of drugs on the fetus, the mother's medical condition is controlled. Therefore, there is a responsibility on the non-medical pre-scriber, when obtaining a history from the patient, to consider pregnancy from a variety of perspectives:

- Those non-medical prescribers prescribing any drug for a female patient must ascertain whether or not the patient is pregnant and, if so, the safety of the drug must be considered in relation to potential harm to the fetus as well as the mother.
- Where the patient requires drug therapy to stabilise a medical condition, such as epilepsy, and where the drug is considered harmful or potentially harmful in pregnancy, the non-medical prescriber must counsel the patient about commencing, or perhaps continuing, the treatment. This may include supporting the patient to avoid unplanned pregnancy by providing contraceptive advice or referral.
- Non-medical prescribers responsible for monitoring and reviewing patients with conditions requiring drug treatments considered harmful or potentially harmful in pregnancy must consider the patient's current position in relation to pregnancy.

Unfortunately, as a result of the general advice being to avoid prescribing in pregnancy, the data available on specific drugs are often sparse, and most manufacturers' SPCs are written from the medicolegal view which may not help with the decision on whether a drug is suitable in pregnancy (Lee et al 2000). The current BNF provides a table of drugs to be avoided or used with caution in pregnancy, together with the tri-mester of risk; however, absence from the list does not imply safety. Specialist text-books on prescribing in pregnancy are also available and midwife non-medical prescribers, in particular, should develop comprehensive personal formularies that equip them with the necessary knowledge to prescribe safely and effectively in pregnancy. Of course, it could be argued that all non-medical prescribers should have this knowledge. However, it must be recognised that most non-medical prescribers will rarely prescribe for pregnant women and would normally refer the patient to another relevant health professional, competent to prescribe for this specific group. Nevertheless, it is important that all non-medical prescribers are able to access information about the safety during pregnancy of any of the drugs they prescribe.

 Activity box 8.4

All UK drug information centres can provide information on drugs in pregnancy, and their contact details are listed in the front of the BNF. In addition, information on drugs and pregnancy is available from the National Teratology Information Service, the contact details of which are also in the BNF.

Use the resources above to identify information about the safety in pregnancy of three drugs that you commonly prescribe for women of child-bearing age.

Consider if, during your consultation, you are providing adequate and appropriate information on potential risks related to the use of those drugs in pregnancy.

A holistic approach to prescribing for patients in pregnancy

Adopting a holistic approach to non-medical prescribing in pregnancy is as important as with any other specific group. However, to ensure that holism is truly achieved, the non-medical prescriber must consider pregnancy from all perspectives: confirmed, potential, planned and unplanned. This is important not least because the UK abortion rates indicate that a significant proportion of pregnancies are unplanned (Information Services Division Scotland 2007, DH 2008). It is also important to recognise that a significant number of abortions were in women aged 45 years and over (Information Services Division Scotland 2007, DH 2008. This age group did represent the smallest group in terms of numbers of abortions, but still equated to 660 abortions in 2008 in England and Wales alone. These data serve to reiterate the need for non-medical prescribers to consider pregnancy in age groups in which they may not automatically consider it. In addition, it highlights the need to discuss contraception with patients, recognising it as a public health issue. Importantly, drugs such as antibacterials can have an effect on the effectiveness of some oral contraceptives (BMA and RPSGB 2010). Therefore, non-medical prescribers must not only be aware of such issues with regard to any drugs that they may prescribe but they must also be equipped to advise patients.

It is essential at this juncture to highlight that consideration of pregnancy-related issues is not exclusive to female patients. Indeed, although the drugs that require caution or avoidance in pregnancy obviously refer to female patients, it must be remembered that some drugs used by male patients can impact on fertility and pregnancy. Fertility concerns can have a significant impact on both women and men, with the potential to cause significant psychological and psychosocial problems (Cousineau and Domar 2007). Therefore, where there is potential for drug treatments to cause fertility problems, it is essential that the non-medical prescriber is not only able to explore these issues with the patient but also able to make referral to other services, such as counselling, as appropriate.

Activity box 8.5

Read case study 3 and answer the questions below. It will be useful to read the guidance in the BNF and at the Electronic Medicines Compendium available at www.medicines.org.uk/emc:

- What are the risks/considerations for this patient?
- What advice and information would you give?

Another pertinent public health issue is the prevention of neural tube defects. Folic acid supplements taken before and during pregnancy can reduce the occurrence of neural tube defects (BMA and RPSGB 2010). All women should be advised to take a medicinal or food supplement of 400 mcg folic acid daily before conception until week 12 of pregnancy. Women at higher risk should take a higher dose according to BNF (BMA

Table 8.8 Considerations of pregnancy

A full and holistic assessment to determine actual pregnancy, potential pregnancy
   or planning for pregnancy (including men where appropriate)
Assessment to include consideration of patient's perception and concerns about
   drugs in pregnancy/fertility
Awareness of the potential risks in each trimester

and RPSGB 2010) advice. Non-medical prescribers are often in an ideal position to tackle public health targets and should consider folic acid use, where appropriate, while exploring pregnancy-related issues with the patient.

In recognition of the complexity of pregnancy and related issues, it is perhaps more appropriate to make reference to the considerations 'of' pregnancy rather than limiting them to 'in' pregnancy. Table 8.8 summarises the actions that non-medical prescribers are able to undertake, to ensure that the needs of pregnant women, and those of men and women who are considering starting a family, are met.

Prescribing in breastfeeding

The benefits of breastfeeding in reducing health inequalities, and in improving health, are well recognised within UK health policy (DH 2009). Breast milk contains nutritional and immunological properties superior to those found in infant formulas (Briggs et al 2008). The benefits of breastfeeding are vast, and include reduction in the risk of infection, allergic disease and sudden infant death syndrome, as well as enhancing cognitive and sensory development (Unicef 2006). Furthermore, women who breastfeed reduce their risk of developing ovarian and breast cancer in later life (World Health Organization (WHO) 2010). Therefore, there is clear recognition of the need for health professionals to work to increase breastfeeding rates (DH 2009), a responsibility that is equally relevant to professionals in a non-medical prescribing capacity.

Concerns about drugs and breastfeeding

Although there is concern that drugs taken by the mother might affect the infant, there is very little information available to support or dispute this. Manufacturers' literature often contraindicates prescribing in breastfeeding but this may be due a lack of evidence rather than known adverse effects. In the absence of published data, prescribing decisions should take into account the pharmacokinetic and pharmacodynamic properties of the drug and its side-effect profile (Lee et al 2000).

The most important question to ask is whether or not a breastfeeding mother needs the medication. If drugs were required, it would be logical to choose drugs that would have the least effect on the breastfed baby or child. With careful selection and appropriate advice, the mother may be able to continue breastfeeding. It is seldom necessary to deny the infant the known benefits of breastfeeding, but it is sometimes necessary to temporarily stop breastfeeding (by expressing and discarding the milk), e.g. after radiopharmaceuticals. If the mother is on long-term medication with drugs known to harm the infant, it may be possible to minimise exposure by timing breastfeeding to coincide with trough blood concentration, which is just before taking a dose.

Factors determining the amount of drug in breast milk

Most drugs penetrate into breast milk in quantities too small to be of concern (BMA and RPSGB 2010). However, this knowledge may not be adequate reassurance to those taking drugs while breastfeeding or to those prescribing them. Unfortunately for the health professional prescribing for a breastfeeding mother and for the mother and infant, there is no reliable method of predicting how much of a drug will appear in the breast milk (Larsen 2003). The reason for this uncertainty is that there are a number of factors that can impact on the presence (and amount) of drugs in breast milk.

Maternal factors

There is a direct correlation between the dose of drug taken by the mother and the subsequent milk levels (Briggs et al 2008). The route of administration affects maternal blood levels, and also the concentration present in milk. A parenteral formulation will give higher plasma concentrations than an oral formulation, whereas topical or inhaled routes (for local application) generally lead to lower plasma levels. Importantly, dose frequency affects the ability of the breastfeeding mother to time feeds to avoid maximum concentrations in milk. The mother's ability to excrete the drug will also affect drug concentration in milk and therefore maternal renal or hepatic impairment may be significant factors when considering prescribing options.

Characteristics of the drug

Absorption of drugs is enhanced if more of the drug is ionised, and this characteristic is affected by pH. The pH of breast milk is more acidic than plasma so basic drugs will be more ionised and their passage into milk will be greater. Conversely, acidic drugs are less easily passed into milk. The degree of maternal protein binding affects the passage of drugs into breast milk and highly protein bound drugs such as warfarin appear in breast milk in only small quantities.

The lipid solubility of a drug affects its passage into breast milk. Drugs with low lipid solubility do not achieve significant levels in milk because they are unable to penetrate lipid barriers. The lipid content of milk changes over time so variation in drug levels can be expected at different stages of lactation. Drugs with a low molecular weight, such as alcohol and lithium salts, appear in breast milk rapidly.

Infant factors

Neonates and premature infants are at greatest risk from exposure to drugs because they are less able to excrete them. Hepatic and renal function are immature in neonates (Simonsen et al 2006). As a result, the half-life of drugs can be prolonged, and this can lead to accumulation and adverse effects.

Once drugs are present in breast milk, the impact that these will have on the infant will depend, in part, on the volume of milk ingested (although some drugs may cause hypersensitivity reactions regardless of the amount ingested), and the extent of absorption from the gastrointestinal tract. Some drugs that are normally given parenterally to avoid first-pass metabolism, such as insulin and heparin, are not well absorbed by the infant. The risk of adverse drug reactions in infants after ingestion of drugs via breast milk may depend on the tissue receptor sensitivity of the infant.

Drug safety profile

In general, drugs licensed for use in children can be safely given to the breastfeeding mother (the side-effect profile will indicate any potential hazards to the infant). However, the BNF advises using only essential drugs in breastfeeding. If medication has to be used, drugs with a short half-life are preferable because they are less likely to accumulate. When considering prescribing for a breastfeeding mother, it is important to consult specialist literature for further information, because drugs are classified into one of three groups according to their safety: unsuitable; use with caution and monitoring; appear safe.

A holistic approach to prescribing breastfeeding mothers

As discussed earlier, breastfeeding has many advantages, for both mother and infant. In view of this, the non-medical prescriber has a public health responsibility to support breastfeeding mothers to enable them to continue for as long as possible. Therefore, using a holistic approach to non-medical prescribing with breastfeeding mothers must aim to allow them to continue to breastfeed safely while ensuring that they themselves receive effective treatment. This requires consideration of both the safety of drugs on the infant when ingested through breast milk and the ability of the mother to continue to breastfeed. Measures to ensure safety for the infant have been identified, yet consideration of maintenance of breastfeeding needs further exploration.

There is a potential for some breastfeeding mothers to avoid accessing treatment because of fears of the harmful effects on the infant of any drugs they may be prescribed. An extreme consequence of this could be that a mother becomes too ill to breastfeed. However, it is important to recognise that some drugs can cause a reduction in lactation. These drugs include bromocriptine, high dose thiazides and oestrogens and progestogens (Winstanley and Walley 2002, BMA and RPSGB 2010). Difficulties in breastfeeding resulting from a drug-induced reduction in lactation could have a psychological impact on a mother. There is evidence to suggest that early cessation of breastfeeding is associated with an increased risk of maternal postpartum depression (Ip et al 2007). Therefore, in seeking to achieve concordance, the non-medical prescriber must explore the possible impact of any prescribing decision on the mother's ability to breastfeed. Table 8.9 summarises the actions that non-medical prescribers are able to undertake, to ensure that the needs of breastfeeding mothers are met.

Table 8.9 Considerations in breastfeeding

A full and holistic assessment to include consideration of patient's perception and concerns about drugs in breastfeeding
Use of drugs only when there is a definite indication and use drugs that will have the least effect on the infant, considering the influences on concentrations in breast milk

Activity box 8.6

Read case study 6 and critically analyse the prescribing decision. It will be useful to read the guidance in the BNF and at the Electronic Medicines Compendium available at: www.medicines.org.uk/emc

Prescribing for older people

Medicines are a fundamental part of healthcare for older people, and although many are fit and healthy, many others are frail or have co-morbidities that can make prescribing challenging and complex. The National Service Framework for Older People (DH 2001a) identified medicines as a key issue in relation to older people's health, so much so that the supporting document, *Medicines and Older People: Implementing medicines-related aspects of the NSF for Older People* (DH 2001b) was introduced. Older people are at greater risk from the adverse effects of medicines due to the altered ability of the body to handle medicines and drug interactions as a result of polypharmacy (Kairuz et al 2008), e.g. the sedating effects of drugs such as antidepressants and benzodiazepines have been shown to increase the risk of falls (Leipzig et al 1999, Fonad et al 2008). Physical problems such as poor nutritional status can affect the body's response to drugs (Greenstein 2004).

Pharmacokinetics

Absorption
The following changes in the gastrointestinal tract may occur with advancing age:

- Reduced acid secretion in the stomach
- Reduced total surface area for absorption
- Slower emptying of stomach contents
- Slowed intestinal motility
- Reduced blood flow to the liver can increase the bioavailability of some drugs as first-pass metabolism is reduced.

Although these changes may occur, it is not usually necessary to avoid medication or adjust doses based on these factors alone, unless the older person has other problems such as diarrhoea or malabsorption syndromes.

Distribution
Body composition changes with age. Older people have less muscle and more fat compared with younger adults. The percentage of body water decreases and this can affect the volume of distribution of some drugs. Water-soluble drugs such as digoxin will have higher plasma concentrations, leading to increased pharmacological effects and

lipid-soluble drugs will have lower plasma concentrations leading to reduced pharma-cological effects. The half-life of lipid soluble drugs may be prolonged if they are eliminated more slowly.

Metabolism

Enzyme activity per hepatocyte (predominant liver cell type) is unchanged by age, but the size of the liver and its blood flow are reduced. This decreases the capacity for metabolism of some lipid-soluble drugs, and some drugs may stay in the body for longer and cause toxicity with repeated doses.

Excretion

This is the most important pharmacokinetic factor that is affected by age. Renal function is reduced in older people due to a reduction in the GFR and renally excreted drugs are eliminated more slowly. Acute illness, especially if associated with dehydration, can lead to a rapid reduction in renal clearance. Drugs with a narrow therapeutic index, such as lithium, digoxin and gentamicin, are more likely to lead to toxicity (Waller et al 2005).

Altered pharmacokinetics can lead to a 50% increase in plasma concentration in older people and patients who are debilitated may show even larger increases (Livingston 2003).

Pharmacodynamics

Pharmacodynamic changes may occur due to the change in responsiveness of the target organ or altered receptor sensitivity, and examples include the following:

- Increased sensitivity to drugs acting on the CNS, possibly due to changes in receptor numbers or changes in the efficiency of the blood–brain barrier
- Decrease in numbers of β-adrenoceptors, reducing the response to drugs that act as agonists or antagonists at these receptors
- Impaired baroreceptor function: vasodilators are more likely to cause postural hypotension, and this may lead to falls
- Sensitivity to diuretics is increased due to impaired homeostasis mechanisms, also with the possibility of leading to falls
- The side effects of slowed gastrointestinal motility and retention of urine tend to be greater with anticholinergic drugs such as tricyclic antidepressants, e.g. amitriptyline
- Enhanced sensitivity to warfarin due to greater inhibition of vitamin K-dependent clotting factors; in addition, the outcome of bleeding tends to be more serious in older people
- Impairment of thermoregulatory mechanisms can increase risk of hypothermia with drugs such as phenothiazine, antipsychotics or opioid analgesics.

Drugs to be used with caution

Some drugs are frequently associated with adverse drug reactions in older people, including:

- **Hypnotics**, particularly those with a long half-life, because they can cause drowsiness, confusion, slurred speech and unsteadiness, leading to falls. If a hypnotic must be used, one with a short half-life should be chosen.
- **Diuretics**, which are overprescribed in elderly people (BMA and RPSGB 2010). They should not be prescribed on a long-term basis to treat simple gravitational oedema. A few days of diuretic treatment may be sufficient to clear the oedema, which can then often be treated non-pharmacologically with increased mobility, support stockings and raising the legs.
- **NSAIDs**: elderly people are particularly susceptible to their side effects which include bleeding, heart failure and renal impairment – the last is more common in elderly people so their use in this population is more hazardous. For this reason, non-pharmacological treatments (warmth, exercise, use of walking stick or weight loss if applicable) should be tried first for osteoarthritis, back pain and soft-tissue disorders. Paracetamol is the drug of choice in these conditions because it is safer.
- Other drugs cited as commonly causing adverse effects in elderly people are antiparkinsonian drugs, antihypertensives, psychotropics and digoxin (Livingston 2003).

Activity box 8.7

From the drugs that you commonly prescribe, make a list of those that should be carefully monitored in older people.

Points to consider when prescribing for elderly people

Elderly people often take several drugs for multiple diseases. This increases the chance of adverse effects and drug interactions, and can affect compliance. The following points should therefore be taken into consideration before prescribing.

Limit range
It is sensible to become thoroughly familiar with the effects in elderly people of the drugs that you commonly prescribe.

Reduce dose
Elderly people often require a lower dose and it is common to start with about 50% of the usual adult dose.

Regular medication review
At each medication review check that drugs are still indicated because it may be possible to withdraw unnecessary items. Ensure that dosages are appropriate for an elderly person, reducing the dose if necessary.

Simplify regimens
Simple treatment regimens are easier to adhere to, with medications given just once or twice a day if possible.

Explain clearly

Write full instructions on prescriptions so that containers can be labelled properly. Avoid the instruction 'as directed' on prescriptions. Compliance among those older people at greater risk of adverse effects from medicines can be improved by ensuring that communication is effective and promotes patient education, while incorporating regular medication reviews (Kairuz et al 2008).

Repeats and disposal

Explain to patients what to do when medicine runs out, and how to dispose of medicines that are no longer needed (usually they should be returned to the pharmacy for destruction). Try to arrange for individual items prescribed to be issued on the same date of the month and to prescribe matching quantities.

 Activity box 8.8

Identify an older person for whom you would have recently prescribed. Check whether the above guidelines for safe prescribing were applied.

A holistic approach to prescribing for older people

The recognition that older people have specific needs has been recognised in the standards set in the *NSF for Older People* (DH 2001), together with the standards reiterated in *Better Health in Old Age* (DH 2004c). Specific needs in relation to the consultation process are discussed at length in Chapter 4. However, there are some key health needs worthy of exploration at this juncture.

Coronary heart disease and cerebral vascular disease are identified as key health targets (DH 2001). Targeting individuals (and groups) at risk should be seen as an integral part of the non-medical prescriber's role, particularly as many of the problems associated with the ageing process, respond positively to physical activity and healthy eating (DH 2001a). This intervention may help prevent prescribing in the future.

Accidents have also been identified as a national health target (DH 2004c), with accident prevention in older people focusing on falls (DH 2001a, 2004c). Older people are at greater risk of accidents due to both intrinsic factors, resulting from the ageing process and medication, and extrinsic environmental factors (Ewles 2005, Kulmala et al 2008). Therefore, the non-medical prescriber should be aware of factors, such as sensory impairment, incontinence, alcohol misuse, environmental hazards and restricted mobility, that would increase the risk of accidents among older people (NICE 2004).

Another common health concern in older people is that of mental illness. Unfortunately, this is often poorly managed or goes unrecognised (DH 2004c). Non-medical prescribers, who are in contact with older people, must incorporate mental wellbeing into their holistic assessment. This will help early detection and timely referral to specialist services, both seen as essential in tackling mental health issues effectively (DH 2001a, NICE 2008).

Table 8.10 Considerations in older people

A full and holistic assessment to include consideration of social issues, mental health and accident risk
Reduction in drug dosage as appropriate
Simplified treatment regimens
Clear explanations accompanied by written instructions
Advice about safe disposal of medicines
Review and monitoring
Consideration of public health issues: accident prevention, mental health, cardiovascular disease and stroke risk
Referral to other agencies where appropriate (e.g. social support, psychological support, carer support)

Therefore, using a holistic approach to non-medical prescribing with older people requires consideration of both the safety of drugs in relation to the physiological changes of ageing and the ability of the patient to take or use any prescribed treatment safely. This will require consideration of issues such as social support, mental health and accident risk. Concordance can be achieved only if consideration is given to the specific issues of older people and that these are incorporated into any treatment plan. Table 8.10 summarises the actions that non-medical prescribers are able to undertake, to ensure that the needs of older people are met.

Activity box 8.9

Read Case study 2 and consider the holistic needs of the patient. What actions would you take to improve the management plan for this patient?

Prescribing for children and young people

Defining children and young people

To ensure that guidance regarding prescribing for children is clearly understood, it is essential that the non-medical prescriber is familiar with the terminology used in relation to children and prescribing. The National Prescribing Centre (NPC 2000) identified the recognised stages of childhood that are summarised in Table 8.11. The various organs, body systems and enzymes develop at different rates throughout childhood and, because of this, children's dosages should always be taken from a paediatric dosing text and should not be extrapolated from the usual adult dose.

Table 8.11 Distinctions in childhood

Term	Age	Comments
Neonate	Birth to 27 days	Covers the changes immediately after birth to 1 month; however, infants under 37 weeks' gestation require special consideration
Infant	1-23 months	Covers the early growth spurt
Child	2-11 years	Covers the gradual growth spurt
Adolescent	12-18 years	Covers the adolescent growth spurt to final height

Source: NPC (2000).

Altered pharmacokinetics

Absorption

The absorption of oral medicines is variable and unreliable due to several reasons. From birth until the age of 2-3 years, the gastric mucosa is immature and gastric acid reduction is reduced. For drugs such as penicillins, which are usually partly broken down by acid in the stomach, this can lead to increased absorption. Peristalsis is reduced for the first 6 months and gastric emptying is relatively slow. This can depend on age, feeding patterns and the nature of the feed. Reduced production of bile means that fat-soluble medicines are absorbed more slowly. Other factors include posture, disease states, variation in the amounts of gut microflora, vomiting and the spitting out of medicines (Conroy 2003).

Intramuscular injections are less well absorbed in neonates because of low muscle mass and reduced blood flow to the muscles. In addition, intramuscular injections are painful and should be avoided if possible. Topical absorption is often higher in neonates and infants because of their thinner skin, and the large surface area relative to body weight can lead to adverse effects through increased absorption. However, this method of absorption may be used more in the future because it avoids the problems of other methods, e.g. erratic absorption from oral medicines and difficult venous access. The rectal route is sometimes used if oral or intravenous administration is not possible, but rectal absorption may be slow or incomplete in neonates (only a limited range of drugs and dosages is available in suppository formulation).

Distribution

Several factors that determine drug distribution within the body are subject to change with age. These include vascular perfusion, body composition, tissue-binding characteristics and the extent of plasma protein binding (Walker and Whittlesea 2007). Compared with adults, total body water is relatively high at birth and decreases with age. This is significant for water-soluble drugs, particularly those with a narrow therapeutic range such as gentamicin, where a higher dose per milligram will be required in order to reach a therapeutic serum concentration.

Metabolism

Most enzyme systems responsible for drug metabolism are undeveloped at birth, and the various pathways do not mature at the same time. This reduced ability to metabolise is followed by a rapid increase in the metabolic rate of children aged 1–9 and the metabolic clearance of drugs in this age group can exceed that of adults – this is thought to be due to the relatively larger size of the liver (Conroy 2003).

Renal excretion

GFR and tubular secretion are reduced in infants, and clearance of renally excreted drugs is reduced. Therefore, a longer dose interval may be required.

 Activity box 8.10

Read case study 7 and identify the pharmacokinetic factors that would impact on the non-medical prescriber's treatment choice.

Dose

The dose should always be calculated on an individual basis using a reputable source such as the *BNF for Children* (BNFC) or by seeking advice from a medicines information centre. The doses of some drugs with a wide therapeutic range may be based on age ranges, but most drug doses are based on weight.

Although age, weight and height are easy to measure, using body surface area (BSA) to calculate drug dosages is more accurate because it reflects cardiac output, fluid requirements and renal function (Conroy 2003). Nomograms are available to calculate the BSA (BNFC) and these are often used to calculate dosages in cytotoxic regimens where the dose is critical.

Licensing

For a medicine to be marketed in the UK, it has to have a marketing authorisation (MA) (formerly known as a product licence) to ensure that it is safe, effective and of suitable quality (NPC 2000). The MA states the indication(s), contraindications and usually the age range in which the medicine may be used. All medicines should ideally be prescribed according to the MA, and if this is the case the MA holder (usually the manufacturer) shares some of the responsibility with the prescriber if a patient comes to harm as a result of using the medicine. If the medicine is used outside the terms of the MA, this is referred to as 'off-licence' or 'off-label' use. A great deal of prescribing in paediatrics is 'off-label' but this does not necessarily indicate poor practice – it usually shows that there is a lack of suitably licensed medicines available for children in the UK. There are several reasons for this, e.g. there may be proven safety issues that contraindicate or caution against prescribing in children, but more commonly it reflects the absence of clinical trials providing the evidence necessary to support licensing applications for paediatric use. There are ethical, practical and technical difficulties in carrying out clinical trials with children, and sometimes the relatively small market for the medicine may not balance the additional expense that the manufacturer will incur in conducting pae-diatric trials.

When prescribing an unlicensed medicine for a child, it can be difficult to obtain the necessary prescribing information to ensure safety because there may be no paediatric dose listed in the usual reference sources, e.g. BNF or SPCs. It is important to consult specialist literature and both the BNFC and UK medicines information centres or local hospital pharmacy medicines information departments are easily accessible and can provide advice on drug use in children. In addition, it is important to consider the infor-mation that is provided to the parent or child, because the patient information leaflet may be inappropriate if the medicine is to be used off-label.

It can also be difficult to find a suitable formulation for a child, e.g. a medicine that is available only in tablet form will not be suitable for a child who cannot or will not swallow tablets. The pharmacy will need to consider a range of options in deciding how to dispense such prescriptions. This may involve arranging for the product to be made up by a 'specials' manufacturer, i.e. manufactured by a commercial or hospital licensed manufacturing unit; importing the medicine; or adapting existing adult formulations, e.g. splitting tablets, or diluting a concentrated solution. All of these options have drawbacks (Conroy 2003).

Activity box 8.11

Consider the potential drawbacks of using an unlicensed medicine for a child if it has to be:

- purchased from a 'specials' manufacturer
- imported from abroad
- a tablet dissolved in a volume of liquid and an aliquot taken (a proportion of it used).

What discussion would take place between yourself and the patient/parent if you were prescribing an unlicensed medicine?

Excipients

Medicines contain other ingredients in addition to the active drug, and these are known as excipients. When prescribing for children, non-medical prescribers should be aware of the excipients within the drugs that they prescribe so that they can identify the associated risks, which in turn should, in part, inform the prescribing decision. The pres-ence of excipients associated with problems is identified within the monographs of drugs in the BNFC. Examples of excipients and some of their uses and problems can be found in Table 8.12.

Considerations (Table 8.13)

To meet the specific needs of children and young people, consideration should be given to the formulation, taste and appearance of the medicine, and also the ease of admin-istration of treatment. A simple regimen should be prescribed with as few medicines as

Table 8.12 Excipients: considerations when prescribing for children and young people

Excipient	Comments
Lactose	Used as a bulking agent and should be avoided in lactose intolerant patients
Chloroform and other alcohols	Used as preservatives
Colouring agents	Can lead to hyperactivity
Sorbitol	Often used as a sweetener though this can cause diarrhoea. Sugar-free preparations should be prescribed where possible to avoid dental decay

Table 8.13 Considerations in children and young people

A full and holistic assessment to include consideration of parent and patient expectations and health beliefs

Consideration of formulation, taste, appearance and ease of administration and dispensing of medicine

Calculation of drug dosage on an individual basis using the appropriate method, e.g. age, weight

As few medicines as possible

Simplified treatment regimens tailored to routines and limited to waking hours where possible

Clear explanations accompanied by written instructions

Advise regarding safe disposal of medicines

Reporting all adverse drug reactions in children to the MHRA

Consideration of public health issues, e.g. safe storage of medicines, including the specific health issues of adolescents, e.g. sexual health, smoking and alcohol

Referral to other agencies where appropriate (e.g. social support, psychological support, carer support)

possible, tailored to the child's routine, with doses scheduled to waking hours where possible. Clear instructions should be provided, reinforced with written information where necessary. Liquid medicines with doses in multiples of 5 mL will be dispensed with a spoon; doses of other volumes, or less than 5 mL, will be dispensed with an oral syringe. All adverse drug reactions in children should be reported to the Medicines and Healthcare products Regulatory Agency (MHRA) on a Yellow Card.

Activity box 8.12

You wish to prescribe an antihistamine to an infant that is available as 2 mg/5 mL liquid. The recommended dose is 1 mg every 4–6 h up to a maximum of 6 mg.

Consider the practical instructions that you would give to the parent about administration of the medicine.

Professional responsibilities

All non-medical prescribers have a responsibility to ensure that the care provided to children is appropriate, while ensuring that they practise within their competence. For many, this responsibility will promote a decision not to prescribe. The ethical codes of the professional bodies have competence at their core (RPSGB 2007, HPC 2008, Nursing and Midwifery Council (NMC) 2009, Pharmaceutical Society of Northern Ireland (PSNI) 2009) and it is clear that the necessity for practitioners to practise within their competence carries equal significance when prescribing for children. In other words, unless, as a professional, you have sufficient clinical experience and expertise with children and young people, to ensure that you are competent to prescribe for them, you must not do so. The NMC (2007, p. 2) recognised the particular importance of this issue and responded by making it a requirement that, within the assessment processes of educational programmes for non-medical prescribing, nurses and midwives must demonstrate:

> ... recognition of the unique implications and developmental context of the anatomical and physiological differences between neonates, children and young people ...

Indeed, this reiterated the message that children and young children are not just small adults (RPSGB 2004) but instead demonstrate more complex physiological and anatomical differences.

Although it is clear that, unless non-medical prescribers are competent to prescribe for children, they must not do so, there remains a responsibility to ensure that a child in need of treatment receives it. It was established in Chapter 1 that prescribing practice goes beyond writing a prescription and, as such, the non-medical prescriber may be in a position to use some prescribing skills to ensure that the child is referred appropriately, e.g. a non-medical prescriber may be able to recognise the symptoms of a particular condition and establish that it requires immediate treatment. This may be based on his or her expertise in assessing and treating adult patients with the same condition, yet he or she is not competent to prescribe for children. On the other hand, it may be the situation that it is inappropriate for the non-medical prescriber to make any assessment of the child because it is outside of his or her competence. It is essential therefore, that the non-medical prescriber is able to recognise the appropriate use of prescribing skills to ensure the safety of children and young people.

A holistic approach to prescribing for children and young people

The importance of establishing an effective rapport is particularly relevant when dealing with children, where the dynamics within the consultation can be very varied. Depending on the age of the child, involvement will vary (see Chapter 4). In prescribing for infants, for example, the history will be obtained from the parent or carer. As the child gets older, the opportunity for involvement of the child will increase. The contribution that all healthcare professionals can have on ensuring better outcomes for children and young people was recognised by DH (2004a) in the *NSF for Children, Young People and*

Maternity Services: The mental health and psychological wellbeing of children and young people. This philosophy should therefore, influence the non-medical prescriber's practice. The experiences of contact with healthcare professionals can adversely affect children psychologically (Campbell et al 1988, Kirkby and Whelan 1996) and there is a potential that, for some, the impressions acquired as a child can last a lifetime, so care is required to ensure a 'safe' consultation and relationship.

Naturally, parents and carers often feel anxious about their child's health during a consultation and the non-medical prescriber's response to this anxiety can prove crucial. The parent/carer is, in most instances, acting as the child's advocate and will have expectations that reflect this role. However, this may not always reflect the expectations of the child, requiring non-medical prescribers to remember that the patient, i.e. the child, is their priority and to ensure that the needs of the child are being appropriately identified and addressed.

Teenagers/adolescents, as a specific subgroup of children and young people, have their own 'health profile' which indicates that obesity, smoking, alcohol and drug misuse, sexual health and teenage pregnancy are issues of particular relevance to them (DH 2007). Although many of these issues reflect the health profile of the UK as a whole, the manifestation of these health issues within this group shows a 'distinct pattern of health and illness' (Viner and Booy 2005). Mental health issues among young people are a major UK concern, with one in ten children and young people having some kind of diagnosable mental disorder (DH 2007), including depression, attention deficit hyperactivity disorder, schizophrenia and eating disorders (Office of National Statistics 2004a, Viner and Booy 2005). A non-medical prescriber with an awareness of these issues will be better equipped to ensure that a relevant and effective assessment is undertaken with both increased accuracy and sensitivity. However, awareness of the health issues for this group is only part of the process. Williams et al (2007), in studying the health beliefs of 11-12 and 14-15 year olds, identified that health was not seen as a priority when considered alongside other relevant issues such as school and relationships. The challenge for the non-medical prescriber is, therefore, to elicit the young person's perception of health in order to achieve concordance in any related intervention.

Communication is key to any consultation and has been considered earlier in relation to children. However, special skills are required when communicating with young people. Macfarlane and McPherson (2007) identified two issues that can impact on the effectiveness of communication in health settings. The first issue relates to the involvement of adults, who often accompany young people, resulting in three-way consultations. Although tact is paramount, this issue can often be readily addressed, where appropriate, by arranging to undertake the consultation without the adult present. Less easily resolved is the second issue, which relates to the differences between the young person and the practitioner, resulting from a difference in understanding or values. Training has been shown to be effective in improving consultations with young people (Macfarlane and McPherson 2007) and should be considered as part of the non-medical prescriber's continuing professional development, should repeated problems arise.

Confidentiality is an issue identified as a major concern for adolescents/teenagers accessing health services (Churchill et al 2000). They are often unaware of the practitioner's responsibilities with regard to this and fear information will be disclosed.

Therefore, clearly identifying the position on confidentiality at the outset will go some way to address this.

The non-medical prescriber must also consider the social implications of any treatments prescribed for a child or young person. It is most likely that, when prescribing for children, a parent or carer will be involved in administration or supervision of the medicine. The non-medical prescriber therefore has a responsibility to ensure that parents/carers are educated on the appropriate use of the medicine and, importantly, that they are able to administer it using the routes and methods of administration prescribed. It is important to recognise that, for some treatments, and for some parents/carers, a period of training may be necessary and other health professionals may be referred to in order to assist in this process. In some instances, it may be necessary for medicines to be taken or administered in a school or college environment. This again may require training and support for those involved. In addition, the need to receive medicines in settings outside the home may be a potential source of embarrassment for the child or young person. This can result in children and young people failing to take their medication (Penza-Clyve et al 2004). It is essential therefore that the non-medical prescriber considers the settings in which the child or young person may have to receive medicines and chooses the most appropriate treatment to minimize the social impact. Such strategies may include consideration of administrations times, appliance usage and type, arrangement of facilities within the setting or advice on discreet administration.

One consideration when working with children and young people must be that of safeguarding. The Department for Children Schools and Families (2010) reiterate the message of the Children Act 1989 and the Children Act 2004, in that safeguarding children and young people is everyone's responsibility. 'Working together' is seen as fundamental in safeguarding. The non-medical prescribing consultation provides an ideal example of a situation in which the practitioner should be aware of safeguarding issues and be able to respond appropriately. This requires that the non-medical prescriber is vigilant in identifying safeguarding issues, is able to initiate the appropriate action and can liaise with other agencies to work together to safeguard children and young people.

 Activity box 8.13

Consider the child in case study 8.

Would you prescribe for the child?

Provide a rationale for your answer (making reference to relevant standards and guidance and reflecting and critically analysing your expertise and knowledge base).

Develop an action plan to address any personal and/or professional development issues that you identify.

Other groups

Although the more obvious groups have been considered, there are a number of other groups to whom it is worthwhile giving some thought. It is indeed possible to split the population for whom the non-medical prescriber may prescribe into numerous groups, all of whom will have their own issues and needs. However, there are some groups of particular significance when considering prescribing practice.

Develop an action plan to address any personal and/or professional development issues that you identify.

Activity box 8.14

Access the following link:
www.dcsf.gov.uk/everychildmatters/safeguardingandsocialcare
Take some time to look through the documents and update/refresh your knowledge.
Write down what you would do if you suspected a non-accidental injury on a child who presented to you in your practice area.

Men

It has been recognised that UK men's use of health services differs to that of women (ONS 2001) and in fact, that they are often reluctant to access services. The concern regarding this issue is compounded by the fact that more men than women die from cancer and ischaemic heart disease (ONS 2008), with fewer surviving for 5 years or more post-diagnosis (ONS 2008). This culturally embedded reluctance to access health services must be acknowledged by non-medical prescribers because not only does it impact on the likelihood of men accessing their services in the first place but also it may affect the likelihood of men returning for review. However, although this may appear to be indifference from men over their health, this is not the case in most instances. In fact, Smith et al (2008) identified that men undertake a period of self-monitoring before reaching a decision on whether or not to seek the help of health services. There would therefore appear to be a need for practitioners to target this practice and make it more effective. Smith et al (2008) identified important factors in this process of self-monitoring, which included the individual's perception of the severity of the health problem, previous experiences and the ability to continue with daily activities. In other words, men have a need to legitimise seeking health services (Robertson 2007). Much of this can be addressed by providing services which are accessible and by providing relevant information which enables them to undertake this self-monitoring more effectively.

Black and minority ethnic (BME) groups

The UK has a very diverse population, with almost 8% being from a non-white ethnic group (ONS 2004b). In view of this, it is essential that the non-medical prescriber have an awareness of the cultural health issues relating to the BME groups within his or her practice area. The impact and influence of culture on prescribing are explored in detail in Chapter 3. However, in considering those patients from BME groups as a specific group or groups, it is important to highlight some of the key health issues.

One aspect of particular importance to the non-medical prescriber must be the link between ethnicity and health. In acknowledging and understanding the specific health risks known to affect specific BME groups, the practitioner is better placed to provide relevant, holistic and effective care. Table 8.14 summarises the links between specific groups and identified health issues based on data collated by the Health Protection Agency (HPA 2006). This highlights that not only are some BME groups at greater risk than the general UK population of specific diseases, indicating a need for practitioners to target these issues, but that some diseases are specific to certain BME groups.

Table 8.14 Prevalence of health issues in black and minority ethnic (BME) groups in the UK

BME group	Higher incidence	Population-specific condition
Indian (whole)		Thalassaemia
Pakistani men	Myocardial infarction	
Pakistani women	Myocardial infarction	
	Stroke	
Pakistani boys	Childhood obesity	
Pakistani (whole)		Thalassaemia
Bangladeshi women	Stroke	
Asian (whole)	Diabetes	
Black Caribbean men	Diabetes	
Black Caribbean women	Diabetes	
Black Caribbean boys	Childhood obesity	
Black Caribbean girls	Childhood obesity	
Black African boys	Childhood obesity	
Black African girls	Childhood obesity	
Black African (whole)		Sickle cell disease
		Thalassaemia
African (whole)	Glaucoma	
African–Caribbean (whole)	Glaucoma	
Irish men	Stroke	
Roma		Thalassaemia
Middle Eastern (whole)		Thalassaemia
Eastern Mediterranean (whole)		Thalassaemia
All ethnic minority groups	Mental health problems	

Information sourced from Health Protection Agency (2006).
Whole refers to the UK population of the specific group as a whole rather than gender or age specific.

In order for health professionals to provide appropriate, effective and accessible services for BME groups, the HPA (2006) recommended that non-UK-born communities should have access to health services that are culturally appropriate and that these services should have language support. This of course is equally relevant to patients from BME groups who were born in the UK. The challenge for individual non-medical prescribers is to provide culturally appropriate consultations for all patients while working within the boundaries of their often limited resources. Many clinical areas make effective use of interpreters, language services and link workers but there are huge variations in their availability. Assessment of individual cultural needs will go some way to support forward planning but this in itself may be limited by the availability of language support. Therefore, the non-medical prescriber may be required to develop a full assessment over a number of contacts with the patient.

Mental health problems have been identified as significant in the UK BME population as a whole (HPA 2006) and, as such, the non-medical prescriber has a responsibility to ensure that this is incorporated into the holistic assessment (as is the case for all patients). However, it is important to consider this issue of mental health and ethnicity in context. Hatloy (2010) identified that differences within some BME groups can increase the likelihood of them receiving a diagnosis and treatment. These differences can manifest in the expression of symptoms, and in the amount and type of contact with other services. Again, increased awareness of cultural differences and a holistic assessment are essential to enable the non-medical prescriber to identify and appropriately address any mental health needs.

Gypsies and travelling families

The need to consider gypsies and travellers as a specific group stems from both their specific health profile and the social and cultural issues that result in increased health inequalities. The use of the terms 'gypsies' and 'travellers' in the UK context requires inclusion of Romany gypsies, Roma, Bargees, Irish travellers, English gypsies, Welsh gypsies, Scottish gypsy travellers and circus and fairgound/showmen (NHS Primary Care Contracting 2009). A Department of Health-commissioned quantitative study exploring the health issues of gypsies and travellers (DH 2004b) identified that gypsy travellers have a higher prevalence of self-reported chest pain, arthritis, respiratory problems and anxiety. These findings supported the suggestion made by Van Cleemput (2000), based on data relating to Ireland's traveller community, that travellers have specific health needs and that these are reflected in their reduced life expectancy. As with other specific groups, the health profile of gypsies and travellers indicates the need for the non-medical prescriber to have an awareness of their specific health needs and to target these as appropriate.

Significantly, the DH (2004b) study identified a cultural 'self-reliance' and tolerance of chronic illness' within this group. This, of course, may impact on their likelihood of accessing non-medical prescriber services and influence the strategies used in achieving concordance. Difficulty in accessing health services is a problem common to gypsies and travellers, not only because of the changes in location but also because of the perceived prejudices of health professionals (DH 2004b). This again reflects the need for the non-medical prescribing consultation to be culturally sensitive.

Although neither of the studies discussed in relation to gypsies and travellers included new travellers, due to the fact that they do not share the Romani cultural characteristics, it is important to acknowledge that the problems relating to access to health services may still present a problem for all travellers. Therefore, non-medical prescribers working with new travellers will need to consider these issues and employ appropriate strategies to address them.

Activity box 8.15

Many local authorities and trusts within the UK, particularly those for whom gypsies and travellers are a regular component of the patient population, have developed policies and specialised roles to address the health needs of this specific group more effectively. An example of this can be found using the following link: www.gypsy-traveller.org/health/health-project

Search your trust intranet to identify any policies or strategies that aim to address the health issues of gypsies and travellers.

Consider how these policies and strategies could impact upon your prescribing role.

Key themes: conclusions and considerations

Public health	Specific groups have health issues that are particularly prevalent within them and most of these reflect national and international health targets. Awareness of the health issues relevant to specific groups will enable the non-medical prescriber to ensure that a holistic approach can be effectively adopted
	Consider the specific groups for whom you will prescribe and identify how you can incorporate the public health issue of accident prevention into your consultations
Social and cultural issues	For all specific groups, there will be potential for illness to have some social and cultural impact. This impact may be as a consequence of their condition or their treatment. Alternatively, it may be as a result of cultural issues and their influence on health beliefs and perceptions
	Consider your clinical practice area and identify the facilities and policies that support and/or hinder accessibility for the specific groups with which you work
Prescribing principles	The prescribing principles support the non-medical prescriber in safe and effective prescribing for specific groups
	Consider a specific group for whom you may prescribe and identify the factors taken into account and the strategies used to agree an appropriate strategy

References

Ashley C, Currie A (2008) *The Renal Drug Handbook*, 3rd edn. Oxford: Radcliffe Medical Press.

Barber N, Willson A (2007) *Clinical Pharmacy*, 2nd edn. Edinburgh: Churchill Livingstone Elsevier.

Briggs G, Freeman R, Yaffe S (2008) *Drugs in Pregnancy and Lactation*, 8th edn, Philadelphia: Lippincott Williams & Wilkins.

British Medical Association and Royal Pharmaceutical Society of Great Britain (2010) *British National Formulary 58*. London: BMA and RPSGB.

Campbell IR, Scaife JM, Johnstone JMS (1988) Psychological effects of day case surgery compared with inpatient surgery. *Arch Dis Childh* **63**: 415-17.

Churchill R, Allen J, Denman S et al (2000) Do the attitudes and beliefs of young teenagers towards general practice influence actual consultation behaviour? *Br J Gen Pract* **50**: 953-7.

Conroy S (2003) Paediatric pharmacy - drug therapy. *Hosp Pharm* **10**: 49-57.

Collis I, Lloyd G (1992) Psychiatric aspects of liver disease. *Br J Psychiatry* **161**: 12-22.

Cousineau TM, Domar AD (2007) Psychological impact of infertility. *Best Pract Res Clin Obstet Gynaecol* **21**: 293-308.

Davison SN (2007) Chronic kidney disease: psychosocial impact of chronic pain. *Geriatrics* **62**: 17-23.

Department for Children, Schools and Families (2010) *Working Together to Safeguard Children: A guide to inter-agency working to safeguard and promote the welfare of children*. London: DfCSF.

Department of Health (2001a) *National Service Framework for Older People*. London: The Stationery Office.

Department of Health (2001b) *National Service Framework: Medicines and Older People - implementing medicines-related aspects of the NSF for Older People*. London: The Stationery Office.

Department of Health (2004a) *National Service Framework for Children, Young People and Maternity Services: The Mental health and psychological wellbeing of children and young people*. London: The Stationery Office.

Department of Health (2004b) *The Health Status of Gypsies and Travellers in England*. London: TSO.

Department of Health (2004c) *Better Health in Old Age: Report from Professor Ian Philp*. London: The Stationery Office.

Department of Health (2007) *Children's Health, Our Future: A review of progress against the National Service Framework for Children, Young People and Maternity Services 2004*. London: HMSO.

Department of Health (2008) *Abortion Statistics, England and Wales: 2008*. London: The Stationery Office.

Department of Health (2009) *Commissioning Local Breastfeeding Support Services*. London: The Stationery Office.

Department of Health (2010) *Improving the Health and Well-Being of People with Long Term Conditions. World class services for people with long term conditions: Information tool for commissioners*. London: The Stationery Office.

Elliott J (2007) Thalidomide legacy lives on. *BBC News Bulletin* 8 April 2007.

Ewles L (2005) *Key Topics in Public Health, Essential Briefings on Prevention and Health Promotion*. London: Elsevier Churchill Livingstone.

Fonad E, Wahlin TR, Winbald B, Emami A, Sandmark H (2008) Falls and fall risk among nursing home residents. *J Clin Nurs* **17**: 126-34.

Greenstein B (2004) *Trounce's Clinical Pharmacology for Nurses*, 17th edn. Edinburgh: Churchill Livingstone.

Hatloy I (2010) *Statistics 3: Race, Culture and Mental Health* (online). Available at: www.mind.org.uk/help/people_groups_and_communities/statistics_3_race_culture_and_mental_health#rates (accessed 30 April 2010).

Health Professions Council (2008) *Standards of Conduct, Performance and Ethics*. London: HPC.

Health Protection Agency (2006) *Migration: A Baseline Report*. London: HPA.

Hutchinson TA (2005) Transitions in the lives of patients with end stage renal disease: a cause of suffering and an opportunity for healing. *Palliat Med* **19**: 270-7.

Information Services Division Scotland (2007) *Abortion Statistics* (online). Available at: www.isdscotland.org/isd/1919.html (accessed 30 April 2010).

Ip S, Chung M, Raman G et al (2007) Breastfeeding and maternal and infant health outcomes in developed countries. *Agency for Healthcare Research and Quality (AHRQ) Evidence Report 153*. Rockville, MA: AHRQ.

Kairuz T, Bye L, Birdsall R et al (2008) Identifying compliance issues with prescription medicines among older people: a pilot study. *Drugs Aging* **25**: 153-62.

Kirkby RJ, Whelan TA (1996) The effects of hospitalisation and medical procedures on children and their families. *J Family Stud* **2**: 65-77.

Kulmala J, Era P, Parssinen O et al (2008) Lowered vision as a risk factor for injuries accidents in older people. *Aging Clin Exp Res* **20**: 25-30.

Larsen LA (2003) Prediction of milk/plasma concentration ratio of drugs. *Ann Pharmacother* **37**: 1299-306.

Lee A, Inch S, Finnigan D (2000) *Therapeutics in Lactation*. Oxon: Radcliffe Medical Press Ltd.

Leipzig RM, Cumming RG, Tinetti ME (1999) Drugs and falls in older people: a systematic review and meta-analysis: I. Psychotropic drugs. *J Am Geriatr Soc* **47**: 30-9.

Lewis P (2008) *Drugs and the Liver*. London: Pharmaceutical Press.

Livingston S (2003) NSF for older people. (2) The older patient. *Pharmaceut J* **270**: 862-3.

Long Term Conditions Alliance Northern Ireland (2008) *Response to Proposals for Health and Social Care Reform in Northern Ireland*. Belfast: LTCANI.

Macfarlane A, McPherson A (2007) Getting it right in health services for young people. In: Coleman J, Hendry LB, Kloep M (eds), (2007) *Adolescence and Health*. Chichester: John Wiley & Sons Ltd.

Martin LM, Sheridan MJ, Younossi ZM (2007) The impact of liver disease on health-related quality of life: A review of the literature, *Current Gastroenterology Reports* **4**(1): 79-83.

National Health Service Primary Care Contracting (2009) *Primary Care Service Framework: Gypsy and traveller communities* (online). Available at: www.pcc.nhs.uk/uploads/primary_care_service_frameworks/2009/ehrg_gypsies_and_travellers_pcsf_190509.pdf (accessed 30 April 2010).

National Institute for Health and Clinical Excellence (2004) *The Assessment and Prevention of Falls in Older People*, NICE: London.

National Institute for Health and Clinical Excellence (2008) *Public Health Guidance: Occupational therapy and physical activity interventions to promote the mental wellbeing of older people in primary care and residential care*. NICE: London.

National Institute for Health and Clinical Excellence (2009) *Depression with a Chronic Physical Health Problem*. London: NICE.

National Prescribing Centre (2000) Prescribing for children. *MeReC Bull* **11**(2): 5-8.

Nursing and Midwifery Council (2007) *NMC Circular 22/2007 Prescribing for Children and Young People*. London: NMC.

Nursing and Midwifery Council (2009) *The Code Standards of Conduct, Performance and Ethics for Nurses and Midwives*. London: NMC.

Office of National Statistics (2001) *Use of Health Services: by Gender and Age, 1998-99: Social Focus on Men* (online). Available at: www.statistics.gov.uk/StatBase/ssdataset.asp?vlnk=4457&Pos=&ColRank=2&Rank=272 (accessed 13 September 2010).

Office for National Statistics (2004a) *The Health of Children and Young People* (online). Available at: www.statistics.gov.uk/children/default_print.asp (accessed 30 April 2010).

Office for National Statistics (2004b) *Ethnicity and Identity: Population size* (online). Available at: www.statistics.gov.uk/cci/nugget.asp?id=455 (accessed 30 April 2010).

Office of National Statistics (2008) *Focus on Gender – September 2008* (online). Available at: www.statistics.gov.uk/STATBASE/Product.asp?vlnk=10923 (accessed 13 September 2010).

Penza-Clyve, SM, Mansell C, McQuaid EL (2004) Why don't children take their asthma medications? A qualitative analysis of children's perspectives on adherence. *J Asthma* **41**: 189–97.

Pharmaceutical Society of Northern Ireland (2009) *Code of Ethics*. Belfast: PSNI.

Robertson S (2007) *Understanding Men and Health, Masculinities, Identity and Well-Being*. Maidenhead: Open University Press.

Royal Pharmaceutical Society of Great Britain (2004) *Medicines for Children, Fact Sheet*. London: RPSGB.

Royal Pharmaceutical Society of Great Britain (2007) *Clinical Governance Framework for Pharmacist Prescribers and Organisations Commissioning or Participating in Pharmacist Prescribing*, London: RPSGB.

Scottish Government (2009) *Improving the Health and Wellbeing of People with Long Term Conditions in Scotland: A national action plan*. Edinburgh: Scottish Government.

Simonsen T, Aarbakke J, Kay I, Coleman I, Sinnott P, Lysaa R (2006) *Illustrated Pharmacology for Nurses*. London: Hodder Arnold.

Smith JA, Braunack-Mayer A, Wittert Gand Warin M (2008) 'It's sort of like being a detective': Understanding how Australian men self-monitor their health prior to seeking help. *BMC Health Serv Res* **8**: 56.

Unicef (2006) *The Baby Friendly Initiative: Benefits of Breastfeeding* (online). Available at: www.babyfriendly.org.uk/page.asp?page=111 (accessed 18 April 2010).

UK Medicines Information (2010) *What Factors Need to be Considered when Dosing Patients with Renal Impairment* (online). Available at: www.ukmi.nhs.uk/activities/specialistServices/default.asp?pageRef=5 (accessed 26 April 2010).

Van Cleemput P (2000) Health Care Needs of Travellers. *Arch Dis Childh* **82**: 32–7.

Vickers MA, Brackley K (2002) Drugs in pregnancy. *Curr Obstet Gynaecol* **12**: 131–7.

Viner R, Booy R (2005) ABC of adolescence, epidemiology of health and illness. *BMJ* **330**: 411–14.

Walker R, Whittlesea C (2007) *Clinical Pharmacy and Therapeutics*, 4th edn. Edinburgh: Churchill Livingstone.

Waller D, Renwick A, Hillier K (2005) *Medical Pharmacology and Therapeutics*, 2nd edn. Edinburgh: Elsevier.

White Y, Grenyer BF (1999) The biopsychosocial impact of end-stage renal disease: the experience of dialysis patients and their partners. *J Adv Nurs* **30**: 1312–20.

Williams SJ, Bendelow GA, France A (2007) *Beliefs of Young People in Relation to Health, Risk and Lifestyles*, MCH 18-03(online). Available at: www.dh.gov.uk/en/Researchanddevelopment/A-Z/Motherandchildhealth/DH_4015169 (accessed 30 April 2010).

Winstanley P, Walley T (2002) *Medical Pharmacology*, 2nd edition. Edinburgh: Elsevier Science Ltd.

World Health Organization (2010) *Ten Facts about Breastfeeding* (online). Available at: www.who.int/features/factfiles/breastfeeding/facts/en/index.html (accessed 18 April 2010).

Wright J, Gray A, Goodey V (2006) *Clinical Pharmacy*. London: Pharmaceutical Press.

Chapter 9
Enhancing Non-medical Prescribing

Jean Taylor and Anne Lewis

Learning objectives

After reading this chapter and completing the activities within it, the reader will be able to:

1 critically analyse the strategic infrastructures that support non-medical prescribing practice
2 critically analyse the processes in place to support continued professional development in non-medical prescribing in relation to practice
3 identify your individual learning needs and develop an action plan to address these

Medicines are the most common healthcare intervention

National Prescribing Centre (NPC 2007a, p. 1)

Since its introduction in the 1990s, non-medical prescribing has continually evolved, with increasing groups of professionals able to prescribe. The scope of prescribing has increased in tandem. To enable non-medical prescribing to continue to develop and progress, it is vital that there is a robust infrastructure in place. This chapter initially considers the current level of non-medical prescribing practice in the UK and other parts of the world, followed by its impact on practitioners, doctors, patients and organisations. Subsequently the infrastructures that support non-medical prescribing activity and related continuing professional development are explored.

Current practice in prescribing

The NHS Plan (Department of Health (DH) 2000) heralded a new phase for the NHS where emphasis was placed on the organisation, development and delivery of services around the needs of patients. This modernisation required practitioners to work more

The Textbook of Non-medical Prescribing, edited by Dilyse Nuttall and Jane Rutt-Howard.
© 2011 Blackwell Publishing Ltd

flexibly, thus breaking down traditional roles and barriers between healthcare profes-sionals. One key way of achieving this was already under way within nurse prescribing (Daly 2006). In 1994 trained district nurses and health visitors were able to prescribe for the first time, albeit from a limited formulary. By 2004 training had been extended to all nurses along with pharmacists and consideration of some allied health profession-als (Daly 2006, Camp 2008). This was accompanied by an extension of the medicines formulary from which they could prescribe. The introduction of non-medical prescribing is an integral part of the greater agenda to modernise the NHS. However the uptake of prescribing courses was lower than the Government anticipated in the early years of inception. The time frame for reaching targets of 10 000 extended formulary independ-ent prescribers by 2004 had to be extended to 2006 with additional central funding to support this (Ryan-Woolley et al 2007).

UK history of prescribing

The history of non-medical prescribing in the UK is identified in more detail in Chapter 1, and is summarised in Table 9.1. This demonstrates a rather gradual and restrained development (Courtenay and Griffiths 2004). However, Hemingway and Ely (2009) suggest that there should be little surprise at the slow, cautious roll-out of non-medical prescribing, for two reasons. First, the successful implementation of non-medical pre-scribing is often dependent on local championing but this is in direct competition with other initiatives and priorities. Second they suggest that the NHS has a 'boom–bust' resource approach and, in the micro-world of local service planning, other issues become greater priorities. Thus, a short-term response is taken to issues rather than considering the long-term benefits of such a change in practice.

Table 9.1 The history of non-medical prescribing in the UK

1994	Limited formulary health visitors (HVs) and district nurses (DNs) (eight project sites)
1998	National for all HVs and DNs
2001	Extended nurse prescribing
2002	Supplementary nurse and pharmacist prescribing
2005	Supplementary prescribing for allied health professionals
2005	Controlled drugs allowed via supplementary prescribing for nurses
2006	Independent prescribing for pharmacists (ENPs titled independent prescribers)
2006	Independent prescribing from the full *British National Formulary* with the exception of certain controlled drugs
2007	Independent prescribing for optometrists
2009	Medicine regulation changes enable mixing of medicines before administration
2010	Consultation re other professions prescribing medication, e.g. paramedics

Department of Health statistics gained from the regulatory bodies in December 2009 suggest that there are:

- Nurse independent prescribers – over 15 000 registered on the Nursing and Midwifery Council (NMC) register
- Pharmacist independent prescribers – over 900 registered with the Royal Pharmaceutical Society of Great Britain (RPSGB)
- Allied health professionals – 295 registered with the Health Professions Council (HPC).

However, when the above data are compared with the NHS Prescription Services data, this shows that the numbers of prescribers is lower:

- Nurse independent prescribers – 12 280
- Community practitioner prescribers – 21 330
- Pharmacists – 664
- Allied health professionals – 87 (NHS Prescription Services 2009).

The difference in these figures can be explained partially by the fact that only primary care prescriptions are collated by NHS Prescription Services and thus do not include those prescribed in an acute care setting. It is also known that some practitioners who undertake a non-medical prescribing programme register with their professional body do not then go on to prescribe. This may be for a variety of reasons; some may change their job to one in which prescribing is not required, e.g. management or education; others may choose not to prescribe due to personal or organisational reasons (see Chapter 3 for a detailed exploration of these issues).

The NHS Business Authority reported that the NHS Prescription Services (2009) received 12.2 million items prescribed by nurses for processing in the year 2009 (a 13.4% increase on the previous year), 201 789 items for processing from pharmacist prescribers (an increase of 67% on the year) and 831 items from physiotherapists and chiropodists/podiatrists registered on their database.

In Scotland, the 'Information Services Division (ISD) Scotland' state that, although nurse prescribing is small in relation to GP prescribing, it has grown from fewer than 2000 prescription items in 1996-7 to over 888 000 by 2008-9. This is a volume increase of 23.8% and a cost increase of 21.6% within 2 financial years – 2007-9 (ISD Scotland 2009). This rapid increase in prescription writing indicates that prescribing is becoming integral to the role of a number of professionals other than just doctors.

Although non-medical prescribers make a significant contribution to healthcare in the UK, there is a variation in their practice and impact. Numbers will rise but, in order to meet this expansion, the provision of a responsive, supportive and facilitative learning organisation needs to be in place (Ring 2005, Avery et al 2007a, Hacking and Taylor 2010). Organisational structures are vitally important for the expansion of non-medical prescribing to provide the supportive environment that perceives this as an integral part of service development. The appointment of a non-medical prescribing lead in trusts has assisted the professional development and prescribing activity of an organisation. Non-medical prescribers who have consolidated their practice and demonstrated they are able to integrate their role within mainstream practice offer excellent role models to others (Bissell et al 2008).

Non medical prescribing signifies a major challenge to the traditional medical hierarchy with the potential to cause conflict (Bradley, Campbell and Nolan 2005) and the extension of non-medical prescribing is not without criticism (Avery el al 2007a; Ryan-Woolley et al 2007). McCartney et al (1999) suggest that prescribing has been used by the labour government to challenge the power of the medical profession. Doctors have traditionally been the only profession who had prescribing powers but by removing their control their dominance over other professions is removed. Others argued that, by allowing other professions to prescribe, the inherent expertise in prescribing is being 'dumbed down'. James et al (1999) suggest that its development is part of the quest for professional enhancement whereas Jones (2004) argues that the prescribing issue lies in the gender division territory. McCann and Baker (2002) claim, however, that it highlights the care versus cure debate, suggesting that those who prescribe place too great an emphasis on diagnostic activity and pharmacological cures rather than paying attention to caring. A counter argument to this is the suggestion that having the ability to prescribe enables practitioners to approach the care of a patient in a far more holistic way than they have done previously (Hacking and Taylor 2010).

Department of Health-funded evaluations have proclaimed prescribing as a success (Luker et al 1997, Latter et al 2005, Norman et al 2007, Bissell et al 2008). However, a central issue for the medical profession concerns the adequacy of the training received by non-medical prescribers to enable them to diagnose medical conditions, which is seen as the basis for appropriate prescribing (Ryan-Woolley et al 2007). Latter et al (2007) evaluated the clinical appropriateness of nurses prescribing by using an expert panel to analyse their clinical prescribing decisions. A medication appropriateness index (MAI) was developed, piloted and used by seven medical prescribing experts to rate the transcripts of nurse prescriber consultations. In the majority of assessments made by the expert panel, nurses' prescribing decisions were rated as clinically appropriate on all nine items of the MAI. In most instances experts considered that there was an indication for the medicine prescribed, it was effective for the condition, the dosage was correct and there was no unnecessary duplication with other medicines. Ryan-Woolley et al (2007) suggest that the evaluation studies have legitimised prescribing and have encouraged an expansion of the range of drugs that can be prescribed.

Despite all the debate, non-medical prescribing in this country is gathering momentum. Avery et al (2007b) note how the change in 'cultural philosophy' has resulted in restrictions that were first imposed being lifted and changes being introduced more frequently. The most recent amendment in December 2009 was the change to the medicines regulations to enable mixing of medicines before administration in clinical practice (DH 2010). The introduction of nurses being able to prescribe controlled drugs independently and the inclusion of paramedics in non-medical prescribing are two of the items currently being debated in the arena of non-medical prescribing. Hemingway and Ely (2009) suggest that this rapid progression of non-medical prescribing from the limited formulary in the 1990s to today's situation represents a major professional development but that it also presents new challenges, temptations and burdens for professional integrity.

Non-medical prescribing in other countries

Internationally, several healthcare systems now include some form of prescribing by non-medical healthcare professionals (Cooper et al 2008a, Creedon et al 2009). Hemingway and Ely (2009) identify a number of countries around the world where professionals, other than doctors, are prescribing, such as Africa, Australia, Canada, Ireland, New Zealand, Sweden and the USA. There is a range of prescribing models worldwide due to the international differences between legislative procedures and professional bodies responsible for regulating clinical practice (Creedon et al 2009). The UK's model of non-medical prescribing that has a nationally recognised and accredited educational programme is in contrast with other countries, such as the USA, where prescriptive authority varies from state to state in terms of independence given and competence is assessed locally (Cooper et al 2008c, Creedon et al 2009).

In Sweden, prescribing was introduced for nurses in the early 1990s, with the aim of improving patient services, reducing doctors' workload and ensuring the continuity of care by a mix of healthcare professionals in a community setting (Courtenay and Carey 2008). Swedish nurses are now able to prescribe from a restricted list of medicines and for a limited number of conditions. Prescribing in Canada and several states in Australia has been predominantly in rural areas, where there is a shortage of doctors, and where nurses work independently (Courtenay and Carey 2008) but it is restricted to nurse practitioners and they have limited prescribing rights. In New Zealand, initially as a pilot, some nurses working in child family health or care of older people were granted prescriptive authority (Lockwood and Fealy 2008). Later this was extended to nurses who worked in diabetes or asthma care, mental or occupational health, family planning or palliative care. In the USA nurse prescribing varies across the 50 states with regard to requirements, standards and practices. Courtenay and Carey (2008) suggest that there is very little evidence evaluating nurse prescribing in any of these countries, except the USA, where there is an indication that nurses are prescribing effectively, improving patient outcomes and reducing healthcare costs.

The impact of prescribing

The motivation for non-medical prescribing was quicker access to medicines, increased patient choice, more efficient delivery of services, and better use of practitioner skills and knowledge (Hawkes 2009). A number of studies have highlighted the impact that prescribing has had on prescribers, patients, doctors and the organisation as a whole.

Prescribers

The majority of studies have shown a positive impact on those practitioners who choose to prescribe (Latter et al 2005, Bradley and Nolan 2007, 2008, Drennan et al 2009, Stenner and Courtenay 2008, Carey et al 2009). Avery et al (2007b) found that practitioners had increased autonomy and job satisfaction. Watterson et al (2009) identified improved professional satisfaction and better use of staff time, whereas Pontin and Jones (2007) found relationships with pharmacists and doctors improved. Courtenay and Berry's (2007) study of 30 GPs and 31 nurses identified time/convenience, job satisfaction and professional development as advantages for the prescribers. Studies that have focused specifically on specialist nurses who prescribe have shown improvement in quality of care and patient safety (Latter et al 2005, Stenner and Courtenay 2008, Carey et al 2009).

Although nurses' evaluations of nurse prescribing have been generally positive some concerns have been identified by mental health nurses (Nolan et al 2001); student nurse prescribers (Bradley et al 2005) and early independent prescribers (Latter et al 2005). These concerns included increased responsibility and administrative workload as found by Watterson et al's (2009) national Scotland study. Courtenay and Berry's (2007) study identified the disadvantages perceived by nurses to include the lack of remuneration, limited formulary to prescribe from and increased workload, whereas doctors said that disadvantages included limited training for nurses, restricted formulary and not giving a complete service. Cooper et al (2008a, 2008b) found that pharmacists identified a number of barriers and delays after qualifying as supplementary prescribers. They reported lack of access to patients' records and information technology, time and financial limitations, and problems developing relationships with doctors.

Doctors

Initially there was a variable response by doctors to the introduction of non-medical prescribing but now doctors are generally more positive. Avery et al (2007b) found, in GP practices with a non-medical prescriber, that non-medical prescribing resulted in fewer interruptions to GP clinics and a redistribution of workload from which they benefited. Drennan et al (2009) also noted savings in time for doctors. In Watterson et al's study (2009) they noted that doctors found non-medical prescribing to be safe, that it helped patients and made their workloads more manageable, with rural GPs being particularly appreciative of this. Courtenay and Berry (2007) reported improved professional relationships, fewer interruptions, reduced workload, fewer delays in waiting for prescriptions to be signed and more detailed information about medicine. Their study also found improved time management, teamwork and delegation, leaving them free to deal with more complex cases.

However, the disadvantages identified included the level of commitment and time required to undertake the designated medical practitioner role that is required while a non-medical prescriber undertakes the qualification (Avery et al 2004, Latter et al 2005). Watterson et al (2009) found that GPs had more reservations than the national medical stakeholder group. From the evidence reviewed it seems that, if a doctor knows and works with a non-medical prescriber, he or she is more in favour of its development than general development of non-medical prescribing!

Patients

For patients, the introduction of non-medical prescribing has been perceived as generally positive, although there are few studies that actually illicit the direct views of patients having access to a wider range of practitioners other than doctors who can prescribe medication. Two studies that were completed during the first wave of non-medical prescribing (health visitors and district nurses) indicated that the initiative was largely successful. Luker et al (1997) interviewed 148 patients and Brooks et al (2001) interviewed 50 patients; both concluded that they were overwhelmingly positive about non-medical prescribing. O'Connell et al's (2009) literature review identified nine studies that investigated the patients' perspectives on nurse prescribing between 1998 and 2008. Eight of these had been carried out in the UK and one in Australia. O'Connell et al (2009) note that the findings of these studies were generally positive with most patients approving the introduction of nurse prescribing. Watterson et al (2009) completed an omnibus study in Scotland with approximately 156 people and found that respondents commented on the ease and rapidity of seeing a nurse and how this resulted in a key area of satisfaction. In addition respondents commented that they had a more in-depth conversation with nurses compared with the 'remoteness' of GPs. All the groups interviewed within Watterson et al's (2009) study noted that the perceived benefits to practice far outweighed the perceived difficulties.

Most studies reflect the views of professionals and the impact that they perceive non-medical prescribing has on patients' care. Avery et al (2007b) suggest that there tends to be universal acknowledgement of significant advantages for patients, particularly with regard to the speed of access to treatment, along with the facilitation of access for marginalised groups. Other benefits identified by Latter et al (2005), Bradley and Nolan (2007, 2008), Courtenay and Berry (2007), Stenner and Courtenay (2008), Cooper et al (2008a) and Watterson et al (2009) were the increase in patient continuity of care and access to medicines, improved compliance, fewer drug reactions, reductions in patient waiting times and less fragmentation of care. Ryan-Woolley et al (2007) found that prescribing led to patients receiving medicines more quickly and this was seen as an improvement in patient care. Watterson et al (2009) also found improved access for patients to medicines, better patient care and experiences, and that patients had confidence in this group of prescribing practitioners. In support of these findings, Latter et al (2005) note that patient satisfaction surveys suggest that non-medical prescribing is a positive step because patients identified accessibility to medicine, treatment and management as major advantages.

Organisation

The findings in relation to the organisational impact are complex and variable. The initial studies tended to highlight the difficulties associated with the lack of structures to support the implementation of non-medical prescribing, whereas later studies have identified some of these ongoing issues but have also tried to consider the economic impact of introducing this new way of working.

A number of factors have been identified as preventing independent prescribing, including limitations of formularies, local arrangement restrictions, knowledge, inability to computer generate prescriptions, lack of prescription pads, lack of access to prescribing budgets and PACT (prescribing analysis and cost tabulation) data (Latter et al 2005, Hall et al 2006, Courtenay et al 2007, Courtenay and Carey 2008, Cooper et al 2008a, 2008b, Watterson et al 2009). Whereas factors limiting supplementary prescribing identified by Courtenay and Carey (2008) in their national survey included problems implementing clinical management plans (CMPs), due to hospital policies time required to set CMPs up, and difficulties accessing records, restrictions to local arrangements, inability to generate computer prescriptions and accessing doctors. Courtenay and Carey (2008) suggest that the fact that a high percentage of nurses use supplementary prescribing despite implementation problems and the availability of independent prescribing demonstrate that there is a need for supplementary prescribing. They suggest that it may be a result of nurses gaining confidence re prescribing, treating patients with multiple pathologies, but this requires further exploration.

Avery et al (2007b) found that there was some evidence of cost savings. Cooper et al (2008a) noted the organisational benefits in terms of better utilisation of economic and human resources, e.g. the introduction and expansion of non-medical prescribing in community clinical practice has led to time saving for community nurses who no longer need to wait outside GP surgeries for prescriptions to be signed. Their time and skills are used more appropriately. Patients are seen, their needs assessed and prescribing decisions made in a timely manner (Drennan et al 2009, Watterson et al 2009). There are fewer repeat prescriptions or medications wasted because non-medical prescribers prescribe in amounts appropriate to the patient's needs and explain and engage with patients, leading to better understanding and concordance. There is improved patient safety due to regular review and adherence to agreed local joint formularies. This has enabled rationalisation of products prescribed to promote safe and cost-effective prescribing by non-medical prescribers.

Trusts review the proportion of qualified non-medical prescribers who are actively prescribing in any period of time, aiding the identification of potential barriers to prescribing so adequate support can be provided. In primary care trusts (PCTs) prescribing data are analysed at prescriber or locality level to identify reasons for high cost prescription items. Expenditure trends for non-medical prescribing can also be determined. Although PACT data are not available for secondary care settings, many acute trusts have developed strategies to monitor non-medical prescribing activity.

Issues emerging from the introduction of non-medical prescribing

With the inception of non-medical prescribing a number of topics are discussed regularly in journal articles, including the following:

- Numeracy and prescribing errors
- Lack of writing prescriptions once qualified as a non-medical prescriber
- Ageing workforce
- Infrastructures to support non-medical prescribing – including clinical governance, clinical audit, PACT data and clinical guidelines
- Continuing professional development – including reflective practice, clinical supervision and appraisal.

Numeracy and prescribing errors

Poor numeracy among healthcare staff has been a concern to healthcare providers for many years (Warburton et al 2010). These problems with numeracy have led to medication errors among healthcare staff. Griffiths and Courtenay (2007) comment that 'everyday about 2.5 million medicines are prescribed in the community and in hospitals in England'. National Patient Safety Agency (NPSA 2007) noted that 72 482 medication incident reports occurred between 1 January and 31 December 2007. Incidents involving medicines was the third largest group (9%) of all incidents reported. Most of the medicines incidents (96%) had actual clinical outcomes of no or low harm. Acute care remains the highest reporter of all incidents (73%). Next highest is primary care (14%) and mental health is the third highest with 9%.

Dornan et al (2009) also note that prescribing errors are common and can result in adverse events and harm to patients. This research reviewed 124 260 medication orders by first year foundation trainee doctors (FY1) across 19 hospitals in the north west of the UK. Of these, an error rate of 8.9% was noted (i.e. 11 077 medication orders contained errors). Potentially lethal errors were found in fewer than 2% erroneous prescriptions. The report stressed that very few prescribing errors caused harm to patients because almost all were intercepted and corrected before reaching them. Dornan el at (2009) noted that the intervention of nurses, senior doctors and, in particular, pharmacists was vital in picking up errors before impacting on patients.

The implementation of non-medical prescribing and the safety concern of medication prescribing errors have led to the introduction of entry standards and assessment criteria for all nursing programmes (Nursing and Midwifery Council (NMC) 2006). However, Warburton et al (2010) note that there is no national approach to numeracy assessment and the application of the NMC (2006) standards varies across higher education institutions. In response to this the NHS in the north west established a numeracy consortium and developed an online numeracy assessment tool for use in the region by all practitioners who wanted to access a non-medical prescribing programme (Warburton et al 2010). The use of this numeracy assessment tool, since its introduction in June 2007, has resulted in the identification of poor numeracy skills, thus enabling practitioners to be given appropriate support. In addition its usage has resulted in increasing the awareness of the importance of numeracy skills and also reducing anxiety in the non-medical prescribing students (Warburton et al 2010). The specific significance of sound numeracy skills in prescribing is explored in Chapter 7.

Lack of writing prescriptions once qualified as a non-medical prescriber

A number of studies have highlighted the number of practitioners who undertake the non-medical prescribing education programme, enabling them to prescribe, but choose not to actually write a prescription. Larsen (2004) found that 40% were not prescribing after completion of a non-medical prescribing programme. Ryan-Woolley et al's (2007) study of Macmillan nurses found that almost 50% of those who undertook and successfully completed an extended formulary independent nurse prescribing education programme did not prescribe. Gray et al (2005) found that only 51% of mental health nurses trained were actually practising as prescribers. This low uptake of prescribing in practice is much higher than other studies where the percentage has been less than 20%. Latter et al (2005) found that 14% of those who had qualified did not go onto to prescribing whereas Hacking and Taylor (2010) found that 17% of respondents did not prescribe once qualified. In the latter study although a number of those respondents clarified that, even though they were not actually prescribing, they were using their skills and knowledge in providing holistic care to their patients.

Ageing workforce

A number of studies show that the typical prescriber is a mature and highly experienced professional (Avery et al 2007a, 2007b, Courtenay and Carey 2008, Watterson et al 2009, Hacking and Taylor 2010, Kelly et al 2010). Kelly et al (2010) found that a third of their 151 sample of practice nurses were aged 50 years or over and so would be expected to retire within 15 years, thus having significant implications for future service delivery. Watterson et al (2009) also suggest that the age profile of the nurse prescribing workforce may prove problematic and be more difficult to address, but acknowledge that this is part of a wider debate about the workforce planning in Scotland.

Considering the ageing workforce from the specific perspective of community specialist practitioners and V100 prescribers, workforce projections reflect this depletion which has led to the advent of the V150 prescriber. The entry requirements for the V150 education programmes, coupled with the lack of community specialist practitioner prescribing mentors means that there is considerable preparation and support required to develop this workforce. However, the increasing shift to care in the community, with more complex care required, as well as the introduction of the case care management model, mean there is a greater need for practitioners with prescribing skills than ever before.

Although there is a need for V150 prescribers to support community nursing teams, there is increasing requirement to develop V300 prescribers. Community trusts are charged with keeping people out of hospital, with a particular focus on those with long-term and chronic conditions. This requires increased development of specialist roles across all disciplines, and will require appropriate marketing and recruitment strategies with relevant support structures.

The Department of Health's *Transforming Community Services* (DH 2009a) agenda, with the focus on managing long-term conditions, will lead to the expansion of many existing roles as well as new developments. These roles will include community matrons, prison practitioners and diabetes specialist nurses, all requiring prescribing skills. The introduction or expansion of community assessment centres, walk-in centres and one-stop shops (multipurpose buildings offering a range of services) will require first-contact practitioners who are multiskilled in order to increase access and improve patient experience and safety, in line with Lord Darzi's (DH 2008) quality agenda. The skills required will include advanced diagnostic and assessment skills, as well as the ability to make prescribing decisions.

The NHS Operating Framework for England 2010/11 (DH 2009b) and the accompanying document *NHS 2010-15: From good to great* (DH 2009c), with the focus on productivity, prevention and people-centred care, has led organisations to embark on extensive pieces of work to introduce a care and case management model into community services. This will provide a systematic and coordinated approach to managing patients, in particular those with long-term conditions, and maintaining them in the community setting. It will involve delivery of integrated care across organisational boundaries and require a mix of practitioners able to respond to the varying needs of the client groups based on the principle of ensuring 'right skills, right place, right time'. It is envisaged that a full complement of clinicians and support practitioners will be required to provide the integrated case and care management approach planned for community services. A detailed projection has demonstrated the need for non-medical prescribers with both nursing and therapy skills to support this model.

These changes in care provision, roles and ways of working are not restricted to primary care. Reductions in hospital admissions must be supported by efficient and effective care for those patients who do require secondary care-based services. Non-medical prescribing is a key instrument in achieving this, with many hospital-based practitioners developing extended and advanced roles.

Infrastructures

There are a plethora of structures present in the area of non-medical prescribing, ranging from local to national, from individual to organisational, from general to specific. For some individual non-medical prescribers, the range of available support processes and tools can be overwhelming, whereas for others they feel unsupported and isolated (Kelly et al 2010).

From an organisational perspective, non-medical prescribing will come under the umbrella of the trust's clinical governance frameworks. Often though there are additional mechanisms available to support practitioners who undertake prescribing as part of their clinical practice. Each trust has a named non-medical prescribing lead. The amount of time that this lead may have dedicated to this post is variable (Hacking and Taylor 2010). Some prescribing leads are very involved in offering support either individually to practitioners or through a group mechanism. Some of these group sessions are about providing current information in relation to policy and procedures, sharing good practice and experiences, and supporting newly appointed prescribers whether independent, supplementary or community nursing practitioner prescribers. In addition, on a national basis, health authority representatives regularly meet with Department of Health representatives to consider policy development and discuss professional/practice issues re prescribing.

At an individual level, practitioners may access support from a wide range of resources including their colleagues, medical practitioners/mentors, medicines management team, managers and databases (e.g. Department of Health, NHS Clinical Knowledge Summaries (CKS), National Prescribing Centre).

The Department of Health (2006) clearly identified that non-medical prescribers should be supported through local support forums. It is just that this support varies across the country. Bradley et al (2005) highlighted how the success of non-medical prescribing may depend on organisational support coupled with a robust continuing professional development (CPD) strategy for all prescribers. While and Biggs (2004) noted the importance of a supportive environment and associated infrastructure for nurturing the role of non-medical prescribing. Regular discussions with other members of the care team, clinical supervision and employer-circulated information have also been identified as helpful support mechanisms (While and Biggs 2004). Ryan-Woolley et al's (2007) national survey of specialist Macmillan nurses found that having a supportive organisational and team network were key factors in assisting practitioners to prescribe within a cancer and palliative care area. In addition, having appropriate arrangements put in place by their employing trust was another notable factor, particularly because, on completion of a non-medical prescribing education programme, some practitioners had been unable to prescribe due to the necessary mechanisms not being in place.

McKay (2007) found that in 2004 only 30% of non-medical prescribers had access to a support forum within the Kent and Medway Strategic Health Authority. In response to this, the provision of support became a priority and, by 2005, 65% of non-medical prescribers had access to support forums. Despite this, however, the biggest challenge was getting staff to attend, given the other demands that they had. Those who attended recognised the benefits of such mechanisms including the opportunity to network and exchange ideas, which McKay (2007) argues can be a powerful initiator of change. If facilitated well, support forums can enable non-medical prescribers to reflect on their prescribing practice with their peers, network and address common issues that impact on prescribing practice (McKay 2007).

Clinical governance

There is a vast array of literature with regard to the concept of clinical governance. Information can be accessed at national, strategic and local levels. Although services have developed in the NHS since its inception, it was recognised that there were no formal structures to ensure the quality of services. Focus initially was upon quantities, e.g. waiting times, numbers of operations. The emphasis on outcomes did not acknowledge the subject of processes and thus was highlighted as missing (McKinnon 2007). The main political shift through the introduction of clinical governance was the change from making management decisions to that of service provision based on quality and clinical need (McKinnon 2007).

Clinical governance was first introduced in 1998 with the Government's policy document *A First Class Service: Quality in the new NHS* (DH 1998). Its central issue in clinical governance is the enhancement of patient outcomes at least cost. The clinical governance agenda is associated more closely with the term 'quality'. The National Clinical Governance Support Team put patient professional partnership as the pinnacle of their 'temple model'. The seven pillars holding the temple up are the elements of clinical governance identified as:

1 Clinical effectiveness
2 Risk management
3 Communication effectiveness
4 Resource effectiveness
5 Strategic effectiveness
6 Learning effectiveness
7 Patient experience.

Traditionally clinical governance has been defined using these seven key pillars. More recently it has been refined but this approach remains the easiest way to remember and describe clinical governance.

Professionals could not ignore this particular document because each trust had to produce an annual report on clinical governance issues. Although chief executives were made accountable for assuring the quality of the service, clinical involvement was secured by the requirement for a designated senior clinician to take responsibility for ensuring that clinical governance systems were in place and their effectiveness monitored. By placing this high on the agenda, it was apparent that quality reports on clinical care should be given the same importance as financial reports in the aims and management of every trust (Morris and Footit 2003). Consequently within each trust, processes have been developed for the continuous monitoring and improvement of the quality of healthcare that is delivered.

In addition to trust structures to support clinical governance, the establishment of the National Institute for Health and Clinical Excellence (NICE), Social Care Institute for Excellence (SCIE) and the production of National Service Frameworks (NSFs) are the tools by which standards for much of the clinical care are set throughout the country. The Care Quality Commission (CQC) was established in April 2009 and is the independent regulator of health, mental health and adult social care services in England. The CQC replaces previous regulatory functions carried out by the Healthcare Commission, the Commission for Social Care Inspection and the Mental Health Act Commission. The CQC regulates **all** health and social care providers whether NHS, local authorities, private companies or voluntary/third sector organisations, and is focused on ensuring that people get better care. This is achieved by (CQC 2009a):

- driving improvement across health and adult social care
- putting people first and championing their rights
- acting swiftly to remedy bad practice
- gathering and using knowledge and expertise, and working with others.

The legislative background for compliance is the Health and Social Care Act 2008 (Regulated Activities) Regulations 2009, and the CQC (Registration) Regulations 2009. Further information on the role and function of the CQC can be found at the website: www.cqc.org.

All providers of health and social care must be registered with the CQC in order to deliver services. If registration is not approved, organisations cannot operate as providers of healthcare. Therefore, it is imperative that organisations can demonstrate that they meet the requirements of registration.

The CQC has produced the essential standards for quality and safety (CQC 2009b), which organisations are expected to achieve in order to be registered as providers. The standards focus on respecting patients' dignity and protecting rights, and on outcomes of care rather than systems and processes. The views and experiences of people who use services are central to the system. Each provider will be reviewed for compliance formally every 2 years, but unannounced visits can occur at any time with little or no notice. Failure to meet the registration requirements can result in a range of enforcement actions, including: warning notices; applying conditions of registration; suspension of registration (pending action/improvement); and cancellation of registration. This represents a radical change to the regulatory framework surrounding the provision of healthcare and will require a more stringent approach to the way that organisations demonstrate the standard of care delivered.

The regulations that must be met are contained within the Health and Social Care Act 2008. They are reflected as 28 outcomes grouped into six key areas:

1 Involvement and information
2 Personalised care, treatment and support
3 Safeguarding and safety
4 Quality and management
5 Suitability of staffing
6 Suitability of management.

Not all outcomes relate to NHS providers. Of the 16 outcomes relevant to the NHS, outcome 9, management of medicines, is key to provision of safe and effective care for non-medical prescribers. Outcome 9 that states people who use services:

- Will have their medicines at the times they need them, and in a safe way.
- Wherever possible will have information about the medicine being prescribed made available to them or others acting on their behalf.

This is because providers who comply with the regulations will:

- Handle medicines safely, securely and appropriately.
- Ensure that medicines are prescribed and given by people safely.
- Follow published guidance about how to use medicines safely.

CQC (2009b, p. 104)

Community providers are also required to meet the requirements of the NHS community contract agreed with their commissioners. This covers a comprehensive set of requirements including: CQC registration requirements, national targets and vital signs; quality (patient safety, experience and clinical outcomes); business delivery targets; strategic enablers; assurance; and accreditation. Detailed specifications for every service commissioned, which includes service descriptions, models, activity, key performance indicators, targets, finance and reporting requirements, underpin and drive the contract. Medicines management and non-medical prescribing are among many elements that will be performance managed as part of the contract.

The Commissioning for Quality and Innovation (CQUIN) payment framework allows all local health communities to develop their own schemes to encourage quality improvement, and recognise innovation by making a proportion of provider income conditional on locally agreed goals. The CQUIN payment framework aims to support a cultural shift by embedding quality improvement and innovation as part of the commissioner-provider discussion everywhere. It was introduced in April 2009, requiring a proportion of provider contract value to be linked to the achievement of locally agreed ambitious quality improvement goals (or, in the first year, a simpler quality improvement plan for non-acute providers). Locally agreed CQUIN schemes are required to include goals in the three domains of quality - safety, effectiveness and patient experience - and to reflect innovation. An example of CQUIN indicators for medicines management for community providers include: compliance with medicines policy and patient group direction training; uplift in the ratio of non-medical prescribing; medical prescribing for wound management and other dressings; and reduction on net ingredient cost/item for wound management and other dressings.

Clinical governance is now viewed as a well embedded tool which the government uses to achieve the aims of *The NHS Plan* (DH 2000) to ensure that there is safe, effective, high-quality care that is patient centred. Organisations and their employers are responsible for ensuring that all care conforms to the principles of clinical governance and this provides the basis on which trusts will evidence compliance with CQC registration requirements. Thus, there are clear implications for non-medical prescribing practice, involving risk management (e.g. critical incident reporting), audit, evaluation of clinical effectiveness, quality assurance mechanisms, and research and development. It is also expected that non-medical prescribers achieve and maintain appropriate skills and knowledge and that they are supported by their employing organisation because they have a duty to support their staff in maintaining and building on their competence. Halligan (2006) refers to clinical governance as being the 'organisational conscience'. It is expected that there is a partnership between employer and employee to improve patient care based on evidence-based practice. Non-medical prescribing is a particularly difficult field to work in, because new evidence is emerging constantly and the cost implications are becoming increasingly more important in the current economic climate.

In addition the government has introduced the NHS Quality, Innovation, Productivity and Prevention Challenge (QIPP). This charges organisations to seek local solutions to improving productivity and eliminating waste while focusing relentlessly on clinical quality. The NHS needs to identify £15-20 billion of efficiency savings by the end of 2013-14 (DH 2009b) that can be reinvested in the service to continue to deliver year-on-year quality improvements. This is a huge challenge that will require everyone in the NHS to focus on maximising the quality of care provided through efficient use of resources, as well as improving the experience of patients and public. The government believes that focusing on the four components of quality, innovation, productivity and prevention will enable us to meet that challenge. A national programme of work streams has been set up to support clinical teams and NHS organisations to succeed. Work streams focusing on long-term conditions, urgent care and end-of-life pathways are looking at improving quality and productivity across care pathways. Innovation and prevention will be key enablers for achieving the quality and productivity gains required. The introduction of new roles and ways of working, including the case and care management model, will require an increasing role for non-medical prescribing that can and will provide a key element in achieving these gains.

Activity box 9.1

Using the CQC document *Essential Standards of Quality and Safety* (CQC 2009b) (available at www.cqc.org.uk) as a guide, consider your own prescribing practice against outcome 9, management of medicines:

- How do these outcomes relate to your practice?
- How do you as a non-medical prescriber meet these requirements?
- What systems and processes support you to demonstrate the outcomes?

The Department of Health have also produced guidelines for both independent (DH 2006) and supplementary (DH 2005) prescribers to follow. Both these guidance documents require that organisations underpin non-medical prescribing with a robust clinical governance framework (Mills 2008). These frameworks aim to ensure that non-medical prescribing will:

- ensure that patient safety is paramount
- benefit both patient and the NHS
- ensure good communication between all prescribers and access to shared records
- include voluntary partnerships with patients as partners in their care
- provide appropriate educational preparation and CPD to ensure maintenance of competency.

The clinical governance framework is embedded in the non-medical prescribing policy to which all non-medical prescribers must adhere. The following are examples of strategies that can be incorporated into non-medical prescribing policy to support clinical governance and contribute to the provision of safe, effective, appropriate high-quality healthcare.

Non-medical prescriber database
A live register of all non-medical prescribers, giving contact details, prescribing status, scope of practice, CPD and review status.

Intention to prescribe, scope of practice statement
Completed by all non-medical prescribers and agreed by the service manager on qualification and reviewed annually thereafter. This describes prescribing areas, how competency is maintained, details of supervision and audit/evaluation of practice.

NHS Knowledge and Skills Framework (KSF)
Personal development review (PDR): an annual requirement for all staff, which includes review of the scope of practice statement and ePACT data.

Are you still prescribing statements?
An annual review of all prescribers to determine those who are and are not prescribing, CPD undertaken or needed, and barriers to prescribing. Subsequent action to support those not prescribing can be taken as appropriate.

Analysis of PACT data
On an individual, service/discipline and by product or cost basis.

Partnerships with education providers and strategic health authorities
To ensure and enable robust selection procedures and programmes that are fit for purpose and meet service needs.

CPD provision
The organisation has responsibility for supporting identification of development needs through KSF review and provision of CPD opportunities according to needs identified,

including provision of opportunity for peer support and clinical supervision. Individual non-medical prescribers are responsible for identifying needs, participating in CPD opportunities and maintaining competency through self-directed learning.

Clinical supervision

This process assists with the ongoing development of individual non-medical prescribers and can also be used as a useful support mechanism for newly qualified non-medical prescribers through a 'buddy' system approach.

Non-medical prescribing forums at non-medical prescribing leads and practitioner levels

Networking, discussing lessons learnt, sharing of information and good practice have been found to be very beneficial (Hacking and Taylor 2010).

Standard operating procedures

For example, for handwriting a prescription, ordering and obtaining prescriptions, security and safe handling of prescription pads, dealing with lost or stolen prescriptions, reporting medicine-related incidents, prescribing errors.

Audit of practice

The NHS North West has developed the non-medical prescribing e-audit. This is a computer system designed to measure a trust's readiness to embrace non-medical prescribing policy implementation. It does so by allowing trusts to carry out an open self-assessment of non-medical prescribing systems and progress at a given time. The self-assessment, or audit, comprises six sections that cover areas ranging from organisational strategies to non-medical prescriber communication:

1 Trust information/responsibilities
2 Policies/strategies/risk management and liability
3 Prescriber information
4 Reports/data/systems
5 Communication and support groups
6 CPD/mentorship and support/peer review/training/selection.

By completing the audit and producing the reports, organisations can understand their strengths and weaknesses. The audit also helps to build a growing non-medical prescribing evidence base, which enables organisations to benchmark performance, articulate demand and identify priorities.

Healthcare professionals have a duty of care and a responsibility for the wellbeing of their patients. Clinical governance is one of the frameworks that are in place to support them to do this successfully.

Clinical audit

Clinical audit is seen as a central component of clinical governance. According to the National Clinical Audit Advisory Group (2009) it is:

The assessment of the process (using evidence-based criteria) and/or the outcome of care (by comparison with others). Its aim is to stimulate and support national and local quality improvement interventions and, through re-auditing, to assess the impact of such interventions.

The audit cycle outlines the various stages that a practitioner needs to undertake to ensure that it is carried out in a systematic manner. Initially standards are identified and then data is collected on current practice. The collected data is analysed and compared to the identified standards. This may result in the necessity to change and improve practice. Once a plan has been agreed this should be implemented and the practice is reaudited again a few months later. Detailed guidance of the audit process is provided by NICE who published *Principles for Best Practice in Clinical Audit* in 2002. This process is summarised as follows:

- Prepare for audit
- Select criteria
- Measure performance
- Make improvements
- Sustain improvement.

The Healthcare Quality Improvement Partnership (HQIP) was established in April 2008 to promote quality in healthcare, and in particular its overall aim is to increase the impact that clinical audit has on healthcare quality in England and Wales. The use of the clinical audit process is a valuable tool for non-medical prescribers because it can be used to justify and evaluate the individual's prescribing practice, as well as highlighting practice around the use of specific medication usage and its impact on patient outcomes.

Activity box 9.2

Look at a recently completed audit report within your clinical area:

- Can you identify the criteria and standards used to compare current practice against?
- Is it evidence based?
- What impact has the completion of the audit had upon practice?

PACT data

Monitoring of prescribing habits is expected by governing bodies such as the NMC and DH (2006). Within primary care, this is facilitated by the provision of prescribing analysis and cost tabulation (PACT) data. At an organisational level this data is used to monitor and control prescribing cost and also to set prescribing budgets. At an individual practitioner level it is used by practitioners to audit and improve their prescribing practice (Lovejoy and Savage 2001). PACT reports provide feedback to individual prescribers on the data on quantities and cost of items prescribed as a comparison of prescribing performance against quality indicators such as the prescribing of drugs of limited clinical value. Such feedback is disseminated via PACT reports which can also be supplemented by visits from a professional prescribing adviser on behalf of the PCT. As a result of PACT data health authorities and PCTs have introduced local formularies that have helped to control costs by limiting prescribing to those items that are considered to be cost-effective, and promote quality by familiarising prescribers with a restricted range of products (Hall et al 2004).

However, PACT data is unavailable for most people prescribing within an acute care setting. Morran (2007) identifies why they have difficulties collating such data:

- Paucity of electronic prescribing to support the gathering of data in hospital settings
- Use of inpatient drug cards creates difficulties identifying non-medical and medical prescribing.

Prescriptions within secondary care are commonly documented on hospital drug cards, which accommodate multiple prescriptions often by multiple prescribers. Therefore the use of PACT data to analyse and monitor individual prescribing habits is not possible. Although pharmacy units within hospitals can monitor the quantity of drugs used by different departments through their ordering schemes, they are unable to track individual prescribing activity. As a result some areas have introduced their own audit schemes to monitor prescribing activity of non-medical prescribers. Morran (2007) documents the approach taken by Derby Hospitals NHS Foundation Trust.

Clinical guidelines

Hall et al (2004) suggest that there has been a proliferation of guidelines produced to assist practitioners in a wide variety of clinical roles. Clinical guidelines can be defined as 'recommendations for the care of individuals by healthcare professionals; they are based on the best available evidence' (NICE 2010). Hall et al (2006) suggest that these guidelines can be seen as attempts by the government and professional bodies to improve the quality of patient care.

Many healthcare organisations support the introduction of clinical guidelines in order to improve patient care, reduce variations in patient care and control costs. Hall et al (2006) refer to a number of studies that clearly show that practitioners do not adhere to these frequently. In their study they found that the more inexperienced used them more.

Activity box 9.3

Identify the specific guidelines that you use to guide your prescribing practice.

Choose one of these guidelines and critically analyse its application to your practice area. Consider the factors that support your ability to adhere to the guidelines and those which hinder it.

Continuing professional development

The introduction and roll-out of non-medical prescribing are part of the Government's aim to modernise the health service in making it accessible and responsive to patient needs. As greater numbers of professionals across a wide range of healthcare settings, with an increasing range of medicines, are able to use acquired prescribing powers, this increases the points of access that patients have to obtaining medicines (Latter et al 2005). It is imperative that safety and efficacy are paramount in this context. However, health professionals would argue that these are essential principles that underpin their practice as a whole. Individual health professionals have a responsibility to engage in CPD capabilities in order to maintain and enhance skills and knowledge. CPD helps individual practitioners to turn that accountability into a positive opportunity to achieve career objectives. In addition, the credibility of any profession is based on the willingness of individuals to embrace new skills, knowledge and experiences (Chartered Institute of Personnel and Development (CIPD) 2009).

CPD is also about a personal commitment to keeping professional knowledge up to date and improving one's abilities. It focuses on what you learn and how you develop through your career. CPD isn't a fixed process but should involve setting objectives for development and then recording progress towards achieving these. It can involve questioning where you want to be and how you plan to get there. The focus is based on reflecting on how the objectives were achieved rather than the 'time spent' on achieving them (CIPD 2009).

The importance of CPD is emphasised by all the professional bodies involved in non-medical prescribing (i.e. Health Professions Council (HPC), NMC, General Pharmaceutical Council (GPhC), Pharmaceutical Society of Northern Ireland (PSNI) and the College of Optometrists) in order to maintain competence and enhance patient safety.

The HPC (2009) define CPD as:

> ... a range of learning activities through which health professionals maintain and develop throughout their career to ensure that they retain their capacity to practice safely, effectively and legally within their evolving scope of practice.

Put simply, CPD is the way that health professionals continue to learn and develop throughout their careers so that they keep their skills and knowledge up to date and are able to work safely, legally and effectively. PSNI introduced CPD as a professional requirement in 2005 as 'part of a system of good clinical governance' (PSNI 2010). The importance of CPD is also reflected in the recently published GPhC (2010) standards for mandatory CPD for pharmacists. There is a variety of different ways of achieving CPD, which can include self-directed study, attending workshops or educational programmes, visiting other clinical areas, sharing good practice with other practitioners and support forums. Latter et al (2005) found that nurses used a variety of resources to keep up to date with clinical developments, e.g. conferences, support groups, journals. Courtenay and Gordon (2009) found that the preferred method of learning was e-learning (60% of 546 respondents), followed closely by day time meetings (55%) and 36% distance learning. The key to CPD is that individuals capture useful experiences and reflects on the benefits of what they have learned (CIPD 2009).

A wide range of evidence-based resources exists for non-medical prescribers to use. Various websites are available, such as www.cks.nhs.uk (Clinical Knowledge Summaries, formerly Prodigy), which is an online source of evidence-based information about common conditions managed in primary care and first contact care. The site provides practical guidance on how to reach a diagnosis, available treatment options and when to refer to a specialist for assessment or management. Clinical Knowledge Summaries is commissioned by NHS Evidence, which is provided by NICE. In addition national service frameworks that support good practice in a range of areas such as cancer services, coronary heart disease and care of older people can be used. At a local level trusts also provide formularies and clinical guidelines for practitioners to use. Many non-medical prescribers have contributed to the development of such tools within their own employing organisation. In addition the National Prescribing Centre (NPC) also provides learning support to newly qualified practitioners.

Courtenay et al (2007) found that 58% reported that they had accessed CPD since qualifying as a non-medical prescriber whereas 32% had reported CPD to be inaccessible. In a later study, however, Carey and Courtenay (2010) found that over 80% had accessed CPD to support their prescribing role and only 20% had no access to CPD due to lack of facilities, funding or workload. Bradley et al (2005) found that 16% of 91 respondents undertaking a non-medical prescriber's programme identified concerns about the availability of support for CPD once they had qualified. Stenner and Courtenay (2008) found the difficulties included accessing support at an appropriate level, lack of funding and protected learning time. Franklin (2009) found that a lack of supervision and CPD was one of the main areas identified as limiting community practitioner nurse prescribers' prescribing practice. Carey and Courtenay (2010) found over 40% of nurses had CPD needs in relation to prescribing policy and pharmacological knowledge (32% of 439 participants surveyed). Courtenay and Gordon (2009) found that over 50% (of 546 nurses) identified assessment and diagnosis as a need. Assessment and diagnosis skills are prerequisites for prescribing education (NMC 2006) and so the reason for such large numbers requiring this type of CPD is unclear. Courtenay and Gordon (2009) go on to suggest that this may reflect the government's policy (DH 2006) that nurses continue to develop their prescribing practice once qualified and therefore require additional education and support.

Burnham (2006) argues that it is imperative that non-medical prescribers maintain and develop their skills as prescribers because poor prescribing costs the NHS billions of pounds annually. Kelly et al (2010) suggest that the professional lead for practice nurses is crucial for raising the local profile of nurse prescribing and facilitating training needs. Training would include CPD and clinical supervision for practice nurses who already hold the prescribing qualification.

In addition, Bradley et al (2005) suggest that prescribing may represent a way of advancing the health professional's role and increasing the morale within the workforce. CPD is vital to support this role and it is imperative that organisations make time available for health professionals to update their knowledge. Future research is required to examine the nature and extent of CPD required for this purpose (Bradley et al 2005, p. 446).

Activity box 9.4

How do you maintain competency in prescribing practice?

List the CPD activities that you have undertaken in the past 3 years.

Reflect on the different approaches that you have taken and identify those that have had the most impact on your practice.

Maintaining competence in practice and CPD

Prescribed medicine is the most common form of medical intervention, accounting for almost 15% of all health expenditure. The NHS spent £8 billion on medicines in England *in* 2005.

NPC (2007b, p. 5)

Competency can be described as a mix of knowledge skills and attitudes. Competencies enable individuals to assess and review how they perform in their role. By developing and enhancing role competencies, individuals can improve their performance and work more effectively (NPC 2007b). The NPC have developed a number of competency frameworks to enable prescribers to do this and these can be found at the website: www.npc.co.uk/prescribers/competency_frameworks.htm.

Reflective practice

Non-medical prescribers are encouraged to reflect on their practice at both an individual level and within their teams. Reflection is a process of learning from different life experiences. It helps us to learn about ourselves, others, our job and the employing organisation. Professional bodies highlight the benefits of reflective practice in their learning strategies (McClure 2005). This reflection can be achieved by using a reflective model to assist a structured approach to reflection, enabling practitioners to evaluate their own practice, and identify gaps in knowledge and areas for further development. There is whole range of models to choose from and practitioners are advised to use one that suits them best (Bulman and Shutz 2008).

Activity box 9.5

Choose a reflective model to think about a recent prescribing event, incidence or experience.

Follow the prompters of the model to guide your reflection. These prompters may include:

- Describe the event, incident or experience
- What happened?
- How did you feel?
- What did you do and why?
- What went well?
- What could have been better?
- What would you do different next time?
- What have you learnt from this experience?
- How will it impact on your future practice?

Clinical supervision

Clinical supervision helps practitioners to expand their knowledge base, become clinically more proficient and gain confidence in their practice settings. Studies have shown that workplace peer support, mentoring and clinical supervision are key factors in maintaining practitioners prescribing competence in practice (Humphries and Green 2000, Hacking and Taylor 2010). By joining in with other groups or accessing non-medical prescribing forums to assess evidence, critical skills are further honed.

Appraisal

McKay (2007) noted that 78% of prescribers felt that their prescribing practice should be appraised. The process of feedback, reflection and learning can be seen as an improvement tool in changing practice and behaviour. The use of PACT data can also be part of this process too. McKay (2007) found that the respondents suggested a number of models of appraisal including formally with a manager, informally with a prescribing lead, peer appraisal, by a medical prescriber or by another designated medical practitioner. These findings suggest that there are many ways to consider appraisal and it may be based on an individual's choice, although this needs to be balanced with the needs of the organisation that has a responsibility to manage their staff performance in a constructive and supportive manner. Appraisal is an essential part of clinical governance. The difficulty is whether the line manager is the most appropriate individual to undertake this activity. The NHS KSF (DH 2004) and its accompanying process are already in place in a number of organisations, but it needs to be acknowledged that it is difficult to feed the relationship of prescribing with performance into the appraisal process (McKay 2007).

Medicines management

Medicines management is defined as 'a system of processes and behaviours that determines how medicines are used by the health service and patients' (NPC 2008). Reports have indicated that 6.5% of patients admitted to hospital and up to 9% of those who stay in hospital experience medication-related harm (Crocker 2009). Medicines management can be seen as a broad concept that includes a comprehensive range of activities and procedures, from the development of new drugs through to the choice of medication by a prescriber to the use of medicines by a patient. This is explored in more depth in Chapter 5.

Patients have their care delivered by a range of healthcare professionals and therefore, in order to ensure that medicines are well managed across a health community that covers a range of healthcare organisations, the NPC (2007a) strongly advise that all stakeholder organisations are involved in a collaborative approach. The NPC recommend that, as there are clinical and financial risks and benefits associated with medicines, they are best managed using a collaborative approach. Area prescribing and medicines management committees (APCs) or their equivalents were introduced in an attempt to manage more effectively the entry of new drugs into the NHS. As time has progressed the NPC acknowledge that the environment in which they were first introduced has changed considerably and there is a significant variation in the way that APCs operate across the country today. The National Audit Office (NAO 2007a) concluded that a coordinated approach to prescribing across primary and secondary care sectors is one of the key ways of improving the value for money of prescribing. They reported that PCTs could save more than £200 million a year without compromising patient care if GPs prescribed cheaper, generic medicines (NAO 2007a). These findings have now been confirmed by Keele University who calculated that almost £400 million has been saved by the Department of Health, the NHS and PCTs in England, through more cost-effective prescribing as recommended in the NAO (2007b) report.

Bradley et al (2005) found that, although the literature highlights that nurses are well placed to monitor the impact of prescribed medication on their patients, only 14% of their respondents identified that they had a role in medication management, monitoring side effects and early signs of relapse. They suggest that, if medicines management does not become part of the prescribing role, there is a possibility that prescribing will be seen as an isolated technical skill.

Conclusion

This chapter has considered the current level of non-medical prescribing in this country and its subsequent impact on practitioners, doctors, patients and organisations. In addition the infrastructures that have supported this development have been addressed. The introduction of non-medical prescribing in the early 1990s was initially slow, whereas now it has become a fast moving field of practice, and those who work in this arena constantly have to adapt and meet the new challenges on a daily basis.

The future may see prescribing as integral to a range of pre-registration programmes such as pharmacists, nursing and allied health professionals. This is an exciting time for healthcare professionals as they are developing new roles. As long as these new roles benefit patients, expansion will continue.

Key themes: conclusions and considerations

Public health	Non-medical prescribing relies on robust policy and support mechanisms. These non-medical prescribing policies and frameworks can be effective in supporting wider public health targets and the associated policy
	Consider how the strategies used to support non-medical prescribing within organisations delivering health services can support the following public health targets:
	• Accident prevention • Antimicrobial resistance
Social and cultural issues	The development of non-medical prescribing has relied on changes within the culture and attitudes of health service staff. The NHS can be seen to have its own social and cultural expectations which have had to be challenged and changed in order to enable non-medical prescribing
	Consider how the establishment of robust support mechanisms can influence the acceptance of, and reduce resistance to, non-medical prescribing
Prescribing principles	Reflection (prescribing principle 7) is a key tool in the development of safe and effective prescribing. It supports continuing professional development by enabling the non-medical prescriber to identify strengths and learning needs
	Consider how reflective practice can be supported by the NPC competency frameworks

References

Avery A, Savelyich B, Wright L (2004) Doctors' views on supervising nurse prescribers. *Prescriber* **5**: 56–61.

Avery G, Todd J, Green G, Sains K (2007a) Non-Medical prescribing: the doctor-nurse relationship revisited. *Nurse Prescrib* **5**: 109–13.

Avery G, Todd J, Green G, Sains K (2007b) The impact of non-medical prescribing on practice. *Nurse Prescrib* **5**: 488–92.

Bissell P, Cooper R, Guillaume L et al (2008) *An Evaluation of Supplementary Prescribing in Nursing and Pharmacy*. University of Sheffield, University of Nottingham, Flinders University and University of South Australia.

Bradley E, Campbell P, Nolan P (2005) Nurse prescribers: who are they and how do they perceive their role? *J Adv Nurs* **51**: 439–48.

Bradley E, Nolan P (2007) Impact of nurse prescribing: a qualitative study. *J Adv Nurs* **59**: 120–8.

Bradley E, Nolan P (2008) *Non-Medical Prescribing*. Cambridge: Cambridge University Press.

Brooks N, Otway C, Rashid C, Kilty L, Maggs C (2001) Nurse prescribing what do patients think? *Nurs Stand* **15**: 33–8.

Bulman C, Shutz S (2008) *Reflective Practice in Nursing*, 4th edn. Oxford: Blackwell.

Burnham A (2006) *NHS Urged to 'Reduce Drugs Bill'*. BBC News, Health (online). Available at: http://news.bbc.co.uk/1/hi/health/6212133.stm (accessed 6 May 2010).

Camp J (2008) Public policy implementation of nurse prescribing. *Nurse Prescrib* **6**: 252-7.

Care Quality Commission (2009a) *Guidance about Compliance: Judgement framework*. London: CQC.

Care Quality Commission (2009b) *Guidance about Compliance: Essential standards of quality and safety*. London: CQC.

Carey N, Courtenay M (2010) An exploration of the continuing professional development needs of nurse independent prescribers and nurse supplementary prescribers who prescribe medicines for patients with diabetes. *J Clin Nurs* **19**: 208-16.

Carey N, Stenner K, Courtenay M (2009) Adopting the prescribing role in practice: exploring nurses' views in a specialist children's hospital. *Paediatr Nurs* **21**(9): 25-9.

Chartered Institute of Personnel and Development (2009) *Continuing Professional Development* (online). Available at: www.cipd.co.uk/cpd/aboutcpd/whatiscpd.htm (accessed 30 December 2009.

Cooper R, Anderson C, Avery T et al (2008a) Nurse and pharmacist supplementary prescribing in the UK - a thematic review of the literature. *Health Policy*, **85**: 277-92.

Cooper R, Anderson C, Avery T et al (2008b) Stakeholders' views of UK nurse and pharmacist supplementary prescribing. *J Health Serv Res Policy* **13**: 215-21.

Cooper R, Lymm J, Anderson C et al (2008c) Learning to prescribe - pharmacists' experiences of supplementary prescribing training in England. *BMC Med Educ* **8**: 57.

Courtenay M, Berry D (2007) Comparing nurses' and doctors' views of nurse prescribing: a questionnaire survey. *Nurse Prescrib* **5**: 205-10.

Courtenay M, Carey N (2008) Nurse independent prescribing and nurse supplementary prescribing practice: national survey. *J Adv Nurs* **61**: 291-9.

Courtenay M, Gordon J (2009) A survey of therapy areas in which nurses prescribe and CPD needs. *Nurse Prescrib* **7**: 255-61.

Courtenay M, Griffiths M (2004) Non-medical prescribing - an overview. *J Commun Nurs* **18**(8): 18-20.

Courtenay M, Carey N, Burke J (2007) independent extended and supplementary nurse prescribing practice in the UK: A national questionnaire survey. *Int J Nurs Studies* **44**: 1093-101.

Creedon R, O'Connell E, McCarthy G, Lehane B (2009) An evaluation of nurse prescribing: Part 1: A literature review. *Br J Nurs* **18**: 1322-6.

Crocker C (2009) Following the patient journey to improve medicines management and reduce errors. *Nursing Times* **105**(46): 12-15.

Daly G (2006) Non-medical prescribing: a discussion on practice implications. *Work Based Learning in Primary Care* **4**: 236-42.

Department of Health (1998) *A First Class Service: Quality in the new NHS*. London: The Stationery Office.

Department of Health (2000) *The NHS Plan: A plan for investment, a plan for reform*. London: The Stationery Office.

Department of Health (2004) *The NHS Knowledge and Skills Framework and the Development Review Process* (online). Available at: www.dh.gov.uk/prod_consum_dh/groups/dh_digitalassets/@dh/@en/documents/digitalasset/dh_4090861.pdf (accessed 6 May 2010).

Department of Health (2005) *Supplementary Prescribing by Nurses, Pharmacists, Chiropodists/ Podiatrists, Physiotherapists and Radiographers within the NHS in England* (online). Available at: www.dh.gov.uk/prod_consum_dh/groups/dh_digitalassets/@dh/@en/documents/digitalasset/dh_4110033.pdf (accessed 5 May 2010).

Department of Health (2006) *Improving Patients' Access to Medicines: A guide to implementing nurse and pharmacist prescribing within the NHS in England*. London: The Stationery Office.

Department of Health (2008) *High Quality Care For All: NHS next stage review final report* (online). Available at: www.dh.gov.uk/prod_consum_dh/groups/dh_digitalassets/@dh/@en/ documents/digitalasset/dh_085828.pdf (accessed 21 May 2010).

Department of Health (2009a) *Transforming Community Services: Enabling new patterns of provision*. London: The Stationery Office.

Department of Health (2009b) *The NHS Operating Framework for England for 2010/1* (online). Available at: www.dh.gov.uk/en/Publicationsandstatistics/Publications/PublicationsPolicy AndGuidance/DH_110107 (accessed 20 May 2010).

Department of Health (2009c) *NHS 2010-15: From Good to Great. Preventative, People Centred, Productive* (online). Available at: www.dh.gov.uk/en/publicationsandstatistics/ publications/publicationspolicyandguidance/dh_109876 (accessed 20 May 2010).

Department of Health (2010) *Changes to Medicines Legislation to Enable Mixing of Medicines Prior to Administration in Clinical Practice* (online). Available at: www.dh.gov.uk/en/ Healthcare/Medicinespharmacyandindustry/Prescriptions/TheNon-MedicalPrescribing Programme/DH_110765 (accessed 18 April 2010).

Dornan T, Ashcroft D, Heathfield H et al (2009) *An In Depth Investigation into Causes of Prescribing Errors by Foundation Trainees in Relation to their Medical Education. EQUIP* (online). Available at: www.gmc-uk.org/FINAL_Report_prevalence_and_causes_of_ prescribing_errors.pdf_28935150.pdf (accessed 6 May 2010).

Drennan J, Naughton C, Allen D et al (2009) *National Independent Evaluation of the Nurse and Midwife Prescribing Initiative*. University College Dublin.

Franklin P (2009) Prescription to practise. *Community Practitioner* **82**(6): 34-5.

General Pharmaceutical Council (2010) Standards for continuing professional development (online). Available at http://www.pharmacyregulation.org/pdfs/continuingprofessional development/gphcstandardscontprofdevlo.pdf (accessed 8 November 2010).

Gray R, Parr A, Brimblecombe N (2005) Mental health nurse supplementary prescribing: mapping progress one year after implementation. *Psychiatr Bull* **29**: 295-7.

Griffiths M, Courtenay M (2007) Opinion: Nurses lead the way on medication safety. *Independent Nurse* 17 September: 17.

Hacking S, Taylor J (2010) *An Evaluation of the Scope and Practice of non-Medical Prescribing in the North West*. University of Central Lancashire.

Hall J, Cantrill J, Noyce P (2004) Managing Independent prescribing: the influence of primary care trusts on community nurse prescribing. *Int J Pharm Pract* **12**: 133-9.

Hall J, Cantrill J, Noyce P (2006) Why don't trained community nurse prescribers prescribe? *J Clin Nurs* **15**: 403-12.

Halligan A (2006) Clinical governance assuring the sacred duty of trust to patients. *Clin Governance An Int J* (online). Available at: www.emeraldinsight.com/Insight/ ViewContentServlet?Filename=Published/EmeraldFullTextArticle/Articles/2480110101. html (accessed 5 May 2010).

Hawkes N (2009) Handing over the prescription pad. *BMJ* **339**: b4835 (online). Available at: www.bmj.com/cgi/content/extract/339/nov27_2/b4835 (accessed 7 December 2009).

Health Professionals Council (2009) *Continuing Professional Development* (online). Available at: www.hpc-uk.org/registrants/cpd (accessed 21 April 2010).

Hemingway S, Ely V (2009) Prescribing by mental health nurses. *Perspect Psychiatr Care* **45**: 24-34.

Humphries J, Green E (2000) Nurse prescribers: infrastructures required to support their role. *Nurs Stand* **14**(48): 35-9.

Information Service Division Scotland (2009) *Nurse Prescribing* (online). Available at: www.isdscotland.org/isd/information-and-statistics.jsp?pContentID=2232&p_applic =CCC&p_service=Content.show& (accessed 18 April 2010).

James V, Sheppard E, Rafferty A (1999) Nurse prescribing: essential practice or political point? In Jones M (ed.), *Nurse Prescribing: Politics to Practice*, London: Ballière Tindall.

Jones M (2004) Case report: Nurse prescribing: a case study in policy influence. *J Nurs Manag* **12**: 266-72.

Kelly A, Neale J, Rollings R (2010) Barriers to extending nurse prescribing among practice nurses. *Community Practitioner* **83**: 21-4.

Larsen D (2004) Nurse practitioners not using their prescribing qualifications. *Nurs Stand* **19**(2): 33-9.

Latter S, Maben J, Myall M, Courtenay M, Young A, Dunn N (2005) *An Evaluation of Extended Formulary Independent Nurse Prescribing. Final report*. Policy Research Programme, Department of Health and University of Southampton, UK.

Latter S, Maben J, Myall M, Young A (2007) Evaluating the clinical appropriateness of nurses' prescribing practice: method development and findings from an expert panel analysis. *Qual Safety Health Care* **16**: 415-21.

Lockwood E, Fealy G (2008) Nurse Prescribing as an aspect of future role expansion: the views of Irish clinical nurse specialists. *J Nurs Manag* **16**: 813-20.

Lovejoy A, Savage I (2001) Professional issues. Prescribing Analysis and Cost Tabulation (PACT) data: An introduction. *Br J Commun Nurs* **6**(2): 62-7.

Luker K, Ferguson B, Austin L (1997) *Evaluation of Nurse Prescribing: Final report*. London: The Stationery Office.

McCann T, Baker M (2002). Community mental health nurses and authority to prescribe medication the way forward? *J Psychiatr Mental Health Nurs* **9**: 175-82.

McCartney W, Tyrer S, Brazier M, Prayle D (1999) Nurse prescribing: radicalism or tokenism? *J Adv Nurs* **29**: 348-54.

McClure P (2005) *Reflection on Practice* (online). Available at: www.practicebasedlearning.org/resources/materials/docs/reflectiononpractice.pdf (accessed 6 May 2010).

McKay C (2007) Supporting and developing non-medical prescribing. *Nurse Prescrib* **5**: 263-7.

McKinnon J (2007) *Towards Prescribing Practice*. Chichester: John Wiley & Sons.

Mills V (2008) Clinical governing non-medical prescribing in an NHS Trust - issues for consideration in mental health and learning disability. *Mental Health Learning Disabil Res Pract* **5**: 77-91.

Morran C (2007) Auditing prescribing in an acute setting. *Assoc Nurse Prescrib J* November: 12-3.

Morris E, Footit B (2003) Structured care. In: Pickering S, Thompson J (eds), *Clinical Governance and Best Value Meeting the Modernisation Agenda*. Edinburgh: Churchill Livingstone, 185-98.

National Audit Office (2007a) *Prescribing Costs in Primary Care*. London: The Stationery Office.

National Audit Office (2007b) Press release. Cheaper Generic Drugs Save £400 Million (online). Available at: www.nao.org.uk/publications/press_notice_home/0809/prescribing_savings_in_2008.aspx (accessed 6 January 2010).

National Clinical Audit Advisory Group (2009) *What is Clinical Audit?* (online). Available at: www.dh.gov.uk/prod_consum_dh/groups/dh_digitalassets/@dh/@en/@ps/@sta/@perf/documents/digitalasset/dh_107462.pdf (accessed 18 April 2010).

National Health Service Prescription Services (2009) *Report. Update and Growth in Prescription Volume and Cost in the Year to December 2009* (online). Available at: www.nhsbsa.nhs.uk/PrescriptionServices/Documents/Volume_and_Cost_year_to_Dec_2009.pdf (accessed 18 April 2010).

National Institute for Health and Clinical Excellence (2002) Principles for Best Practice in Clinical Audit (online). Available at: www.nice.org.uk/media/796/23/BestPracticeClinicalAudit.pdf (accessed 5 May 2010).

National Institute for Health and Clinical Excellence (2010) Published clinical guidelines (online). Available at: www.nice.org.uk/Guidance/CG/Published (accessed 5 May 2010).

National Patient Safety Agency (2007) *The Fourth Report from the Patient Safety Observatory. Safety in Doses: Medication safety incidents in the NHS*. London: NPSA.

National Prescribing Centre (2007a) *Managing Medicines Across a Health Community – Making area prescribing committees fit for purpose*. Liverpool: NPC.

National Prescribing Centre (2007b) *A Competency Framework for Shared Decision-Making with Patients. Achieving Concordance for Taking Medicines* (online). Available at: www.npc.co.uk/prescribers/resources/competency_framework_2007.pdf (accessed 6 May 2010).

National Prescribing Centre (2008) *Medicines Management* (online). Available at: www.npc.co.uk/mm/index.htm (accessed 21 April 2010).

Nolan P, Haque S, Badger F, Dyke R, Khan I (2001) Mental health nurses' perceptions of nurse prescribing. *J Adv Nurs* **36**: 527–34.

Norman I, While A, Whittlesea C et al (2007) *Evaluation of Mental Health Nurses' Supplementary Prescribing: Final Report to the Department of Health (England) Kings College*. London: Division of Health & Social Care Research.

Nursing and Midwifery Council (2006) *Standards of Proficiency for Nurse and Midwife Prescribers*. London: NMC.

O'Connell E, Creedon R, McCarthy G, Lehane B (2009) An evaluation of nurse prescribing: Part 2: A literature review. *Br J Nurs* **18**: 1398–402.

Pharmaceutical Society of Northern Ireland (2010) *Continuing Professional Development* (online). Available at: www.psni.org.uk/professionals/continuing-professional-development/cpd-intro-page.php (accessed 5 May 2010).

Pontin D, Jones S (2007) Children's nurses and nurse prescribing: a case study identifying issues for developing training programmes in the UK. *J Clin Nurs* **16**: 540–8.

Ring M (2005) *An Audit of the Organisational Structures and Systems in Place to Support non-Medical Prescribing in Shropshire and Staffordshire*. Shropshire and Staffordshire Strategic Health Authority.

Ryan-Woolley B, McHugh G, Luker K (2007) Prescribing by specialist nurses in cancer and palliative care: results of a national survey. *Palliat Med* **21**: 273–7.

Stenner K, Courtenay M (2008) The role of inter-professional relationships and support for nurse prescribing in acute and chronic pain. *J Adv Nurs* **63**: 276–83.

Warburton P, Sherrington S, Kirkton J, Jinks A (2010) An evaluation of an online numeracy assessment tool. *Nurs Stand* **24**(30): 62–8.

Watterson A, Turner F, Coull A, Murray I, Boreham N (2009) *An Evaluation of the Expansion of Nurse Prescribing in Scotland*. University of Stirling, Scottish Government Social Research.

While AE, Biggs KSM (2004) Benefits and challenges of nurse prescribing, *J Adv Nurs* **45**: 559–67.

Patient Case Studies

The Textbook of Non-medical Prescribing, edited by Dilyse Nuttall and Jane Rutt-Howard.
© 2011 Blackwell Publishing Ltd

Case study 2: Barbara

Barbara is 84 years old, lives alone and has multiple pathologies: osteoporosis, arthritis and chronic obstructive pulmonary disease (COPD).

Barbara is considered 'housebound' and is regularly visited by a practitioner who principally monitors her COPD status.

Due to an increase in pain from Barbara's arthritic joints, the practitioner decides to conduct a thorough review, including history and examination, with the intention of prescribing an increase in analgesia for Barbara. Below is Barbara's current medication list.

Medication list

Ipratropium bromide 500 mcg/2 mL via nebuliser
Qvar 100 mcg two puffs twice daily
Co-codamol 8/500 up to four times daily
Alendronate acid 70 mg weekly
Anastrozole 1 mg daily
Natecal D3 (colecalciferol)
Furosemide 40 mg twice daily
Thiamine hydrochoride 100 mg daily
Salbutamol 100 mcg one or two puffs as required/four times daily
Seretide 500 mcg twice daily
Carbocisteine 375 mg four times daily
Sertraline 100 mg daily
Slo-Phyllin 250 mg twice daily
Dihydrocodeine 30 mg up to four times daily

During the review, the practitioner notices that Barbara is not her usual self. The practitioner is unable to explain her feelings, and there is no objective deterioration in her vital signs on examination, but, nevertheless, there is something 'not quite right'.

Case study 3: Clare

Clare is a 32-year-old primigravida who is 24 weeks' pregnant. She has remained well throughout her pregnancy but now has cystitis-like symptoms of frequency of micturition and discomfort on passing urine. She is very reluctant to take any medication while pregnant due to concerns about the harmful effects on her unborn child.

The practitioner is considering her prescribing decision in light of her hypotheses of cystitis, urinary tract infection, pyelonephritis (unlikely) or usual effect of pregnancy.

Case study 4: Julie

Julie is 16 years old, has learning difficulties and has a 38-year-old boyfriend. They have attended the family planning clinic requesting a pill to stop her getting pregnant.

During the assessment process, including a detailed sexual history, it becomes apparent that Julie's answers are a cause of concern for the practitioner because of her lack of understanding of sexual intercourse.

Case study 5: Annette

Annette is a 64-year-old woman. The history taken from the patient notes the following information:

- Essential hypertension, diagnosed 18 years ago
- Ischaemic heart disease, diagnosed 12 years ago
- Type 2 diabetes mellitus, diagnosed 11 years ago
- Cushing's syndrome, diagnosed 8 years ago
- Osteoarthritis of the hand, diagnosed 5 years ago
- Stage 3 CKD, diagnosed 3 years ago
- Osteoporosis, diagnosed 2 years ago
- Blood pressure 104/64 mmHg
- BMI 25 kg/m^2
- Smokes 10 cigarettes a day.

Current repeat medication

Lisinopril 20 mg tablets daily
Bendroflumethiazide 2.5 mg tablets once in the morning
Aspirin dispersible 75 mg tablets once in the morning
Lansoprazole 30 mg capsules once in the morning
Calcium carbonate and colecalciferol 1.25 g + 10 mcg chewable tablets two daily
Hydrocortisone 10 mg tablets once in the morning
Alendronic acid 70mg tablets once weekly
Metformin 500 mg tablets daily
Simvastatin 40 mg tablets once at night

Case study 6: Yasmin

Yasmin is a 36-year-old new mum. Antenatally she was treated for depression, being diagnosed in her late teens. At this time she was prescribed doxepin and had never had this reviewed or changed, at her request.

Yasmin decided not to take her antidepressants while she was knowingly pregnant. However, 3 weeks postnatally Yasmin realises that she cannot go on any longer without restarting her medication.

This decision of Yasmin's was discovered 2 weeks later when being visited by her community psychiatric nurse.

Case study 7: Amy

Amy is 7 years old and has recently returned from theatre after an appendectomy. She is very nauseous and it is noticed by the practitioner, who is a non-medical prescriber, that Amy has not been prescribed an antiemetic. It is decided that prochlorperazine will be prescribed. Amy weighs 31 kg.

Case study 8: Louis

Louis is 10 days old. His mum, Michelle, reports that he is reluctant to breastfeed. Michelle has recently completed a course of flucloxacillin for mastitis. On examination, it is found that Louis' tongue, gums and hard palate are covered in white spots. A diagnosis of oral *Candida albicans* is made. A prescription for nystatin oral suspension is provided and a clear explanation of application of the suspension to the lesions is given. The issuing of the prescription is supported with health promotion advice about hygiene and sterilisation of soothers.

Case study 9: Callum (with CMP)

Callum is 11 years old and has asthma. He has had asthmatic symptoms since he was 5 years old and is 'controlled' on step 2 of the BTS (British Thoracic Society) and SIGN (Scottish Intercollegiate Guidelines Network) guidelines, using inhalers: salbutamol and beclometasone. About a year ago Callum had a moderate acute asthma attack requiring nebuliser therapy, which was administered via a patient group direction when he attended the walk-in centre. He has since attended on two further occasions requiring similar treatment.

Since these episodes, the practice noticed the repeat attendances and encouraged Callum and his mother to attend the GP surgery for more regular reviews with the practice nurse, Jean.

Eight months ago, Jean completed her non-medical prescribing course and, together with the GP, Callum and his mother, they constructed a clinical management plan (CMP) to facilitate management by Jean. The CMP has specific indications of referral to the GP to help support Jean in her new role as a supplementary prescriber.

Last week, Callum attended for a review of his asthma because his symptoms had deteriorated. On review by Jean, he was able to talk in sentences but his respiratory rate was 33 respirations/min, his pulse 125 beats/min, peak flow 60% predicted and his SaO_2, via pulse oximetry was recording 94%.

TEMPLATE CMP 2

Name of Patient:	Patient medication sensitivities/allergies:
Callum Jones	No known sensitivities / allergies

Patient identification e.g. ~~ID number~~, date of birth:
21st June 1998

Current medication:	Medical history:
Salbutamol 100mcgs 2 puffs BD and PRN Beclometasone 100mcgs 2 puffs BD	Asthma since 5 years of age

Independent Prescriber(s):	Supplementary prescriber(s):
Dr Taylor	Jean Williams
Contact details: [tel/email/address] drtaylor@email	Contact details: [tel/email/address] jeanwilliams@email

Condition(s) to be treated:	Aim of treatment:
Asthma	Control of asthma symptoms, prevention of exacerbations and achievement of best possible pulmonary function, with minimal side effects

Medicines that my be prescribed by SP:			
Preparation	**Indication**	**Dose schedule**	**Specific indications for referral back to the IP**
Inhaled short acting B2 agonists. Inhaled steroids. Inhaled long acting B2 agonists. Leukotriene receptor antagonist	Relief of asthma symptoms, step 1 to 3 of BTS guidelines	Per BNF section 3.1	Uncontrolled symptoms Deteriorating clinical signs Failure to respond to treatment at step 3 Diagnosis in doubt Unpredicted response to treatment

Guidelines or protocols supporting Clinical Management Plan:
British Thoracic Society and Scottish Intercollegiate Guidelines Network (rev. June 2009) at URL http://www.brit-thoracic.org.uk/Portals/0/Clinical Information/Asthma/Guidelines/sign101 revised June 09.pdf

Frequency of review and monitoring by:

Supplementary prescriber 6 monthly minimum	Supplementary prescriber and independent prescriber Annually

Process for reporting ADRs:
SP to report to IP and record in records. Notify by yellow card system if indicated

Shared record to be used by IP and SP:
Computerised record within the practice.

Agreed by independent prescriber(s):	Date	Agreed by supplementary prescriber(s):	Date	Date agreed with patient/carer
Dr Taylor	14th Dec 2010	Jean Williams	14th Dec 2010	16th December 2010

Health Professional Case Studies

The Textbook of Non-medical Prescribing, edited by Dilyse Nuttall and Jane Rutt-Howard.
© 2011 Blackwell Publishing Ltd

Case study B: Mark

Mark is a team midwife, who works both in the hospital and in the community. He originally trained as a children's nurse and has been qualified as a midwife for 4 years, based solely in the hospital for 2 years before becoming a team midwife. As Mark's experience and areas of competence grew, he found that, although he was able to use exemptions and patient group directions (PGDs), he was unable to use his skills effectively because of an inability to prescribe. After discussing his personal development needs with his manager, and with the trust prescribing lead, Mark completed a non-medical prescribing education programme, qualifying as a V300 prescriber. He is now able to prescribe for antenatal women, postnatal women and neonates, for conditions for which he is competent to do so.

Mark has recently been nominated as a 'buddy' to other midwives undertaking non-medical prescribing education programmes. He is supported in this role by his colleague, Dawn, who is also a prescriber and specialises in diabetes in pregnancy.

Case study C: Rebecca

Rebecca is 31 years old and has worked as a community staff nurse for the past 2 years, before which she worked in the accident and emergency department as a staff nurse. A significant aspect of her role is in wound care and since commencing her current position she has undertaken wound care training and completed a level 3 module in leg ulcer management. Rebecca has worked alongside other professionals who have a prescribing qualification, including the community matron, who has undertaken the V300 prescribing programme, and the team leader, who completed the V100 module as part of the community specialist practitioner programme. As Rebecca's expertise in wound care developed, she became more aware of the benefits that prescribing would bring to her own practice and to the experience of her patients. Rebecca was one of the UK's first V150 prescribers and has supported the expansion of prescribing within her team. The holistic approach used in prescribing practice has complemented that already established in her community staff nurse role. She is able to prescribe wound care products and analgesia for her patients and has developed a personal development plan to enable her to develop competence in the assessment and diagnosis of other conditions for which she will be able to prescribe from the community practitioner formulary.

Case study D: Gail

Gail is a PCT-employed pharmacist and is responsible for medicines management for a cluster of six GP practices. As part of this role, Gail runs a hypertension clinic every Tuesday afternoon at one of the busier practices.

Within this role, Gail is able to develop clinical management plans (CMPs), together with her patients and the team of GPs. Once the CMP is agreed by all and in place, she is then able to initiate and/or titrate any of the antihypertensive medication, as listed on the CMP, in response to the effective consultation, including history taking, measurement and recording of the patient's blood pressure, and the interpretation of relevant blood test results.

It is anticipated that, because of the success of Gail's training and subsequent results (an increase in patients' concordance and reduction in blood pressure, and practitioner role satisfaction), two of her colleagues are about to embark on the same training in order to set up similar clinics for patient with chronic obstructive pulmonary disease and heart failure respectively.

Case study E: David

David is a community pharmacist. He has recently undertaken training to be able to assist clients to stop smoking.

In order to complement this new role and to provide a comprehensive and complete service, it was discussed at the pharmacy team meeting that David embark on the non-medical prescribing programme for independent and supplementary qualification. This would enable David to be able to prescribe any of the adjunctive therapies available to clients in their attempts at smoking cessation.

As an independent prescriber, David is able to provide both pharmacological and non-pharmacological therapies to his clients, including: nicotine (nicotine replacement therapy), bupropion or varenicline, as well as adjunctive behavioural therapy.

Case study F: Andrew

Andrew is a pharmacist working within a multiprofessional team of 'admittance staff'. The role of the team is to clerk in new patients from a number of hospital directorates, including acute admissions, cardiology, surgery and orthopaedics.

Andrew is able to obtain a thorough history from his patients, order the relevant tests and investigations, and, because he has undertaken his independent prescribing qualification, he can also prescribe the patient's current and any new medications, within his scope of professional practice.

In order to enhance safety, the team members all have different speciality knowledge and therefore cover the same wards, although, as a team, almost the whole hospital is covered.

There have been many benefits in response to this new service, not just in helping to address the European Working Time Directive, but patients are admitted more quickly and their medication (new and continuing) is prescribed in a timely manner, thus enhancing care delivery. It is anticipated that the longer-term benefits of this service will include shorter periods of stay for some patients.

In the near future, it is anticipated that this team will expand to facilitate the timely writing of prescriptions for patients awaiting discharge and thus enable the quicker throughput of patients.

Case study G: Andrea

Andrea is a newly qualified supplementary prescriber and an experienced physiotherapist. The decision to obtain her prescribing certificate was driven by her frustration at having to wait for her prescriptions to be signed by the consultant or registrar, who was running a parallel pain clinic for patients with chronic lower back pain.

Andrea, and the patient's consultant, have implemented clinical management plans for their patients, with the patient's consent, and are now able to prescribe a vast range of analgesia and adjunctive medication (e.g. antiemetics and/or laxatives) to facilitate the provision of a truly individualised treatment plan that is also implemented in a timely manner.

Case study H: Lisa

Lisa is a radiographer in a busy oncology unit. She qualified as a supplementary prescriber 18 months ago, and by using clinical management plans (CMPs) provides a more efficient service for patients receiving radiotherapy treatment. She has found the main benefit of undertaking the supplementary prescribing education programme to be the ability to address the patient's needs herself rather than referring the patient back to the doctor. She is now able to prescribe treatments for many of the side effects of radiotherapy including nausea, diarrhoea and skin reactions. Lisa feels that supplementary prescribing has allowed her to use her skills and expertise more effectively and efficiently, providing enhanced job satisfaction. It has also impacted on the overall efficiency of the unit.

Case study I: Christine

Working within a diabetic specialist team, Christine has acquired a caseload of patients who predominately see her for ongoing monitoring and treatment of diabetic foot ulcers. Her clinics run alongside the times that the diabetologist is in attendance, so, between them and the patients, CMPs have been drawn up.

The implementation of the CMP enables Christine to prescribe relevant antibiotics and/or dressings in accordance with her own specialist judgement and clinical decision-making skills. Should there be the need to refer to the independent prescriber; the diabetologist is always on site too.

The clinic as a service also benefits from Christine being able to prescribe, because patients are not waiting to see an independent prescriber and hence have greater satisfaction from the service. The diabetic nurse specialists and all other team members gain greatly from the regular multidisciplinary team meetings that occur on a monthly basis.

Case study J: Simon and Janice

Simon has worked as an optometrist for 7 years. He has worked in his own practice for the past 2 years. Simon completed the optometrist prescribing education programme last year, enabling him to prescribe as an independent prescriber. Before this, he often had to refer patients back to their GP to be given a prescription for eye conditions such as infections or dry eye, for which he was competent to prescribe. This was frustrating for both Simon and his patients.

His colleague, Janice, works part time for the NHS as a specialist glaucoma optometrist and is a supplementary prescriber. Janice reviews and monitors patients with glaucoma. After the diagnosis is initially made by the doctor, they agree a CMP with the patient. She is then able to continue, adjust or alter treatment within the boundaries of the CMP.

Index